Ethical Issues in Mental Health Research
With Children and Adolescents

Ethical Issues in Mental Health Research With Children and Adolescents

❖ ❖ ❖

Edited by

Kimberly Hoagwood
Peter S. Jensen
National Institute of Mental Health
Celia B. Fisher
Fordham University

LEA LAWRENCE ERLBAUM ASSOCIATES, PUBLISHERS
1996 Mahwah, New Jersey

Lawrence Erlbaum Associates, Inc., Publishers
10 Industrial Avenue
Mahwah, New Jersey 07430-2262

Cover design by Gail Silverman

Library of Congress Cataloging-in-Publication Data

Ethical issues in mental health research with children and adolescents / [edited by] Kimberly Hoagwood, Peter S. Jensen, and Celia B. Fisher.
       p. cm.
    Includes bibliographical references and index.
     ISBN 0-8058-1952-5 (cloth) 0-8058-1953-3 (paper)
      1. . 2. . 3. . I. Hoagwood, Kimberly. II. Jensen,
Peter S. III. Fisher, Celia B.
LB2822.82.B65 1996
371.2'00973—dc20   96-18769
                                     CIP

Books published by Lawrence Erlbaum Associates are printed on acid-free paper, and their bindings are chosen for strength and durability

Printed in the United States of America
10 9 8 7 6 5 4 3 2 1

Contents

PART II: ETHICAL CHALLENGES ACROSS DIVERSE RESEARCH CONTEXTS

PART III: CASEBOOK

PART IV: BRIDGING SCIENCE AND ETHICS

Preface

Despite its title, this book is not about ethics. It is not about the guiding beliefs, standards, or ideals of a community, people, or ideology. It does not outline major moral principles for guiding ethical behavior, nor does it excavate the moral undergirdings of scientific practice. Instead, this book represents an ethic. It is about the dialectic exchange between ethical thought in our time and scientific practice in studies of children and adolescents with mental disorders.

At the manifest level, this book concerns relations between scientific advancement and social protections. It is explicitly designed to advance research practice and thinking about that practice by outlining the legal, regulatory, and moral parameters that should guide study of mental disorders in children and adolescents.

The impetus for this volume arose amid growing recognition that study of young populations can be pivotal for understanding how to treat and in some cases prevent severe mental illnesses in adulthood. Because study of mental disorders in children has been hampered by many obstacles, including hesitancy to acknowledge the reality of mental illnesses in children, relatively recent development of age-appropriate research tools and measures, and institutional sluggishness, the addition of complicated and unexamined ethical dilemmas to the list of impediments threatened to halt progress in this field altogether.

Thus, it was with some urgency that we set out to examine in detail ethical issues that arise in the study of children and adolescents with mental disorders. As this field of study encompasses multiple scientific approaches—from basic studies of the brain to clinical treatments for specific disorders to applied studies of service delivery—we sought those interfield linkages that represented the widest array of multidisciplinary scientific practices.

However, identifying and applying ethical standards to any scientific practice requires more than a simple matching of regulations or guidelines to static activities. Rather, it requires a dialectical exchange on at least two levels. Ethical practice is ensured only to the extent that there is active engagement among all members of the research community—families, research participants, scientists, and regulators. Moreover, ethical practice requires an ideological engagement between ethical standards and scientific practice—a deliberate and constant tacking back and forth between shifting standards of scientific practice (brought about as new scientific advances occur) and ethical principles that are recognized and embraced as culturally bound and historically specific. This contextualist view of the relationship between science and ethics realigns our ethical perspectives: Ethics becomes a way of reorganizing thought, not simply a way of identifying and applying regulations. Ethical thinking as applied to scientific practice becomes a system of interpretation whereby science is informed and in some cases transformed by the application of ethical standards, and likewise ethical thought is informed by scientific progress.

At a deeper level, this book represents an ethic in the sense that it symbolizes a certain kind of historically significant belief or standard. Its publication arises within a specifiable historical time, wherein science has become administered through layers of complex institutional apparatuses. This book, by the very fact of its publication, acknowledges the contingencies, limitations, and controls of administered science.

The idea for this book began naively, with a simple discussion in a child research consortium at the National Institute of Mental Health about an unexpected response a child had made during a routine interview. As will happen, the issues grew until it became apparent that many more complex issues surrounded the enterprise we call science, especially in its human instantiation.

The numbers of people who have contributed to this book in both intellectual and enduringly pragmatic ways are large. The contributors to the casebook are listed, and for their examples, their cautions, and their thoughtful responses, we are very grateful. It is through their contributed cases that the human reality of the lives that are touched by science is made palpable.

It is a pleasure to record a major indebtedness to Alan Leshner, who even before this project took shape, recognized the moral value of intellectual leadership and exemplified it. His support for the first conference on ethical issues in mental health research with children in May 1993 provided the needed impetus for this project, but it was his careful guidance at an early stage of preparation that brought the project to fruition.

For allocation of time, but more importantly, unerring enthusiasm for the contributions that this volume can ultimately make, we gratefully acknowledge the assistance of Thomas Lalley. His dedication to the project generously facilitated its completion. In addition, this volume could not have been completed without the painstaking technical support of Mike Feil during its final preparation.

We wish also to acknowledge intellectual debts to John Richters, Frank Putnam, and Gene Arnold, whose thoughtful exchanges with all of us lie behind the development of the arguments in this book. Additionally, Hilary Hoagwood provided a critical perspective on early versions of the casebook. Her questioning of the principles undergirding the decisions for some of those cases helped bring into focus the purposes of this volume. Finally, we wish to thank Ann May and other members of the National Alliance for the Mentally Ill for their thoughtful, comprehensive, and humanized responses to an early draft of the cases.

—*Kimberly Hoagwood*
—*Peter S. Jensen*
—*Celia B. Fisher*

Part I

Scientific, Regulatory, and Family Perspectives

1

Toward a Science of Scientific Ethics in Research on Child and Adolescent Mental Disorders

Kimberly Hoagwood
Peter S. Jensen
National Institute of Mental Health
Celia B. Fisher
Fordham University

If, as Adorno (1969) suggested, the psyche is the distillation of history, then the publication of this book at this historical juncture is no coincidence. Evidence of social dysfunction is on a massive scale, too obvious to bear enumeration. Into the midst of this dysfunction, the term *ethics* has entered common parlance. Media accounts of "ethical" transgressions in political, professional, and business practices abound. The sheer number of articles on "professional ethics" listed in psychology journals rose from 25 in 1988 to 224 in 1993—a 900% increase! During this same period, ethics has become associated with intraprofessional specialization: Ethical guidelines have been developed by most major professional organizations, both within and outside of scientific disciplines. Major medical institutions have established guidelines to delineate mandatory practices (Kovenman & Shipp, 1994). The fact that this historical moment—the last decade of the century, a period usually characterized by decadence—has witnessed such a surge in attention to issues of "morality" deserves a moment's reflection.

Why has there been such a proliferation of interest in ethical initiatives? Perhaps contemporary moral discourse and attention to ethical practices are signs of underlying trouble in the functions of institutions whose work has become increasingly questionable. Although it is not the purpose of this volume to investigate the morality of institutions, the sense of ethics implied in a model of rule-making or guideline

3

development deserves to be examined within the larger question of the meaning and value of institutions and professional practices in the social sciences.

The immediate impulse for this book arose from the concerns of families, scientists, institutional review board (IRB) members, and federal research administrators who regulate research involving children. Their concerns centered on the importance of maintaining a balance between two aims: protecting child and adolescent research participants and their families from harm, and promoting opportunities for advancement of knowledge through scientific endeavors. To accomplish these aims, we have, in this volume, assembled the views of scientists, families, bioethicists, and regulators, all of whom have brought their expertise to bear on the central tension between scientific advancement and participant welfare.

The purpose of this book, then, is to surface the key ethical dilemmas that investigators who study child and adolescent emotional, behavioral, developmental, and mental disorders are encountering, and to offer practical suggestions for integrating ethical thinking into such research. Although federal regulations provide the foundation for ethical action, an ability to identify and critically evaluate the moral ambiguities that arise in human subjects research is necessary if science in the field of mental health is to be advanced. Although there are many ethically justified solutions to these dilemmas, and this book outlines a number of them, as with any complex endeavor, no single solution will fit all cases.

Further, complex as these dilemmas are for research involving any human being, when children and adolescents are the focus of study, the ambiguities multiply. Distinctive features of children create unique challenges to the investigator who must balance the requirements of scientific control against the realities of children's developmental fluctuations. When a study involves children, and even more problematically, children who may be at risk for or who manifest emotional or behavioral disorders, troublesome areas such as defining vulnerability, determining the extent of autonomy, obtaining consent, avoiding coercion, to name but a few, require careful thought. Some of the distinctive features of children that present the greatest ethical challenges to scientists are outlined in this chapter.

The field of research on mental disorders in children and adolescents is of recent origin in comparison to the adult field. Despite its recency, however, the field spans a rich variety of research contexts and this volume seeks to encompass all major types. These include studies of services and service systems for children, as well as community epidemiological surveys; studies of clinical interventions, both psy-

chosocial and pharmacological; investigations using biologically invasive techniques and new technologies; and research with vulnerable
populations, such as children who have been maltreated.

The book is organized into four parts. Part I introduces the major
scientific, regulatory, and community principles that guide ethical practices in research on children's mental health. In this introductory chapter, we argue that science and ethics are linked dialectially through a
process of active engagement with child and family research participants. Ethical actions emerge through a process of construction and
negotiation, not through staid or sterile application of prefabricated
rules or precedents. In chapter 2, Porter describes the major federal
regulations that undergird all research involving human subjects. These
regulations establish the basic standards for protecting child participants. In chapter 3, Osher andTelesford, from the Federation of Families, describe the contributions families can make to enhancing the
ethical conduct of research, and the effect of research practices on
families. They also provide examples of ways in which family involvement in all phases of research can circumvent ethical problems.

Part II reviews major ethical issues across diverse research contexts.
Chapter 4 by Attkisson, Rosenblatt, and Hoagwood describes the range
of ethical issues that arise in studies of services and service systems for
children and their families. Ethical challenges in community surveys of
children are also discussed. In chapter 5, Hibbs and Krener describe
major dilemmas in studies of psychosocial treatments and preventive
interventions, where delineation of treatment, intervention, and research responsibilities often intertwine. Leonard and colleagues, in
chapter 6, outline salient issues that arise in clinical efficacy trials of
psychopharmacological agents for children, and review future challenges that will emerge as new drug therapies become available. In
chapter 7, Arnold and colleagues describe major dilemmas in studies
that involve invasive techniques or procedures, including new techniques of genetic therapy and brain imaging. Some of these procedures
are being employed in studies with normal controls, and applying such
procedures raises serious but surmountable ethical challenges. Putnam,
Liss, and Landsverk (chapter 8) outline some of the major ethical issues
involved in studies of children who have been maltreated. In such
research, the potential of increasing the risk to an already vulnerable
population creates special needs.

Part III focuses attention on illustrative cases. Fisher, Hoagwood, and
Jensen developed 61 cases from contributions provided by more than
100 investigators. The casebook is organized into 10 sections, with each
section containing a scholarly review of work on those ethical issues.
The 10 sections address ethical dilemmas such as balancing research

risks and benefits, protecting participants when withholding treatment, identifying and recruiting participants, obtaining informed consent and assent, use of deception, protection of confidentiality, modifying research procedures when needed, offering services beyond those required by the protocol, and dissemination. The cases illustrate how particular investigators or teams handled ethical dilemmas when they arose. The resolutions are not necessarily the only ethically justifiable solutions, but they represent solutions in the ranges of possibilities approved by IRBs.

In Part IV, DeRenzo discusses the important role that bioethicists can play in critically reviewing research proposals and applying ethical principles in a practical way to achieve a balance between protection and scientific progress. Finally, Jensen, Hoagwood, and Fisher in the concluding chapter present a contextualist view of the relationship between science and ethics.

DISTINCTIVE FEATURES OF CHILDREN
AND ADOLESCENTS

As previously noted, research on children entails unique challenges not necessarily encountered in studies involving adult subjects. In part, these challenges are a function of distinctive characteristics of childhood itself; in part they are a function of the dominant societal modes that are erected for handling those with limited decision-making power.

Developmental Continuity and Discontinuity.   Because children undergo major cognitive, emotional, and physiological changes, the risk and potential benefits of any research need to assessed with specific attention to the course of these changes. Because of the recency of efforts to study the course and consequences of psychopathology in children, there remains much uncertainty about long-term outcomes of childhood mental disorders. This uncertainty makes the assessment of risk especially problematic. Thompson (1992) argued for evaluating different domains of research risk independently when estimating their potential effects on children of different ages. For example, a study of peer influences may have little effect on very young children, for whom peers are relatively inconsequential, as opposed to a study of adolescents, for whom peers may figure more prominently. Within a developmental context, vulnerability is not a linear function. However, research is only now beginning to uncover the types, patterns, and course of vulnerabilities across the life span (Anthony & Cohler, 1987; Anthony & Kupernik, 1974). For children at risk for the development of emotional or behavioral disorders, assessment of their vulnerabilities is even more important. Until the vulnerabilities and protective factors for children across the life span are better understood, assessing potential risk of participation in research will be more complicated. However, one cannot assume homogeneous vulnerability or invulnerability. Thus, the IRB function must be instrumental in assuring that assessment of vulnerability occurs at the individual level.

Developmental nonequilibrium in children has other scientific implications. Childhood itself can be characterized as a "system" of unstable equilibrium. Minor disturbances in the conditions surrounding the system can exert unpredictable influences for the course of its development. Because children are bound within their contextual surrounds to a greater extent than are adults, such disturbances may be magnified over time and in unforeseen ways exert an influence on personality development. Meehl (1978) outlined 20 features of the study of human beings that make psychology difficult to "scientize." One of these is the problem of unknown critical events and the difficulty it presents for interpreting causality. Meehl pointed out that critical events in the history of a child may be forever unsusceptible to ascertainment. For example, inner events, such as embarrassment at a young age in response to an experimentally induced, seemingly innocuous event, may influence the course of personality development in ways that are hard to measure. Although the resilience of children should not be underestimated, neither should their unique vulnerabilities.

The implications of the differences between adults and children in terms of developmental plasticity and fluidity are that harms and benefits for children must be calculated differently. The actual risks of children's participation in research are only beginning to be better understood (Kaser-Boyd, Adelman, & Taylor, 1985; Kruesi et al., 1988). Although many risks can be assessed as soon as procedures are established, benefits are usually contingent on the outcomes of the study. Beneficial outcomes of experimentation can be achieved directly or indirectly (Fisher, 1993). For example, clinical trials research has the potential to benefit child participants in the treatment condition directly and immediately. In contrast, children participating as clinical trial controls, or in studies on the physiological correlates of mental disorders, may only benefit indirectly and at a later point in time. As Thompson (1992) pointed out, in these latter contexts, risks are proximal, but benefits are distal. Although the potential for direct participant risks is always an important ethical variable, sacrificing long-term potential good for the avoidance of potential short-term risks may also be ethically unsound. The third part of this volume presents examples of studies in which research risk was minimized. In addition, several of the chapters in Part II include an extended discussion of issues involved in minimizing risk.

Limited Rights and Legal Prerogatives. Children, by definition, have limited autonomy and are legally powerless. Although their abilities are often grossly underrated, nevertheless, children's legal rights and access to decision-making power are limited by law. Some have argued that children constitute the most discriminated legal category (Koocher & Keith-Spiegel, 1990). Legal limitations on minors diminish their autonomy and have necessitated the introduction of special protections and waivers (see chapter 2 for a fuller discussion). For adolescents who are capable of making certain types of personal decisions, contradictory legal limitations pose special problems (Rotheram-Borus & Koopman, 1991). The extent of protection to be afforded children and adolescents depends on a calculation of both the potential risks involved in participating in research and the likelihood of benefit. In some instances, the legal–medical model defining the rights of adolescents to consent to medical treatment has provided a framework for evaluating conditions under which guardian consent for research participation may be waived (Holder, 1981). Researchers should nevertheless guard against simply substituting state laws regarding medical treatment for ethical deliberations about waiving guardian consent (Fisher, 1993).

Cognitive Limitations. Because children's cognitive abilities unfold over time, at certain ages they are less capable of understanding to what they are giving assent. Young children's limited understanding of what constitutes authority may make them more vulnerable than older children to coercion (Fisher & Rosendahl, 1990). The differential and changing cognitive abilities of children require special considerations when obtaining their assent to participate. This is especially true in longitudinal studies, where their understanding of the study and what participation means will change over time. The casebook describes ways to modify consent and assent procedures for children of differing cognitive abilities.

Disparity of Power. There is an unmistakable disparity of power between adults and children, and this power differential governs to a certain extent the relationship between the research investigator and child participant (Fisher & Rosendahl, 1990). This disparity foregrounds two kinds of questions: questions about the responsibilities of the investigator toward the participants, and questions about the balance between immediate and future risk or social benefit. Answers to either of these questions are founded on ascertainment or estimates of harm. Unfortunately, as previously noted, little is known about what actually constitutes harm—potential or actual—for child research participants.

Although it is clear that the decreased cognitive functioning of children may limit their ability to give full and informed consent, we know surprisingly little about the effects of research participation on children and adolescents, nor about their perceptions and experiences as participants in research. Adult attributions about childhood experiences fill the vacuum left by our ignorance.

Exclusionary Research and the Manufacture of Ignorance. As social historians have clearly documented, groups that have been outside the mainstream of social, scientific, or historical study have also been excluded from receiving social benefits (Foucault, 1966; Himmelfarb, 1983). In part because of their legal constraints and diminished autonomy, children have received much less scientific attention than adults in the field of mental health research. The social consequences of excluding children from scientific study, as Leonard et al. (chapter 6) point out, are the creation of "therapeutic orphans," whereby children are unable to accrue the benefits derived from scientific advances. One obvious solution to this is to increase research opportunities for children. Although active recruitment of children can obviate exclusionary practices and strengthen the conclusiveness of scientific evidence (Blanck, Bellack, Rosnow, Rotheram-Borus, & Schooler, 1992), it also poses ethical problems. Questions may be raised about coercive practices, minimization of risk, and so on. These problems respect no boundaries and are found in all the types of research described in this volume.

The literature provides little guidance to determine what actually constitutes harm for child participants, although some studies are beginning to appear on issues such as consent and assent (Appelbaum & Grisso, 1988; Grisso & Appelbaum, 1991; Koocher & DeMaso, 1990), and methods for evaluating risk (Fisher & Rosendahl, 1990; Fisher, Higgins, Rau, Kuther, & Belanger, in press; Freedman, Fuks, & Weijer, 1993; Kaser-Boyd et al., 1985; Kruesi et al., 1988; McGrath, 1993; Wilson & Crowe, 1991). Yet, significant questions remain about the ability of children at different ages and for different procedures to assess personal risks or personal and social benefits of involvement, such as satisfaction with contributing to a larger good. These are some of the questions investigations into which could constitute the core of a science of scientific ethics.

PROTECTIONS FOR CHILDREN
AND ADOLESCENTS

Belmont Principles Applied to Children. In 1979 the National Commission for the Protection of Human Subjects of Biomedical and Behavioral Research laid the foundation for *The Belmont Report: Ethical*

Principles and Guidelines for the Protection of Human Subjects of Research.
The commission formulated three major principles that underpin ethical practice in research involving human beings: respect for persons, beneficence, and justice. The distinctive features of children just described require a reframing of these principles. The principle of respect underscores the importance of individual autonomy, informed, rational, and voluntary consent of those who will be involved in research. As described in this volume, ensuring that children with emotional or behavioral problems understand expectations about their participation in a research study involves additional protections. The requirements for the establishment of IRBs and for determining the hierarchy of risks, descriptions of circumstances under which parental permission is needed, and restrictions on the use of deception and the requirement of debriefing, are examples of ways in which the principle of respect has become operationalized for research involving children. To uphold the principle of beneficence in research with children involves more than mere protection from harm: Research investigators are expected to make efforts to secure the well-being of participants from anticipated risks and from unanticipated factors that may reveal that the child is in potential jeopardy (Fisher, 1994; Fisher, Higgins, et al., in press). Beneficence—producing good—is thus an obligation. The principle of beneficence also extends to research issues of balancing risks and benefits, withholding treatment, and modifying experimental procedures or offering services. Finally, the principle of justice suggests that benefits and burdens of research be distributed fairly and equitably. Participants are to be chosen for reasons related directly to science and not for reasons of convenience. The principle of distributive justice—that is, that all groups should have both equal access and equal exemption from participation in research—has been raised as a concern especially as it relates to participation of children from minority cultures (Fisher, 1993; Fisher, Jackson, & Villarruel, in press; Laosa, 1990; Munir & Earls, 1992; Scott-Jones, 1994). Issues related to noncoercive recruitment procedures and cultural sensitivity are derived from this principle.

Federal Regulations. As discussed by Porter (chapter 2), the Department of Health and Human Services (DHHS) Regulations for the Protection of Human Subjects (Title 45 Code of Federal Regulations Part 46) contains two subparts that address special protections afforded children and adolescents. Subpart A, for example, describes the elements of informed consent, including the necessity of explaining the risks and benefits associated with participation. Subpart D describes the requirements for obtaining assent by children and permission by parents or guardians. It also provides a classificatory framework for categorizing research into four types of risk to which any study is assigned by IRBs. Arnold et al., Leonard et al., Porter, Derenzo, and Fisher et al., in their respective chapters describe these risk categories in detail.

Institutional Review Boards (IRBs).   The most important protection of human subjects is provided through the IRBs. The localization of decision making accorded to a community board that reviews all research protocols has been a source of both comfort and frustration. At the very least, the review boards as a whole are a repository of historic wisdom, and a source of precedent. Although the function of IRBs is not an ethical issue per se, their creation was designed to ensure local attention by members of the participants' immediate community to questions of potential harm.

The variability of IRBs is often cited as a frustration by researchers studying children's mental health. Reviews of children are said to be subject to more extensive analyses and critique, perhaps as a consequence of an overzealous protectionism of children. The presumable vulnerability of child research subjects contributes to the variability in risk assessments among IRBs. In studies involving multiple sites, agencies, populations of children, or institutions, it is not uncommon for multiple IRB reviews to be required. The procedures dictated by one committee sometimes disagree with procedures dictated by other committees. For example, one IRB may want a consent form for 6-year-olds, whereas another does not even raise the issue, and another believes such a procedure might be viewed as coercive. However, this variability, while ungratifying, also reflects the IRB function as a community barometer of local norms, standards, and values. The variability that frustrates is also a protection against hegemony.

CONCLUSION

The unique features of children with mental disorders and the protections available to them create special challenges for the investigator who is trying to conduct ethically justified research. The particularly troublesome areas, such as defining vulnerability, working within the boundaries of legal and cognitive limitations, and maximizing inclusion, suggest that ethics in relation to science is best understood as a dialectic of construction, not as a system of rule interpretation. Ethical thinking guides decision making in science insofar as it involves a continual process of tacking back and forth not rules but principles of action to evolving, changing phenomena. It is through this dialectical process that a science of scientific ethics can be constructed.

Many of the tensions faced by scientists trying to balance scientific standards against human subjects' protection—many of which are documented in Part III—arise from the conflict between competing ethical standards. For example, the duty to debrief or to communicate findings to participants may conflict with concerns about the consequences of such communication. Careful assessment of the risks for each action and the principles of obligation that underlie such actions is needed in order to resolve these issues. Both teleological and deontological factors enter into some research issues, and these factors may be combined integratively to yield ethical approaches.

However, none of the ethical problems that are presented in this book will be understood, much less solved, if ethics is viewed merely as a set of intraprofessional procedures. Rather, the ethical problems and their solutions arise from and are determined by the structure of the social relations within which the problems are embedded. This implies, among other things, that ethical initiatives—including the publication of this book—have a social structure and meaning that need to be interpreted if research participants, especially those diagnosed with mental disorders, are to receive fair and equal treatment. Moreover, if ethical decision making is to be viewed as a process of construction rather than discovery, then the structure of the relationship between ethical thinking and science is more integral than mere intraprofessional specialization would suggest. We return to the relationship between ethics and science in the conclusion to the volume.

This book is an ethical initiative. It arises out of its time and place and is itself historically situated. If this collection is viewed as merely a set of rules for what should or should not be done when studying children and adolescents with mental disorders, then the larger and more important questions of why particular topics are selected for study at any given time become obscured. Within the larger framework of ethical inquiry and its applicability to science, it is important to ask why one wants to study a problem—not only whether a study can be conducted in an ethically defensible manner. When research activities are coupled with professional gain, as is increasingly the case, there is a risk that purposes may become confounded, and that the machinery of funding and promotion may overtake the larger goals for which scientific advancements are pursued.

This volume redefines the reciprocity between scientific practice and ethical thinking. The contributors are a varied lot: They include scientists, who have wrestled often with research's ethical challenges; family members, whose lives have been impacted by their involvement in research; regulators, who develop guidelines to address increasingly complex dilemmas; and bioethicists, who remind us of the principles that undergird all ethical actions. The mutual influence of science and ethics is deepened when the methods of science are informed by ethical perspectives, and when science is linked to the mental health needs of those whom it is designed to benefit. The relationship between ethical inquiry and scientific pursuit can and should be brought into closer alignment. One goal of this volume is to do so.

REFERENCES

Adorno, T. W. (1969). Scientific experiences of a European scholar in America. In D. Fleming and B. Bailyn (Eds.), *The intellectual migration* (pp. 351–363). Cambridge, MA: Harvard University Press.

Anthony, E. J., & Cohler, B. J. (1987). *The invulnerable child.* New York: Guilford.

Anthony, E. J., & Kupernik, C. (1974). *The child in his family: Children at psychiatric risk.* New York: Wiley.

Appelbaum, P. S., & Grisso, T. (1988). Assessing patients' capacities to consent to treatment. *New England Journal of Medicine, 319,* 1635–1638.

Blanck, P. D., Bellack, A. S., Rosnow, R. L., Rotheram-Borus, M. J., & Schooler, N. R. (1992). Scientific rewards and conflicts of ethical choices in human subjects research. *American Psychologist, 47,* 959–965.

Fisher, C. B. (1993). Integrating science and ethics in research with high-risk children and youth. *Social Policy Report, 7,* 1–27.

Fisher, C. B. (1994). Reporting and referring research participants. Ethical challenges for investigators studying children and youth. *Ethics and Behavior, 4,* 87–95.

Fisher, C. B., Higgins, A., Rau, J. M., Kuther, T., & Belanger, S. (in press). Reporting and referring research participants: The view from urban adolescents. *Child Development.*

Fisher, C. B., Jackson, J. F., & Villarruel, F. (in press). The study of ethnic minority children and youth in the United States. In W. Damon (Series Ed.) & R. M. Lerner (Vol. Ed.), Handbook of child psychology: Vol. I. Theoretical models of human development (5th ed.). New York: Wiley.

Fisher, C. B., & Rosendahl, S. W. (1990). Emerging ethical issues in an emerging field. In C. B. Fisher & W. W. Tryon (Eds.), *Annual advances in applied developmental psychology* (Vol. 4, pp. 43–60). Norwood, NJ: Ablex.

Foucault, M. (1966). *The order of things: An archaeology of the human sciences.* London: Tavistock.

Freedman, B., Fuks, A., & Weijer, C. (1993). In loco parentis: Minimal risk as an ethical threshold for research upon children. *Hastings Center Report, 23*(2), 13–19.

Grisso, T., & Appelbaum, P. S. (1991). Mentally ill and non-mentally ill patients' abilities to understand informed consent disclosures for medication: Preliminary data. *Law and Human Behavior, 15,* 377–388.

Himmelfarb, G. (1983). *The idea of poverty. England in the early industrial age.* New York: Vintage.

Holder, A. R. (1981). Can teenagers participate in research without parental consent. *IRB: Review of Human Subjects Research, 3,* 5–7.

Kaser-Boyd, N., Adelman, H. S., & Taylor, L. (1985). Minors' ability to identify risks and benefits of therapy. *Professional Psychology: Research and Practice, 16*(3), 411–417.

Koocher, G. P., & Keith-Spiegel, P. C. (1990). *Children, ethics, & the law: Professional issues and cases.* Lincoln: University of Nebraska Press.

Koocher, G. P., & DeMaso D. R. (1990). Children's competence to consent to medical procedures. *Pediatrician, 17,* 68–73.

Korenman, S. G., & Shipp, A. C. (1994). *Teaching the responsible conduct of research through a case study approach.* Washington, DC: Association of American Medical Colleges.

Kruesi, M. J. P., Swedo, S. E., Coffey, M. L., Hamburger, S. D., Leonard, H., & Rapoport, J. L. (1988). Objective and subjective side effects of research lumbar punctures in children and adolescents. *Psychiatry Research, 25,* 59–63.

Laosa, L. (1990). Population generalizability, cultural sensitivity, and ethical dilemmas. In C. B. Fisher & W. W. Tryon (Eds.), *Ethics in applied developmental psychology* (pp. 227–252). Norwood, NJ: Ablex.

McGrath, P. J. (1993). Inducing pain in children: A controversial issue. *Pain, 52*(3), 255–257.

Meehl, P. (1978). Theoretical risks and tabular askeriks: Sir Karl, Sir Ronald, and the slow progress of soft psychology. *Journal of Consulting and Clinical Psychology, 4,* 806–834.

Munir, K., & Earls, F. (1992). Ethical principles governing research in child and adolescent psychiatry. *Journal of the American Academy of Child and Adolescent Psychiatry, 31,* 408–414.

National Commission for the Protection of Human Subjects of Biomedical and Behavioral Research. (1979). *The Belmont Report: Ethical principles and guidelines for the protection of human subjects of research.* Washington, DC: U.S. Government Printing Office.

Rotheram-Borus, M. J., & Koopman, C. (1991). HIV and adolescents: Special Issue: Preventing the spread of the human immunodeficiency virus. *Journal of Primary Prevention, 12,* 65–82.

Scott-Jones, D. (1994). Ethical issues in reporting and referring in research with low-income minority children. *Ethics and behavior, 4*(2), 97–108.

Thompson, R. A. (1992). Developmental changes in risk and benefit: A changing calculus of concerns. In B. L. Stanley & J. E. Sieber (Eds.), *Social research on children and adolescents: Ethical issues* (pp. 31–64). Newbury Park, CA: Sage.

Wilson, J. R., & Crowe, L. (1991). Genetics of alcoholism: Can and should youth at risk be identified? Special Focus: Alcohol and youth. *Alcohol Health and Research World, 15*(1), 11–17.

2

Regulatory Considerations in Research Involving Children and Adolescents With Mental Disorders

Joan P. Porter
National Institutes of Health

This chapter highlights some of the regulatory considerations in the Department of Health and Human Services (DHHS) regulations for the protection of human subjects at Title 45 Code of Federal Regulations Part 46 (45 CFR Part 46; OPRR Reports, 1994). These regulations are available from the Office for Protection from Research Risks, as well as the Belmont Report, which sets forth the basic guidelines for the conduct of research (OPRR Reports, 1979). As noted in chapter 1, these regulations provide merely the minimum standards for investigators; application of ethical thinking to research issues, on the other hand, is a continual process of reevaluation.

There are additional federal and state laws and regulations that may be applicable and important for those contemplating research to keep in mind when designing and carrying out research involving children and adolescents with mental disorders. For example, the Food and Drug Administration (FDA) has regulations and guidelines that may be applicable. Several laws and regulations applying to activities under the Department of Education and to local schools are relevant to researchers contemplating school-based studies. These directives include (a) Protection of Pupils Rights Act, in the Goals 2000: Educate America Act (Public Law 103-227, Sec. 1017, 108 Stat. 268, 1994), which amends the General Education Provisions Act (20 U.S.C. 1232 g-h); and (b) Protection of Rights and Privacy of Parents and Students Act (20 U.S.C., Sec. 1232g, 1988 as amended Supp. V. 1993).

THE BELMONT REPORT

The Belmont Report was prepared by the National Commission for the Protection of Human Subjects in 1979. The report sets forth the Ethical Principles and Guidelines for Research Involving Human Subjects. The regulations at 45 CFR Part 46 are based on these ethical principles. The "basic ethical principles," which refer to those general judgments that serve as a basic justification for the many particular ethical prescriptions and evaluations of human action, include respect for persons, beneficence, and justice. Respect for persons, sometimes referred to as the principle of autonomy, means that individuals should be treated as autonomous agents, and second, that persons with diminished autonomy are entitled to protection.

The application of the general principle of respect for persons requires that participants, to the degree that they are capable, be allowed to choose what shall happen to them. The process of obtaining adequate consent allows for this choice. Because the participant's ability to comprehend depends on intelligence, rationality, maturity, and language, it is necessary to address the participants' capacities. The Belmont Report also makes clear that special provisions may be appropriate when comprehension is severely limited by conditions of immaturity or mental disability. Respect for these persons requires offering them the opportunity to choose, to the extent they are able, whether or not to participate in research. Respect for persons also mandates seeking permission of other parties to protect the participants from harm. Permission of the parent(s) or the child's legally authorized representative is therefore required.

In addition to the concept of *comprehension*, the concept of *voluntariness* weighs into assessing the adequacy of the consent process. This element of informed consent requires that the circumstances under which informed consent is obtained are free of coercion and undue influence. Those who design, conduct, and authorize research need to make certain that the possibility of coercion or undue influence is minimized.

The principle of beneficence as described in the Belmont Report requires that persons are treated in an ethical manner not only by respecting their decisions and protecting them from harm, but also by making efforts to ensure their well-being. This principle encompasses two parts: do no harm, and maximize possible benefits and minimize possible harms. To accomplish these goals, an assessment of risks and benefits is necessary, which, in turn, is dependent on gathering systematically and evaluating comprehensively information about the proposed research. The Belmont Report indicates that closely related to the principle of beneficence is the requirement that research be justified on the basis of a favorable risk to anticipated benefit assessment.

The institutional review board (IRB) is a key assessment point for determination of the balance of risks and anticipated benefits. In evaluating risks involved in research, the IRB must pay particular attention to the involvement of vulnerable populations to make sure that their inclusion—or exclusion—is justified. The report suggests that variables such as the nature and degree of risk, the condition of particular populations involved, and the nature and level of anticipated benefits be considered.

The principle of justice deals with who should receive the benefits of research and who should bear its burdens. The IRB reviews research to determine if some classes of persons are being systematically selected simply because they are easily available or because they can be easily manipulated. The principle of justice requires that there be fair procedures for selecting research subjects. One consideration is if there are burdens being placed on already burdened populations that could not be borne by other less burdened segments of the population. Some classes of potential subjects of research, such as children or institutionalized populations, may be involved as research subjects only if certain conditions are met. IRBs have a serious balancing responsibility, however, in that they must also make sure that certain classes of subjects for whom possible benefits would accrue are not excluded from the possibility of involvement in research because of considerations of additional costs or inconvenience, for example.

THE DHHS REGULATIONS
FOR THE PROTECTION OF HUMAN SUBJECTS
AT TITLE 45 CODE OF FEDERAL REGULATIONS
PART 46

There are four subparts to this title and part. Subpart A contains the Federal Policy for the Protection of Human Subjects Basic DHHS Policy for Protection of Human Research. In 1991, 15 other federal departments and agencies also adopted the provisions of Subpart A, which is codified at pertinent titles and subparts in their regulations. Subpart B sets forth Additional DHHS Protection Pertaining to Research, Development, and Related Activities Involving Fetuses, Pregnant Women, etc. This subpart is currently under review. Subpart C addresses Additional DHHS Protections pertaining to Biomedical and Behavioral Research Involving Prisoners as Subjects, and Subpart D has Additional DHHS Protection for Children Involved as Subjects in Research. Subparts A and D are those most pertinent to the involvement of children and adolescents with mental disorders, but it is also possible that the protections of Subparts B and C will also pertain in certain circumstances.

Particular provisions of these subparts are discussed in a document issued by the Office for Protection from Research Risks (OPRR), National Institutes of Health (NIH), DHHS in 1993. The book, entitled *OPRR 1993 Protecting Human Research Subjects Institutional Review Board Guidebook,* may be helpful to investigators and others in interpreting the regulations. Discussion of aspects of the FDA regulations is also included in the OPRR *Guidebook.*

OVERVIEW OF SUBPART A—BASIC DHHS POLICY FOR PROTECTION OF HUMAN RESEARCH SUBJECTS

This subpart of the regulations contains key provisions related to the protection of subjects in research. This subpart addresses, for example, the *applicability* of the regulations, key *definitions,* the types of *documentation* institutions that carry out research involving human subjects supported by the department must submit to the OPRR, the department's locus in the NIH that oversees the implementation of the regulations. Also described here are policies for *IRB membership* and *functions and operations,* conditions under which IRB review of research is needed, and *criteria for IRB approval* of research. Other important information contained in this subpart is the general requirements for informed consent, documentation of informed consent, and conditions under which consent may be waived.

The regulations pertain to all research involving human subjects conducted, supported or otherwise regulated by the department in the United States or abroad [Section 46.101(a)].

There are certain *exemptions* to the regulation for some types of research [Section 46.101(b)(1)-(6)]. The general areas of research that might be exempt include certain educational research; research involving educational tests, survey procedures, interview procedures or observations of public behavior, except under certain circumstances where there may be particular risks; research involving the collection or study of existing data, documents, specimens that are not recorded with individual identifiers or linkers; certain types of public benefit assessment projects; and taste and food quality evaluation and consumer acceptance studies, under certain conditions. Note that this is only a list of the general areas of the exemptions. There are certain conditions specified within these exemptions that need to be read carefully in the regulations. Staff or chairs of the IRBs should also be consulted for help in interpretation and to ascertain who can make a decision about what research is considered exempt in an institution. Also note that some of the exemptions do not pertain to research involving children, described later.

The IRB is the entity that carries out important review and enforcement provisions at the institution in which the research is to be conducted. IRBs that review research supported by the department operate under an assurance of compliance that is negotiated with the OPRR [Section 46.103]. At more than 400 major institutions, OPRR has approved assurances to apply the regulations at 45 CFR Part 46 to all research conducted under the auspices of the institution, not just that supported by the department. The influence of the regulations is thus far-reaching.

The IRB has the authority to approve, require modification in, or disapprove all research activities covered by the regulations [Section 46.109(a)]. To approve research, the IRB must determine that risks to the subjects are minimized and that they are reasonable in relation to anticipated benefits, if any, to the subjects. The IRB also must make sure that selection of subjects is equitable; that regulatorily adequate informed consent will be sought from each prospective subject or the subject's legally authorized representative; that informed consent is appropriately documented; that there are adequate provisions for monitoring the data collected to ensure the safety of subjects; and that there are adequate provisions to protect the privacy of subjects and to maintain the confidentiality of data [Section 46.111(a)]. Also, the IRB must decide that when some or all of the participants in the research are likely to be vulnerable to coercion or undue influence, such as children or mentally disabled persons, additional safeguards have been included in the study to protect the rights and welfare of these subjects [Section 46.111(b)].

Subpart A also sets forth general requirements for *informed consent* as well as basic and additional elements for it [Section 46.116]. Consent may only be sought under circumstances that provide the prospective subject or his or her legally authorized representative sufficient opportunity to consider whether or not to participate and that minimize the possibility of coercion or undue influence. The information must be in language that is understandable to the subject or the representative, and no informed consent may include any exculpatory language.

The elements of consent address explanation of risks and benefits; disclosures of appropriate alternative procedures to the research; the extent of confidentiality; explanation under certain circumstances of availability of compensation in the event of research injury; and an explanation of who to contact for answers to questions about the research or in the event of a research-related injury. Also, there must be a statement that participation is voluntary and refusal to participate will not involve a penalty or loss of benefits to which the participants are otherwise entitled. The participant may discontinue participation at any time without penalty or loss of benefits to which he or she is otherwise entitled [Section 46.116(a)]. There are several additional elements found in this Subpart which might also be provided to the participant if the IRB decided that they are pertinent [Section 116(b)]. Again, the regulations bear careful reading to characterize adequately the general requirements and elements of consent.

There are some conditions under which the IRB may find and document that it is acceptable to waive informed consent. Waiver of consent (or alteration of some of the elements of informed consent) is a serious matter about which the IRB must carefully deliberate. To approve an informed consent process that does not include or which alters some or all the elements of informed consent, the IRB must find that four conditions apply: the research involves no more that minimal risk to the subjects; the waiver or alteration will not adversely affect the rights and welfare of the subject; the research could not practicably be carried out without the waiver or alteration; and whenever appropriate, the subjects will be provided with additional pertinent information after participation [Section 46.116(d)]. It is important to remember that the definition of minimal risk is that the probability and magnitude of harm or discomfort anticipated in the research are not greater in and of themselves than those ordinarily encountered in daily life or during the performance of routine physical or psychological examinations or tests [Section 46.102(I)]. There are other requirements of Subpart A not addressed here.

HIGHLIGHTS OF SUBPART D—ADDITIONAL DHHS PROTECTION FOR CHILDREN INVOLVED AS SUBJECTS IN RESEARCH

Federal departments and agencies other than DHHS have not incorporated the provisions of Subpart D into their regulations, but they may have done so by administrative action or cross-reference. The more than 400 institutions that have negotiated assurances with broad coverage with OPRR use these provisions in reviewing all research, regardless of the source of support. Thus, even though these are DHHS provisions, they may apply to research more widely. Understanding of these regu-

latory provisions is particularly important for investigators and institutions conducting research involving children or adolescents with
mental disorders.

This subpart contains, among others, provisions describing the
nonapplicability of provisions found in Subpart A; *key definitions*; several
categories of permissible research based on risk and benefit; explicit requirements for *permission by parents* or guardians and for *assent by children*;
and provisions that pertain to children who are *wards* of the state or
certain other entities.

This subpart makes clear that whereas certain survey and interview
procedures might be exempt from the regulations at 45 CFR Part 46
when adults are participants in research, research involving children is
not exempt from the regulatory requirements. Also, research involving
observation of public behavior when the investigator(s) participate in
the activities being observed is not exempt [Section 46.401(b)].

For purposes of applicability within this subpart, children are persons who have not attained the legal age for consent to treatments or
procedures involved in the research, under that applicable law of the
jurisdiction in which the research will be conducted [Section 46.402(a)].

The terms *permission* and *assent* are used in this subpart instead of the
term *consent*, but the consent requirements described in Subpart A are
applicable here. Permission means the agreement of parent(s) or guardian to the participation of their child or ward in research. Assent means
a child's affirmative agreement to participate in research. It should be
noted that a child's mere failure to dissent should not be taken as assent.
The sick child or the mentally retarded child may have a reduced capacity to dissent. He or she may act passively and compliantly to be
considered cooperative (Grodin & Glantz, 1994). The regulations set no
age specifications on which assent is required; the IRB must make that
determination in the context of the research to be conducted and in
consideration of the capabilities of the child or children.

IRBs have a major responsibility in assessing the risks, possible
benefits, and associated discomforts of the research involving children.
They must make their assessment and justification for approval of the
research in light of the expected benefits to the child who is the subject
of the research or to society as a whole. The federal regulations require
IRBs to classify research involving children into one of four categories
and to document their discussion of the risks and benefits of the research
study. The four categories of research involving children that may be
approved by IRBs, based on degree of risk and benefit to individual
subjects, are as follows:

- Research *not involving greater than minimal risk* [Section 46.404].

- Research *involving greater than minimal risk, but presenting the prospect of direct benefit to an individual subject.* Research in this category is approvable provided (a) the risk is justified by the anticipated benefit to the subject, and (b) the relationship of risk to benefit is at least as favorable as any available alternative approach [Section 46.405].
- Research *involving greater than minimal risk with no prospect of direct benefit to individual subjects, but likely to yield generalizable knowledge about the subject's disorder or condition.* Research in this category is approvable provided (a) the risk represents *a minor increase over minimal risk*; (b) the intervention or procedure presents experiences to subjects that are reasonably commensurate with those inherent in their actual or expected medical, dental, psychological, social, or educational settings; and (c) the intervention or procedure is likely to yield generalizable knowledge about the subject's disorder or condition that is of vital importance for the understanding or amelioration of the subject's disorder or condition [Section 46.406].
- Research that is *not otherwise approvable, but which presents an opportunity to understand, prevent, or alleviate a serious problem affecting the health or welfare of children.* Research that is not approvable under any of these first three categories may be conducted or funded by DHHS provided that the IRB, and the secretary, after consultation with a panel of experts, finds that the research presents a reasonable opportunity to further the understanding, prevention, or alleviation of a significant problem affecting the health and welfare of children. The panel of experts must also find that the research will be conducted in accordance with sound ethical principles [Section 46.408].

OPRR has, to date, convened two panels on behalf of the secretary, DHHS, under this provision to assess if research not meeting the first three categories listed here could be carried out. One concerned juvenile diabetes; one concerned muscular dystrophy. The panels of experts were particularly concerned about the informed consent process and information about the risk and potential benefit balance in the research to be conducted.

OPRR has asked IRBs to make certain that the research to be carried out can be accommodated by the categories of research permitted in Subpart D; this must be documented in the minutes.

When children or minors are involved in research, the regulations require the *assent* of the child or minor and the *permission* of the parent(s), in place of the consent of the subjects. Because children have not reached their full intellectual and emotional capacities and are legally unable to give valid consent, involving children in research requires the permission of their parents or legally authorized representative. The IRB must determine whether the permission of both parents is necessary, and the conditions under which one parent may be considered *not reasonably available* [Section 46.408]. In addition, the regulations require that the IRB determine that adequate provisions are made for soliciting the assent of the children, when in the judgment of the IRB the children are capable of providing assent [Section 46.408(a)].

The regulations provide that an IRB may find that the permission of one parent is sufficient for research to be conducted if the research is minimal risk research or research involving greater than minimal risk but presenting the prospect of direct benefit to individual subjects. When research has other categories of risk and benefit, and permission is to be obtained from parents, both parents must give their permission, unless one parent is deceased, unknown, incompetent, or not reasonably available, or when only one parent has legal responsibility for the care and custody of the child [Section 46.408(b)].

Even if children are not capable of giving informed consent, they may possess the ability to assent to or dissent from participation. In line with the principle of respect for persons, children should be asked whether or not they wish to participate in research, particularly if the research will not be likely to benefit them and if the children can comprehend and appreciate what it means to participate in research. The IRB may choose to review on a case-by-case basis whether assent should be sought from individual children in a protocol.

When the IRB determines that the research presents the possibility of direct benefit to that child that is important to the health or well-being of the child and is available only in the context of the research, the IRB may determine that the assent of the child is not necessary [Section 46.408(a)]. In this case, the child's *dissent* may be overruled by the child's parents, if the IRB find that this is acceptable. When research involves the provision of therapies for life-threatening conditions or other conditions, IRBs need to take into account that parents may wish to try whatever research might have any prospects of success even if that presents considerable discomforts for the child. This may raise some dilemmas for research investigators and IRBs (OPRR *Guidebook,* 1993).

The OPRR *Guidebook* notes that when assent is found to be appropriate, the child should be given an explanation of the research procedures to be conducted in a language that is commensurate with the child's age, experience, maturity, and condition. The assent process should explain the discomforts and inconveniences the child may experience.

Also, a process that invites coercion or undue inducement must be avoided.

Further, for some types of research activities, IRBs may require that an IRB member or an advocate for the child be in attendance during the assent and permission process to verify the child's understanding and to ensure that the child's preferences are honored. In addition, the IRB may require that the parent(s) or a supportive family member be present during the research (OPRR *Guidebook*, 1993).

There are also provisions in this subpart for *not having parental permission*. If consent can be waived under the provisions in Subpart A [Section 46.116(d)], then parental permission need not be sought. Also, if the IRB determines that a research protocol is designed for conditions or for a subject population for which parental or guardian permission is not a reasonable requirement to protect the subjects (e.g., neglected or abused children), it may waive the permission requirements for parents, provided an appropriate mechanism for protecting the children who will participate as subjects in the research is substituted, and provided that the waiver is not inconsistent with federal, state, or local law. The regulations specify that the choice of an appropriate mechanism would depend upon the nature and purpose of the activities described in the protocol, the risk and anticipated benefit to the research subjects, and their age, maturity, status, and condition [Section 46.408(c)].

As noted, there are also special protections for children who are *wards of the state* or of any other agency, institution, or entity [Section 46.409]. If the research involves greater than minimal risk to the subjects with no prospect of direct benefit to individual subjects, or if the research requires secretary of DHHS approval, the research has to be related to the children's status as ward, or it can be conducted in schools, camps, hospitals, institutions, or other similar settings in which the majority of children involved as subjects are not wards. For each child who is a ward, the IRB requires appointment of an advocate in addition to any other individual acting on behalf of the child as a guardian or *in loco parentis*. In line with the principle of justice, it is important that the investigators ensure that children who are wards are not included as participants simply because of their ready availability.

CERTIFICATES OF CONFIDENTIALITY

One of the review criteria of an IRB concerns the extent to which the confidentiality of the participants is adequately protected. Federal Certificates of Confidentiality may be appropriate for investigators to obtain as an extra measure of protection. The research does not have to be supported by the federal or state government in order to be eligible for coverage by the Certificate. Under federal law [Public Health Service Act, Section 301(d), 42 U.S.C. Section 241(d), as added by Pub. L. No. 100-607, Section 163 (November 4, 1988)], all research investigators in the United States may apply for a Certificate of Confidentiality to grant protection against compulsory disclosure of personally identifiable research information. Under the law, the secretary (or designee) may authorize persons engaged in biomedical, behavioral, clinical, or other research (including research on mental health, and research on the use and effects of alcohol and other psychoactive drugs) to protect the privacy of individuals who are the subjects of such research by withholding from all persons not connected with the conduct of such research the names or other identifying characteristics of such individuals.

This authority extends to a broader range of activities an earlier authority that was available only for research on mental health, alcohol, and other psychoactive drugs. The Certificates of Confidentiality may be granted if the research is of a sensitive nature where the protection is judged necessary to achieve the research objectives. Examples of sensitive research include information relating to: sexual attitudes, preferences or practices; the use of alcohol, drugs, or other addictive products; illegal conduct; or information that, if released, could reasonably be damaging to an individual's financial standing, employability, or reputation within the community. Other examples of sensitive research include information that would normally be recorded in a patient's medical record, and the disclosure of which could reasonably lead to social stigmatization or discrimination, and information pertaining to an individual's psychological well-being or mental health.

There are four offices in the Public Health Service that are authorized to issue Certificates of Confidentiality. For further information one may contact the Office of Heath Planning and Evaluation, Public Health Service, U.S. Department of Health and Human Services, Washington DC 20201, or consult the OPRR *Guidebook* (1993, pp. 3-33–3-35).

AN EMERGING ISSUE AREA: GENETIC RESEARCH

The use of genetic technologies holds out great promise for identifying genetic factors that contribute to human health and human disorders. Large recent strides in genetics in the 1980s and 1990s have created intense interest in possible inheritance of mental disorders. A workshop in 1992 sponsored by the Office of Technology Assessment (OTA), on *The Biology of Mental Disorders*, resulted in a report that identified many of the perceptions and social implications of genetics and mental disorder research and ethical issues in that research (U.S. Congress OTA, 1994).The OPRR Guidebook points out some of the particular challenges of involving potentially vulnerable populations of children and persons with mental disorders in genetic research.

The nature of genetic research raises special concerns when the research involves children, or physically or cognitively impaired persons. Not only must the IRB ensure that their participation is fully voluntary and informed, but the IRBs must also be sure to evaluate the risks and benefits of the research as they apply to these special populations. The risk of participation for an adult differs from that of children; persons who suffer from diminished mental capacities may be subject to different risks than persons who do not. If children will be involved in their research, IRB should seriously consider consulting with experts in child development and others knowledgeable about risks to children and families. Similarly, if physically or cognitively impaired persons will be involved in the research, IRBs should consider consulting with experts who can advise them on the special concerns their participation raises (OPRR *Guidebook*, 1993). Further, involving children in genetic research may raise concerns about pressure by family members and potential harm that may result from disclosure of genetic or incidental information (OPRR *Guidebook*, 1993).

The Report of the Institute of Medicine, entitled *Assessing Genetic Risks: Implications for Health and Social Policy* (1994), recommends that children should generally be tested for genetic disorders only when there exists an effective curative or preventive treatment that must be instituted early in life to achieve maximum benefit. The Institute of Medicine committee also recommends that, in the case of predictive tests for mental disorders, results must be handled with stringent attention to confidentiality to protect an already vulnerable population. Predictive testing for mental disorders raise concerns about the potential for stigmatization and discrimination.

Issues of inclusion of children in genetic research involving large pedigree studies are also found in *Ethical and Legal Issues in Pedigree Research* (Frankel & Teich, 1993).

CONCLUSIONS

Children and adolescents with mental disorders represent a population of persons who have several types of vulnerabilities. These vulnerabilities require that those who design, carry out, review, support, and regulate research be particularly diligent to protecting the rights and welfare of these persons.

Because they are children and adolescents, there are limitations on their abilities to comprehend information and thus give autonomous agreement to participation in research. Further, the nature of their mental disability may limit their ability to comprehend and to voluntarily agree to participate in research. The nature of their mental disorder may render them particularly vulnerable to stigmatization and discrimination, necessitating strong protections for privacy and confidentiality. There are certainly also special considerations for involvement of adolescents in research where needs of parents and of adolescents may conflict in terms of concerns over privacy and control. The involvement of an adolescent with a mental disorder may compound these challenges.

Grodin and Glantz (1994), who discussed legal and ethical issues relating to vulnerable children, noted, that some have taken the position that children with limited abilities are owed protection as a moral responsibility of the child's family. When a child is ill there is an even more compelling moral obligation of society to provide protection because of the kind of people we wish to be (Hauerwas, 1970).

Grodin and Glantz further noted that family members may not always be in the best situation to protect the child in research because their judgment may be impaired by the emotional impact of having an ill or handicapped child. The family of a child who is regarded as a burden may become dependent on a therapist, clinician, or research investigator, which might alter their ability to act in the best interests of their child (Grodin & Glantz, 1994).

These authors suggested several safeguards for children with mental disabilities who are participating in research, safeguards that are over and above those offered explicitly in 45 CFR Part 46 for the protection of children. For example, they suggest improved scrutiny in the selection of subjects for research to ensure that the risks and benefits of research are distributed fairly throughout the child population; investigator justification for recruitment of vulnerable children; a consent auditor or parent monitor to examine the quality of the proxy consent; particular scrutiny concerning undue inducements and coercion; nonuse of substitute judgment for this population of younger children; particular attention to assent of children and adolescents; minimization of risks by use of information gained during regular treatment; attention to the milieu in which research takes place; and presence of parents during procedures (Grodin & Glantz, 1994).

This discussion has focused on the regulatory aspects of research involving particularly vulnerable children. There are many dilemmas and ethical issues that arise in the course of particular research situations for which these regulations and the ethical principles described in the Belmont Report will be particularly helpful. Investigators and IRBs also need to be familiar with state and local laws, regulations and institutional policies, as well as laws and regulations pertaining to other federal department and agency programs, such as those of the FDA and the Department of Education.

REFERENCES

Federal Policy of the Protection of Human Subjects; Notices and Rules. *Federal Register*, June 19, 1991, [56FR28002].

Frankel, M. S., & Teich, A. H. (1993). *Ethical and legal issues in pedigree research*. Report on a conference sponsored by the American Association for the Advancement of Science (AAAS) Committee on Scientific Freedom and Responsibility and the AAAS American Bar Association National Conference of Lawyers and Scientists. Washington, DC.

Grodin, M. A., & Glantz, L. H. (1994). *Children as research subjects, science, ethics and law*. New York: Oxford University Press.

Hauerwas, S. (1970). Must a patient be a person to be a patient. Or my uncle Charlie may not be much of a person but he still is my uncle Charlie. *Connecticut Medicine, 39*, 815–887.

Institute of Medicine. (1994). *Assessing genetic risks: Implications for health and social policy*. Washington, DC: National Academy Press.

OPRR. (1993). *OPRR Protecting Human Research Subjects Institutional Review Board Guidebook*. Washington, DC: U.S. Government Printing Office.

OPRR Reports. (1979). *Ethical principles and guidelines for the protection of human subjects of research, the National Commission for the Protection of Human Subjects of Biomedical and Behavioral Research*. Washington, DC: Author.

OPRR Reports. (1994). Protection of human subjects, Title 45 Code of Federal Regulations part 46.

Public Health Service Act, Section 301(d), 42 U.S.C. Section 241(d). Public Law No. 100-607, Section 163. November 4, 1988.

U.S. Congress Office of Technology Assessment. (1994). *Mental disorders and genetics: Bridging the gap between research and society* (OTA-BP-H-133). Washington, DC: U.S. Government Printing Office.

3

Involving Families to Improve Research

Trina W. Osher
Mary Telesford
Federation of Families

Thanks in large part to the Child and Adolescent Service System Program (CASSP) sponsored by the Center for Mental Health Services, the benefits of involving family members as full partners in all aspects of children's mental health service delivery system are widely acknowledged. The concept can effectively be applied to research programs as well. This chapter seeks to unabashedly encourage such collaboration.

Of all the possible stakeholders with an interest in research about children and youth with neurobiological, mental, emotional, or behavioral disorders, it is the children, youth, and families who have the greatest stake. Yet, traditionally, families have played only the narrowest of roles in research. We believe that a family focus is essential to improving the quality of children's mental health research and encouraging attention to the highest standards of ethical conduct.

This chapter explains how to accomplish that goal. The first section sets out the principles of family involvement that apply to research. The second part describes ethical issues that concern families. The third section explores the various ways in which family members can participate in all aspects of the research program. The last section presents best practices for involving family members in research.

PRINCIPLES OF FAMILY INVOLVEMENT

Children and Adolescents Are People First

First and foremost, the research program must acknowledge that children and adolescents who have a neurobiological, mental, emotional, or behavioral disorder are people first and not merely subjects for research. Written and spoken language used in all aspects of the research program must put the children and adolescents before the disability or diagnosis (as in the opening sentence of this paragraph). Phrases like "disturbed children" or "the mentally ill" must be assiduously avoided.

Vocabulary has the great power to label people, places, things, and ideas. Words can be empowering or stigmatizing, flattering or insulting, polite and respectful, or rude and hostile. When language used in a research program is family friendly and jargon free, it respects the diversity, values, language, and culture of all children, youth, and families. To this end, the language of this chapter refers to children, youth, and families who are the focus of research as *participants*.

Children and Adolescents Are Members of Families

Regardless of the nature of their disability, what kind of treatment they are receiving, or where it is provided, children and adolescents are members of a family. Biological, foster, and adoptive parents, siblings, and extended family, and tribal members are the one consistent source of support throughout the life of any child or adolescent with a neurobiological, mental, emotional, or behavioral disorder. Families are the primary decision makers for their children and must be fully informed of and involved in decisions concerning their participation in research.

Researchers must strive for cultural competence and demonstrate that they respect the diversity and varied experiences of families regardless of how they are configured. It is incumbent on professional preparation programs to provide training that will prepare researchers at all levels to collaborate with families as partners in the discovery, analysis, synthesis, and dissemination of new knowledge about the nature, treatment, and prevention of neurobiological, mental, emotional, and behavioral disorders that affect children and youth.

Children and adolescents with these disorders and their families are entitled to treatment and support services that are comprehensive, community-based, and designed to meet their individual needs. Participation in research must never jeopardize their access to or opportunity to benefit from appropriate help to achieve their full potential.

ETHICAL ISSUES AND FAMILY CONCERNS

The number of "interesting questions" for research and study in the area of children's mental health is potentially infinite. Choices have to be made about which investigations will be underwritten with public (federal) funds. There are a number of family-related ethical matters that suggest criteria to use in making these decisions. Space limitations allow only the most overriding matters to be discussed.

Foremost among the ethical questions that must be asked is, "Why would a family want its child or adolescent to participate in a research project?" This goes beyond offering simple incentives (such as cash payments) to the very fundamental issue of what real benefit will accrue to the participants. How will the life of the child or adolescent be enriched by participating in the research project? The benefits to participants can be long or short term and can take many forms depending on the nature of the question being investigated and the research design. Of course, there are risks associated with all benefits. It is incumbent on researchers to ensure that family members fully comprehend these risks before they make a decision to participate. Some examples to illustrate follow.

- Gaining early access to a promising new treatment or service could have concrete, direct benefits. But the family must weigh the risk that the treatment will turn out to be ineffective or possibly harmful.
- Learning more about the origin or life course of a particular condition is a less tangible benefit but, nevertheless, can help a family to understand what they can expect. Having good information or an accurate diagnosis can bring closure to a family's search for answers. Information gained from participation in research can also help a family make decisions about treatments and steer them away from inappropriate alternatives. Despite these benefits, obtaining a diagnosis alone is not a sufficient benefit for most families to undertake the risks associated with participation in research. Families must continue to seek effective treatments and supports for their child. Researchers must make an effort to disseminate findings in such a way that they lead to development of effective follow-up treatment and support for participants.
- The personal satisfaction of being involved in making a contribution to treatment for future generations is an altruistic benefit. This benefit must be weighed against any discomfort participants will experience.

Closely related to issues of benefit to participants is the question, "Why conduct this research at all?" From the point of view of families, there is no moral or ethical justification for research that puts children and youth at even the most minimal risk without a counterbalancing benefit of significance. In other words, there has to be a real need to investigate the question and a high likelihood that the study will result in significant findings.

Research designs must interfere with the lives of participants as little as possible. Gathering information directly from children, adolescents, and families and other intrusive methods should be strategies of last resort. The necessity of including every item on a protocol should be evaluated by first investigating every other possible source of the information and then by determining that without this data the research question cannot be answered. Finally, investigators must repeatedly ask themselves, "Is there a less intrusive way to get this information?"

Research designs that incorporate deceptive strategies such as lying to participants about the procedure in which they are engaged pose a particularly high risk when they involve children and youth with neurobiological, emotional, mental, or behavioral disorders. Deceiving them undermines their capacity to trust adults, including the caregivers who allow them to participate in the research. Lack of trust can contribute to feelings of inadequacy, rejection, insecurity, loneliness, and depression on the part of the children and youth deceived. The implications for therapeutic follow-up that could result from the use of deceptive strategies in research on children's mental health need to be thoroughly explored and planned for before any such studies are approved. From the family perspective, deceptive studies have much to prove before they can gain a legitimate place on the research agenda. It is incumbent on the integrity of the researchers and those who fund research to determine beyond any doubt that there is no alternative way to gather the data and that there is an overwhelming public interest in conducting the research before deceptive studies are conducted where children and youth are the participants.

Designers of research and those who make decisions about funding it as well as family members who agree to participate in it need to address a variety of ethical dilemmas arising from the effect conducting research will have on the participants. Medical risk to children and adolescents participating in clinical trials of a new medication is a classic example. The problem extends to effects on the participants' environments even if there is not direct contact with them. This matter needs attention in services research where, typically, the study design is likely to include observation of participants in a specific setting. This may not seem to be as intrusive a technique as taking a blood sample. But, for adolescents in particular, the invasion of privacy that occurs when outsiders step into their school or other personal space can be very disturbing. The knowledge that they are being studied and the mere presence of observers can be upsetting, thus posing a risk to their well-being.

Studies involving "control" groups also involve ethical issues. Why should a family that is seeking a remedy for a stressful problem be asked to take the risk of being in a nontreatment control group? This is particularly true when existing options are limited, not highly success- ful, or when financial constraints deny families access to treatment. Is there any ethical justification for assigning a group of at risk children or adolescents (e.g., suicidal youth) to a nontreatment control group when clinical intervention is indicated?

The responsibility for demonstrating the benefits of research to the subjects and the community-at-large lies with the research team. The institutional conscience checking on ethics of research involving human subjects is the institutional review board (IRB). Family members and lay persons from the community have to be represented on the IRB to ensure that family perspectives on ethical issues are fully aired and discussed. Family members who sit on IRBs should be representative of the diversity of the community. We recommend that particular efforts be made to include family members from the specific subgroups of the population that are the focus of the study being reviewed. This may mean recruiting new individuals and providing them with background information and training to perform their role with confidence and competence. It may also mean providing supports like transportation and child care, rearranging the IRB meeting schedule, or meeting at a different location to make it possible for family members to participate.

Although its review and approval is a basic condition for conducting research, it is not sufficient to rely exclusively on an IRB to ensure that research is conducted in a manner that is family friendly. The next section discusses a number of other ways to improve research concern- ing children and adolescents with neurobiological, mental, emotional, or behavioral disorders by involving family members.

THE ROLES OF FAMILIES IN RESEARCH

Research can be strengthened when it involves family members every step of the way from the first stages of the research design to dissemi- nation of the findings. This section first describes some roles family members can play and then offers strategies investigators can imple- ment to build collaborative partnerships with the family members on their research team.

Families as Participants

Obviously, family members are the subjects of research. As key participants, they are entitled to be treated with courtesy and respect—not like rats in a maze. Appreciation for their contribution should be clearly and promptly expressed. Research can be improved by getting feedback directly from participants on how they felt about the experience and whether or not they feel it has affected their lives in any significant way—aside from the objectives of the study.

Family members are the largest market for research findings but often have the least opportunity for finding out what research has to say. Research teams should prepare a lay language summary of the results of their work and distribute it through family networks and popular family-oriented magazines. All participants should be given this summary and an opportunity to ask questions and get an in depth explanation of the complete report. Information about their individual participation should be shared when appropriate and particularly if there are implications for treatment, services, or supports to the child, adolescent, or family. Family members and participants should be told how they can receive interventions or treatments that the research has determined to be beneficial.

Families as Advocates

Family members are powerful advocates for research because they and their children stand to gain substantially from the new knowledge it yields. Family perspectives should be included in setting research priorities and in reviewing research grant applications. Research can be improved by asking family members (preferably in small focus or discussion groups) what they think about possible issues, topics, and problems for study as well as how it might affect them.

It is advantageous to include family members on all peer review teams and other procedures used to select projects to be funded. Family members can comment on the broad policy implications and family friendliness of the research proposal. They can contribute to discussion about ethical considerations as well as risks, benefits, and the impact on participants and families. We recommend that research supported with public funds be required to describe how families will be involved in the project. Projects that are not family friendly should not be supported with public funds.

Families can be excellent advocates in support of funding for research. When they are involved, informed, well treated, and satisfied, they will be a stronger voice and they will use their networks to be heard across the land.

Family Members as Research Associates

Family members can be recruited and trained to be excellent research associates. Because they share a common experience with the participants being studied, family members are most likely to gain the trust needed to get accurate information from interviews. Their insights can be useful in reacting to and verifying findings and seeking explanations for unexpected results.

Research can be improved by engaging community leaders and family networks in the design of the research to ensure that the goals of the research are relevant to the community's needs. If a research team cannot find support for its project in the community, they have two options. They can look elsewhere for a community that shares its goals, or they can work with family and community leaders to reframe the research questions. Researchers can gain community good will and support by finding out what additional related questions the families and community want answered and including these in the research design. Research will be improved when investigators use knowledge about the culture of the community and its residents to ensure that the recruitment strategies are appropriate to the population being studied and that they will, in fact, yield accurate and reliable data.

Family Members as Consultants and Advisors

Family participation in the role of consultant or advisor can contribute to improvements in research. Panels of family members or representatives of family organizations can review and give feedback on the clarity and family friendliness of instrumentation. They can review and analyze findings and critique or comment on lay language draft reports.

When using family members as planners, consultants, or advisors, particularly when travel or a fair amount of time is involved, researchers need to fairly compensate them for their time and effort on the same basis as other professionals. Family members are busy people. Involvement with a research project may mean taking time off from work, securing costly child care, loss of vacation or sick pay, paying for travel and meals. These costs should be reimbursed and not be taken for granted.

It is one thing to identify the benefits of involving families and the roles they can play in research but quite another to develop the collaborative partnership necessary to make this really work. There are two primary phases to this task. The first is to identify strategies for reaching out, making contact with family members, recruiting them to your team, and matching the right person to the right role. The second involves developing supports to ensure their effective participation and ongoing commitment to the research project.

Outreach and Recruitment of Family Members

As with all strategic activities, outreach and recruitment of family members to be part of a research team or serve in an advisory capacity requires clear goals and careful planning. Be clear about the specific activities for which family participation is being sought. Prepare a brief notice, similar to a job description, describing the responsibilities the family member will have, the expectations of the research team, and how much of a time commitment the family member will be required to make. Include details about the kind of background and experiences needed. Provide a rough estimate of the time commitment, mention any compensation or other benefit for the family member, and explain any travel requirements.

In any community, there are many family support groups, family advocacy organizations, parent, and community associations with members who are both qualified and interested in collaborating with research teams. Contact as many of them as possible. Most family organizations will be very pleased to allocate a few minutes on their next meeting agenda for a member of the team to explain the research project, circulate the notice, or publish it in their newsletters. Family and community leaders may be able to suggest specific individuals to contact directly.

Families Need Ongoing Support

Once family members have signed on, there are a variety of activities that will ensure they participate as fully franchised members of the team. Investigators and family members should meet informally in a comfortable, nonthreatening atmosphere just to get to know each other and start to develop the mutual respect and trust that characterize effective collaborations and partnerships. Informational briefings may be needed for family members to learn about the project in depth. Family members may need training in using a specific procedure, protocol, or other technique related to the role they will play. Family members should be offered support with logistics such as transportation or child care if needed. Like other members of the team, family members need access to information, technology, and staff support.

When treated with respect and dignity and given training, critical information, and support, family members who are partners in research will contribute substantially to the research process and resulting outcomes. Data accuracy and reliability will increase and the validity of interpretations will improve. Participants will be treated ethically. Findings will be widely available and readable. In short, research will be better able to achieve the highest standards of ethical and scientific integrity when family members are collaborators in the process.

BEST PRACTICES FOR FAMILY-FRIENDLY RESEARCH

It is beyond the scope of this chapter to address all of the best practices for effective and meaningful involvement of family members in research on children's mental health. The topics covered are among the guiding principles for ensuring "family-friendly" research.

The Protection of Privacy and Confidentiality

In order for families to feel free to participate in research activities, there must be some assurance that the data collected, especially personally identifiable data such as social security numbers, names, and addresses, are held in the strictest confidence. Family members do not want "everybody" knowing their business. This is particularly true of families involved with public systems such as child welfare, mental health, public housing, or juvenile justice, where penalties and/or warnings can be issued for the smallest infraction.

Sensitivity to Diversity in Data Collection and Research Design

In designing a research program that includes members of diverse backgrounds, the research team's composition should include family members who are from these diverse backgrounds. This is not to say that all members of the research team should have this background, but that at a minimum there are family members who do. A research team composed in this way is more likely to yield a research design (including assessment and evaluation instruments) that is appropriate for the population being studied.

Diversity is just as important and critical to data collection as it is to research design. In order to get the most positive outcomes from data, collectors need to present themselves in a way that makes family members feel comfortable. This means that data collectors would be culturally sensitive and appropriate in their demeanor, language, and approach of families.

Understanding the Research Methodology

In order to get full support from families, it is important that they fully understand the research methodology. This means explaining the methodology in "plain" language—minus the alphabet soup and PhD jargon. It is also important for families to understand how this research is going to benefit them and, if it is not going to benefit them directly, who will reap the benefit and when.

Another consideration in methodology for families is risk. The risks to the child involved should be fully explored as well as any risk to the entire family. With regard to the child, the following questions need to be addressed at a minimum. If there is a current treatment plan, will the proposed research treatment be compatible with the current treatment plan? Could there be adverse side effects? What would they be? Are there long-term effects or reactions expected beyond the research time span? If so, what are appropriate treatments at that point?

Although the risks to the child are paramount for examination, the risks to the entire family are also important. What types of support does the research program offer families? What types of support are anticipated that the families may need in order to assist in the treatment of the child? If the family is not able to give the child the appropriate supports, what alternatives, including building that capacity in the family, can be exercised? How is the family involved in selecting those supports?

Consent Versus Assent of Families

To maintain the ethical integrity of the research program, efforts should be taken to ensure that it is true consent and not merely assent that is given by families and participants. Many persons who benefit from public systems are reluctant to say no to a research program if it is not made clear in the beginning, by the person introducing the program, that in no way does the potential participant's decision jeopardize any assistance they are currently getting or may seek in the future. Researchers who make such promises must be sure they can be kept.

Research programs that specifically target captive audiences, individuals in detention centers, hospitals, or residential treatment facilities should be careful that program participants are making informed decisions when consenting to participate in a research program or study and, in the case of a minor, that parental consent is also granted. At no time should the family members or the child feel that their decisions would jeopardize the current treatment or placement status.

Put Yourself in the Families' Shoes

Many researchers fail to use their own experiences and instincts with regard to families. The bottom line is that if something is not good for your own family or children, it is most likely not appropriate for someone else's family or children. Before asking others to volunteer their children to participate in a study, researchers should ask themselves, "Would I gladly and willingly subject my own children, my own family, or myself to the procedures to be undertaken by this inquiry?"

CONCLUSION

By establishing meaningful partnerships with families, researchers can ensure high ethical standards, rigorous investigation of significant research questions, reliable data, sound findings, and ongoing advocacy for a research agenda. The justification for spending public money on research is that applying the knowledge gained will improve services, treatments, and interventions as well as the outcomes for children and adolescents who utilize them. Involving families as partners in research not only enhances the quality of life for children and adolescents with neurobiological, emotional, mental, or behavioral disorders, it also strengthens the ethical conduct of the research itself.

Part II

*Ethical Challenges Across
Diverse Research Contexts*

4

Research Ethics and Human Subjects Protection in Child Mental Health Services Research and Community Studies

C. Clifford Attkisson
Abram Rosenblatt
Child Services Research Group, University
of California, San Francisco
Kimberly Hoagwood
National Institute of Mental Health

Research subjects are best viewed as active participants and collaborators in child services research. It is inappropriate and counterproductive to view children, adolescents, and their families as passive objects of study. The relationship between researcher and subject is most respectful and productive when the relationship is structured as a partnership. In this partnership, subjects are fully informed about the goals of the research, specific procedures to be employed by the researcher, requirements and burdens of participation, and risks and benefits pertaining to participation. Subjects enter voluntarily into this partnership, can discontinue participation at will, are entitled to receive reliable information about the project and their own participation, and must be provided information about the scientific findings when they are available or when results at any time could affect their well-being (National Alliance for the Mentally Ill, 1995). The researcher engaged in studies of services or conducting epidemiological investigations is bound by

---

*The Child Services Research Group conducts services research on systems of care for children and adolescents with severe emotional disorders.

legal and ethical responsibility to place the rights and welfare of the research subject above any other consideration pertaining to the research and above the interests of the researcher, including the interests of the institution(s) sponsoring the research activity (American Psychological Association, 1989, 1992; Department of Health and Human Services [DHHS], 1983, 1991; Fisher, 1991, 1993; Fisher & Tryon, 1990).

The role of the research subject as active participant and collaborator stands in stark contrast to the passive stance typical of past and present research involving children, youth, and their families. The active role allows subjects to comprehend more clearly the goals of the research, to participate in setting research goals and identifying methods for obtaining reliable information, to be compensated when possible and appropriate, and to be treated with dignity and respect. Research goals can best be met within a framework of active subject participation as collaborators in implementation of the investigation. However, the role of research subject as active participant is an ideal never fully realized in a specific project. Investigators face many obstacles to the actualization of the ideal.

In this chapter, we identify major ethical and human subjects challenges encountered in conducting research on services for children and conducting research in communities more broadly, including epidemiological surveys. We also identify strategies used by researchers to overcome these obstacles.

MAJOR CHALLENGES AND STRATEGIES

Jurisdiction and Multiple IRB Reviews

The nature of child services research requires the investigator to address and collect data across multiple data domains as well as multiple components of the child services delivery system (Attkisson, Dresser, & Rosenblatt, 1995; Rosenblatt & Attkisson, 1993). This challenge occurs in epidemiological studies as well. Of special importance among the child-serving components are the mental health sector, social services sector, juvenile justice system, the educational system, and pediatric primary care. Frequently, when data are required about the adaptation and social functioning of youth, across all of the domains of the child's life, multiple informants, including providers and administrators within all of these sectors must be contacted. Typically, each sector will require its own individual review of the protocol and often these are stringent reviews. In addition, institutions that serve as the data collection site will also require an independent review of the protocol. These secondary reviews require a presentation of study goals and objectives to groups of providers and administrators and an active process of engaging these individuals in the goals and objectives of the research project.

These multiple reviews can be highly supportive of the ultimate goals of conducting research and yet they can frequently be redundant and overlapping processes. As long as services to children and youth are provided primarily within categorical streams of services, it is highly unlikely that anything can be done about the degree of redundancy and overlap in the review process. One could argue that these requirements encourage necessary critical scrutiny and provide the context for essential oversight to preclude the implementation of superficial studies or invasive and harmful protocols.

Multiple formal and informal reviews are practically a way of life in child services research because of the *balkanization* of categorical programs and the need to include all facets of the child's experience in the clinical services research process. This is a difficult and time-demanding process and one that must be endured with equanimity and a long-range perspective. It is also an opportunity to educate the research participants and sectors of the service system about the goals of the research project and an opportunity for close scrutiny and criticism of the research protocol from various perspectives prior to its implementation. Some of these challenges are, therefore, quite useful and productive for the research process.

Researchers working in communities often have difficulty in securing access to data from the full range of child-serving agencies providing services to research subjects. This is especially true with regard to youth suffering from severe emotional disorders where access to data is needed from multiple social, educational, and health sectors. The history of collaboration and interaction among these child-serving components is a conflicted one and there are countless reports in the literature of lack of collaboration between components during research projects after such collaboration was negotiated well prior to study implementation. In one of our projects, for example, a friendly court intervention was needed to secure access to individual-identified information across component sectors of care. These obstacles are to be expected and often there are appropriate legal constraints on the exchange of information when there is no identified legal need to know or to have access. Investigators need to develop their organizational skills and their documentation skills in order to be able to cope with these problems, and especially need to identify and distinguish when the obstacles that are confronted are realistic and appropriate, and when they mask resistance to the research. Resolution of disguised reluctance often hinges on the identification of *quid pro quo* that include sharing of resources or exchanges of information to create a sound basis for collaboration. Effective research collaboration also requires a commitment to a common vision shared by the research team and the host clinical, service system, or community setting. These shared visions are built over time and sustained by the experience of the utility of scientific information for planning and service system design.

Lack of Local Mechanisms for Protection of Research Subjects

Although multiple institutional review board (IRB) reviews and jurisdictional conflicts are the norm in most large service systems, many smaller service systems suffer from a lack of any mechanism for the protection of research subjects. This is especially the case in smaller communities and more rural areas. Frequently, these systems cannot support the cost and time required to establish even an informal internal review process. Such service systems rarely encounter the need for human subject review committees of any type and may thus be reluctant to establish these mechanisms when the need does arise. In our experience, many of these communities and systems would prefer to rely on IRBs based in universities or other research settings, thereby abdicating both their responsibility for, and their participation in, the human subjects approval process.

We do not contend that all service systems must create formal or informal IRBs to review research projects that have already been formally approved by a university or other research institution. However, we do believe that the service system should have some formal participation in the human subjects' approval process. This may take many forms, including a review of procedures and protocols by professionals and administrators from the collaborating agency. In all these cases, the ultimate responsibility for gaining the full collaboration and knowledge of the participating service system rests with the investigator. We contend that simple presentation of an official IRB letter without further explication to persons of responsibility in the participating agency regarding the potential consequences of the research for human subjects is not acceptable.

In community studies where service agencies will not be involved but rather only household samples, the IRB is likely to be the only body to review the procedures. However, with increasing frequency, investigators are finding that community contexts are important to sample, if one wants to understand human behavior. Consequently, community agencies or providers are increasingly being studied as well.

Resistance to Research

Not infrequently, we have found that reluctance to involvement in research is disguised as concern over breach of confidentiality and the perceived risks of burdening patients, service providers, and the service delivery system. The formal review process in these situations is usually more drawn out and inexplicably delayed while organizational reactions to the prospect of participation in research are worked through. At times, these resistances are due to the perception that academic research is superficial and self-serving; at other times, the operative factor is the control exercised by service providers and administrators seeking to avoid evaluation and public scrutiny. All social systems are cautious about such scrutiny and this situation is made more complex when unions or employee organizations have a vested interest in worker protection or prevention of deviation from work responsibilities and conditions that are negotiated as a part of collective bargaining or union agreements. Most often, one has to work with these restrictions and requirements and substantive accommodation is rarely achieved when such organizational structures are dominant. These resistances can be viewed as individual and group conflicts between the perceived need for control, stasis, and self-protection versus the goal of exploring alternatives to increase organizational efficacy. Such resistances must be understood on their own terms and separated from the absolute requirement that organizations must take all necessary steps to protect children, youth, and families from inappropriate investigations, superficial research, and the overzealous researcher.

Length and Complexity of the Research Protocol

IRBs tend to be highly focused on the length of protocols and are very sensitive to the number of measures proposed for use in a study. This is, of course, an appropriate concern and, at times, child services researchers have had to provide considerable justification on why multiple measures, often measures that index the same trait or state, are necessary components of social science research projects, given the current state of psychometric theory and technique. In our work, we have found that when we provide adequate theoretical and measurement underpinning for our choice of measures and the integration of measures within a specific protocol, the IRB is typically accepting of our strategy and responds with encouragement for us to attempt to minimize or reduce the number of items or measures insofar as possible.

To minimize child and family burden and to prevent intrusive, unethical, or inappropriate interventions, IRBs require stringent review processes for projects involving children and adolescents. There is always extensive concern about minimizing the burden on subjects and family. Frequently, the burden is indexed by the amount of time to be spent with subjects and the extent to which lengthy interview protocols are used.

Time, however, is frequently neither the best nor the only indicator of burden. At this stage in our research activities, we have conducted more than 1,100 interviews with children and adolescents and an additional 1,100 interviews with family members or family surrogate respondents, and we conclude that there is widespread subject acceptance of a relatively demanding interview and diagnostic process, as long as the subjects have ample opportunity to communicate freely their individual histories and their own perceptions. Interviews that are highly structured and that do not allow opportunities for interaction or for sharing perceptions would be likely to constitute a greater burden to the research subject. When subjects experience a choice to discontinue the interview at their own will, they exercise that choice and tend to participate enthusiastically and to experience research interviews as useful and supportive. When the interview content and subject matter is focused on the child or the adolescent, rather than making the parents or parent surrogate the subject of direct inquiry or study, there is greater acceptance of the interview.

Sticking With the Protocol

Given the exigencies and many challenges to studying children in communities and especially services for children and families, it is difficult to maintain the discipline required by an approved protocol. Each case represents a new individual or a new family situation and each case requires an application of the protocol in such a way that the rights and dignity of all concerned are maintained at the highest level. It is legal folly to stray from approved research procedures although the pressures to do so occur constantly. It is frustrating and highly distracting to have to request an IRB modification of an existing protocol because of the time consumed in preparing requests for such changes and the length of time required to obtain a variance or a modification. However, this process must be followed if individual variation necessitates a change from the established protocol.

ART, SKILL, AND PROCESS
IN SUBJECT RECRUITMENT

Child services researchers find that subject recruitment often is an art reflecting a dynamic process requiring judgment and basic clinical skills. There is extensive individual variability in the exercise of these skills. The term *recruitment* itself has a range of connotations. Subjects must be informed and must feel comfortable to choose or not to choose to be participants or continue their participation. When incentives are too high, or the individual sense of power and choice is too low, subjects can be enrolled without freedom of choice. Inducement to research participation in these circumstances can be associated with heightened subject vulnerability (Thompson, 1990). A skillful recruiter provides as much objective information as the potential subject requires or can handle. The skillful recruiter knows how to ask questions, how to answer questions, and how to solicit questions as a part of the decision-making process. The skillful recruiter knows when to withdraw or when to gently press for a decision. Descriptions of this process in the human subjects manuals often make obtaining consent seem cold or impersonal. In contrast, an interactive and personal exchange more accurately reflects the concept of "informed" consent. As in all medical fields, the recruiter's and the investigator's foremost principle should be: First (and always) do no harm!

"Written" Informed Consent

Signed or written informed consent is not always a necessity or a requirement in research. IRBs, however, tend to require investigators to obtain written consent forms to participate and it is always essential to guarantee that subjects are provided with information to guide their decision and to ensure that they are informed. Although the legal stance of the investigator is probably more greatly ensured through the obtaining of a written consent, it is often the case that the written consent process is inappropriately required or unnecessarily burdensome. Investigators should clarify the circumstances where written informed consent is absolutely essential for legal and other reasons. These situations should be distinguished from others where a verbal consent process is sufficient.

Nevertheless, written consent is usually a necessity—particularly in research activities involving interactions with children and youth (Abramovitch, Freedman, Thoden, & Nikolich, 1991; Gaylin & Macklin, 1982; Holder, 1981; Keith-Spiegel, 1983). There are circumstances, however, when collaterals of the child or providers in the service delivery system are interviewed via telephone. In these circumstances, written informed consent may not be necessary except for the initial consent given by the child or parent to conduct such interviews.

Although legal guardians have the right to give consent, assent by the child should also be obtained (Langer, 1985). As Abramovitch et al. (1991) noted, acting on this principle can prove difficult. Children may be able to meaningfully assent to participation but may not make the decision freely. Parental consent, once achieved, may put pressure on the child to participate. Researchers should be sensitive to this problem, and fully acknowledge to the degree possible the right of the child to refuse participation. Concomitantly, researchers must also respect the relationship between the parent and the child and not, in any way, cast aspersions on the authority of the parent.

Supervising Research Personnel

The research investigator must exercise constant vigilance in ensuring objective oversight of the human subjects protection protocol. The primary mechanisms for this are close supervision of data collectors, multiple observers of the behavior of research personnel that allow detection of unethical conduct, and ongoing debriefing about interactions of research personnel with human subjects to allow for understanding and correction of personnel perceptions, choices, and decisions. Data collectors and interviewers require frequent debriefing and supervision that allows them to grow and mature in their work. Frequently, such individuals have only basic levels of professional training and it is unusual that they have had extensive training in ethical principles related to the interaction with clinical patients or human subjects of any type. Obviously, all protocols require such training and ongoing review of the broad and specific principles that relate to the interactions required by the protocol. Because the resources for studies of services are often constrained, it is difficult to obtain highly educated or well-trained personnel for the repetitive and arduous tasks required of ongoing data collection in the laboratory or in the community. This means that there must be ongoing checks of data collector interactions with subjects. This can be achieved, in part, through the use of tape recordings and these tape recordings are maintained for periods of time following the conduct of the interview or data collection process. Such tapes are frequently sampled continuously on a random basis. In the early periods of training, these tapes are monitored extensively by data collection supervisors. Such external monitoring and other quality controls provide reliability checks on the data collection process, structure, and ongoing consultation for the interviewer in the field, and increased vigilance over the rights and well-being of subjects.

Clinical Zeal

Data collectors, especially those at the master's level or those who are inexperienced clinically, regardless of their level of education, often tend to exercise their therapeutic zeal rather than maintaining a work-focused, neutral role as a data collector. Often it is reassuring for the inexperienced data collector to assume a therapeutic stance during the data collection process. Inexperienced or anxious interviewers often revert to providing advice or clinical "interpretations" to interviewees. Consequently, in training of interviewers, it is important to constantly underscore the need to maintain an egalitarian, neutral relationship. Although it is essential in the service of good interviewing skills to be empathic or to acknowledge affect or feelings when needed by the interviewee, it is inappropriate to move beyond the data collection mode into a stance of clinical inquiry or involvement beyond that required by the protocol. This type of behavior is almost always unwarranted and easily harmful to subjects. A calm, objective, and neutral interviewer stance is almost always the most reassuring to subjects who then respond positively and feel more in control of their participation. The separation of clinical from research roles is a challenge in many types of studies especially those involving interviews about services where the need for those services may be acute. This is especially the case for low-income minority children, who may be either over or underidentified as requiring clinical interventions (Scott-Jones, 1994).

Undue Incentives

Compensation of subjects should be an appropriate payment for the individual(s) time spent in contribution to the research project. The use of subject payments at a level that could be considered an undue incentive to participate must be guarded against (Macklin, 1981). Frequently, subjects in child service studies are from impoverished backgrounds and the opportunity to receive a significant payment for time spent in a research project represents an undue incentive leaving the individual little choice but to participate. Whenever possible, undue incentives should be avoided and IRB committees are generally vigilant about this aspect of the research protocol. Assessment of a fair reimbursement is more of an art than a science. Nevertheless, we should continue to struggle for guidelines that allow, insofar as possible, subjects to make a free choice to participate. It is our conviction that this freedom of choice is as highly related to the quality of data and the ultimate success of research than almost any other variable in the administration of a research protocol. Subjects who are coerced through overpayment, or exploited through underpayment, frequently do not constitute the most reliable group of subjects or the most enduring participants in research requiring multiple interviews across time.

In addition to the amount of the payment, researchers must attend to who gets paid. Child services research projects usually include parents, children, and other caretakers as part of the data collection protocols. Human service professionals such as teachers and clinicians may also be included in the data collection process. Establishing, for example, procedures for providing cash payments to the minor rather than the guardian can ensure that all parties see the child as sufficiently compensated (Fisher, 1993). Teachers and other human service professionals may not wish to receive monetary compensation for their participation for a variety of reasons, and in such cases creative solutions can be offered. Teachers, for example, might be compensated in the form of donations or purchase of classroom supplies. Such procedures help all parties feel equitably compensated for their time and effort.

Reporting Child Abuse, Neglect, and Dangerousness

State and federal legislation is quite specific about requirements for reporting abuse and neglect of children and youth when such abuse has not been previously reported and placed under official scrutiny. There are exacting requirements and protocols for such reporting, and these must be included within the human subjects materials and consent forms that are used by research investigators. Specific knowledge of these requirements and the inclusion of conformity with the requirements must be a formal part of our research protocols and disclosed to subjects in our human subjects consent procedure. It is important to understand that procedures and requirements vary by state. Liss (1994) found in a recent review that researchers are currently mandated to report in at least 13 states.

It is not uncommon for researchers to find it necessary to report suspected child abuse or neglect that had not been previously identified or reported (Fisher, 1994). Although the legal requirement for such reports may be clear, the process used to make such reports is all important. For example, in studies in which the youth are either currently in treatment, or have recently been in treatment, one approach is to work with the treating clinician to make the report in a way that minimizes potential damage to the therapeutic relationship between the family and the clinician. In these cases, a report is not made until the clinician of record has been contacted and consulted. In most instances, the clinician knows of the potential abuse and/or neglect and has already filed a report. In other instances, discussion with the clinician is a piece of information that leads the *clinician* to file a report. As a result of this process, it is rare for the research team to file such reports. In community studies, where much of the sample is unlikely to be in treatment and where clinical back-up may not be available, the investi-gator will have to be prepared to respond to reports of abuse when they arise. The casebook in this volume provides several examples of ways in which investigators have handled this kind of situation. In addition, Putnam, Liss, and Landsverk (chapter 8) offer some pertinent examples.

Abuse and neglect are rarely obvious in the course of a research interview, and so a judgment concerning the veracity of the claim virtually always needs to be made. An unfounded report can lead to significant strains for the family and failure to make a needed report usually results in harm to the child. Either event can irrevocably damage the credibility of the research project. This problem is especially relevant to reporting of abuse of children from ethnic minorities and low-income families where overreporting is more likely (Edelbrock, 1994).

Similar tensions exist in the reporting of dangerousness to self or others. California, as the state in which *Tarasoff* was adjudicated, man-dates a duty to warn intended victims of violence, although court cases have yet to apply this directly to researchers (Appelbaum & Rosen-baum, 1989). One approach is to immediately notify the caretaker about the child's potential for harm to self or others. In most cases, the caretaker is well aware of the problem and has already taken steps with the treating clinician to deal with either the suicidal or homicidal statements or potential of the youth. In the remainder of cases, a discussion with a clinician follows contact with the parent.

Although IRBs review procedures for reporting abuse, neglect, and dangerousness, interviewers and senior members of research teams must not only follow protocol but must also exercise decisive judgment on these matters. Even when procedures are closely followed and accompanied by good judgment, mistakes can still be made. Finally, even when a report is accurately made, the research team provides an obvious target for the pain and anger of parents and families. If a research project is to survive, and be helpful to children and families in dealing with such incidents, there needs to be a considerable level of trust and an ongoing working relationship between the research team, the service providers, and the broader community.

Electronic Media

It is increasingly common to use electronic means for maintaining and controlling the large volumes of patient identified confidential data. Often such data are coded with unique subject numbers to prevent disclosure in case data are accessed by unauthorized individuals. But, in some cases in intermediate phases of the research, name identified data are essential to allow for the creation of unique identifiers or integration of multiple data sets where there is no single unique identifier at that stage of the research. Fortunately, most software programs currently allow for password protection of such files and these measures can be used on all confidential data. Nonetheless, such protection is not foolproof, and in all of these situations, the researcher is challenged to work speedily and effectively to reduce risks and at the same time prevent any activity that could minimize the immediate and long-term value of the data. Nonprofessional personnel have to be educated about the risks and ethics pertaining to disclosure of subject data. These personnel must be enlisted in the ongoing effort to maintain security and protect confidentiality. Frequent revisiting of this topic is advisable for all research groups.

Administrators and the Press

Phone calls from administrators or the press regarding individual children and families who independently come to their attention are major challenges to services and epidemiological researchers. All research personnel must be fully informed and frequently reminded of their sole responsibility of preventing any breech in the confidentiality of data provided by human subjects. The mere acknowledgment that an individual has been a subject in the research process can do damage to individuals. Nevertheless, there are frequent pressures from administrators and less frequently from the press to divulge participant information.

Court Orders and Subpoenas

Although many researchers and clinicians comfort themselves with the thought that their records are confidential and protected under the law, such is not always the case. Court records can subpoenaed (Melton, 1990). A Certificate of Confidentiality, issued by DHHS can help protect the privacy and identity of research participants (Hoagwood, 1994). Even this certificate, however, may not necessarily protect the researcher against all reporting requirements. The essential point here is that researchers need to understand the limits of confidentiality in order to represent them accurately to human subjects.

Clinical and Administrative Records

Use of administrative and clinical records is often construed as nonreactive research or as research activities not requiring permission of patients or their families. It is true that administrative records can be used for research purposes as long as such protocols are reviewed and the confidentiality of information is protected by ethical and professional researchers. Nevertheless, the integration of clinical records or service records across service settings, where the identification of subjects is an essential component of the cross use of services, requires that the rights and protection of the individual be given due consideration. Many times, such disclosures can be undertaken without obtaining informed consent. However, those conditions are probably very rare, and consequently the need for permission in a legal and ethical sense is required. This area of research needs considerable thought and analysis. We have very few principles and many precedents that are not necessarily rooted in ethical considerations.

CONCLUSION

Studies of services for children, including studies involving community survey methodologies, necessitate attention to a range of ethical issues that are often unique to the exigencies of service delivery. Studies of this kind arise from, and are responsible to, caregivers, administrators, and community leaders, for whom the results of the study often have great policy relevance. Consequently, issues such as obtaining consent, obtaining multiple IRB reviews, protecting confidentiality, and reporting abuse are fraught with complexities, because they are responsive to the legal and social realities of the natural contexts that surround children's lives. There are creative approaches available for addressing these complex ethical issues, and we have outlined some of these. However, we also need to recognize that there are inconsistencies in the sources of the moral authority that guide our thinking—inconsistencies in regulations, codes, and precedents—and consequently we must be vigilant to apply higher order ethical thinking to all of our research practices (DeRenzo, 1994).

This chapter began with a plea to consider subjects as active participants in the research process. In services research and community studies, much the same needs to be said about service providers and administrators. We are convinced that some investigators eager to enter the applied setting, treat clinicians, administrators, and others in the services systems as research subjects without even according them the basic rights that they accord their actual research subjects. Service system professionals are collaborators, and can be the most powerful agents for assuring that the rights of humans subjects in services research are truly protected.

ACKNOWLEDGMENTS

Work on this chapter was supported, in part, by a research center grant from the Division of Epidemiology and Services Research of the National Institute for Mental Health (MH46122, MH43694, and MH18261); and by evaluation research contracts from the California State Department of Mental Health (89-70225, 90-70195, 91-71106, 92-722091, and 93-73346-A-1. We acknowledge the many contributions of our colleagues and associates: Harold Baize, Karyn Dresser, Rachel Guerrero, Karla Kruse, and Nancy Mills. The views expressed in this chapter represent those of the authors only.

REFERENCES

Abramovitch, R., Freedman, J. L., Thoden, K., & Nikolich, C. (1991). Children's capacity to consent to participation in psychological research: Empirical findings. *Child Development, 62,* 1100–1109.

American Psychological Association. (1989). *Ethical principles in the conduct of research with human participants.* Washington, DC: Author.

American Psychological Association. (1992). Ethical principles of psychologists and code of conduct. *American Psychologist, 47,* 1597–1611.

Appelbaum, P. S., & Rosenbaum, A. (1989). *Tarasoff* and the researcher: Does the duty to protect apply in the research setting? *American Psychologist, 44,* 885–894.

Attkisson, C. C., Dresser, K., & Rosenblatt, A. (1995). Service systems for youth with severe emotional disorder: System of care research in California. In L. Bickman & D. Rog (Eds.), *Creating a children's mental health service system: Policy, research, and evaluation* (pp. 236–280). Beverly Hills, CA: Sage.

Department of Health and Human Services. (1983, March 8). Additional protections for children involved as subjects in research. *Federal Register, 48*(46), 9814–9820.

Department of Health and Human Services. (1991, August). Title 45 Public Welfare, Part 46, *Code of Federal Regulations, Protection of Human Subjects.*

DeRenzo, E. G. (1994, November–December). The ethics of involving psychiatrically impaired persons in research. *IRB: A Review of Human Subjects Research,* 7–9, 11.

Edelbrock, C. (1994). Assessment of child psychopathology. In C. B. Fisher & R. M. Lerner (Eds.), *Applied developmental psychology* (pp. 294–314). New York: McGraw-Hill.

Fisher, C. B. (1991). Ethical considerations for research on psychosocial interventions for high-risk infants and children. *Register Report, 17,* 9–12.

Fisher, C. B. (1993). Integrating science and ethics in research with high-risk children and youth. *Social Policy Report: Society for Research in Child Development, 7*(4).

Fisher, C. B. (1994). Reporting and referring research participants: Ethical challenges for investigators studying children and youth. *Ethics & Behavior, 4*(2), 87–95.

Fisher, C. B., & Tryon, W. W. (Eds.). (1990). *Ethics in applied developmental psychology: Emerging issues in an emerging field.* Norwood, NJ: Ablex.

Gaylin, W., & Macklin, R. (1982). *Who speaks for the child: The problems of proxy consent.* New York: Plenum.

Hoagwood, K. (1994). The Certificate of Confidentiality at the National Institute of Mental Health: Discretionary considerations in its applicability in research on child and adolescent mental disorders. *Ethics & Behavior, 4,* 123–131.

Holder, A. R. (1981). Can teenagers participate in research without parental consent? *IRB: Review of Human subjects Research, 3*(2), 5–7.

Keith-Spiegel, P. C. (1983). Children and consent to participate in research. In G. P. Melton, G. P. Koocher, & M. J. Saks (Eds.), *Children's competence to consent* (pp. 179–211). New York: Plenum.

Langer, D. H. (1985). Children's legal rights as research subjects. *Journal of the American Academy of Child Psychiatry, 24,* 653–662.

Liss, M. (1994). State and federal laws governing reporting for researchers. *Ethics & Behavior, 4*(2), 133–146.

Macklin, R. (1981). "Due" and "undue" inducements: On paying money to research subjects. *IRB: Review of Human Subjects Research, 3*(5), 1–6.

Melton, G. B. (1990). Certificates of Confidentiality under the Public Health Services Act: Strong protection but not enough. *Violence and Victims, 5,* 67–71.

National Alliance for the Mentally Ill. (1995). *Policies on strengthened standards for protection of individuals with severe mental illness who participate as human subjects in research.* Arlington, VA: Author.

Rosenblatt, A., & Attkisson, C. C. (1993). Assessing outcomes for sufferers of severe mental disorder: A conceptual framework and review. *Evaluation and Program Planning, 16*(4), 347–363.

Scott-Jones, D. (1994). Ethical issues in reporting and referring in research with low-income minority children. *Ethics & Behavior, 4,* 97–10.

Thompson, R. A. (1990). Vulnerability in research: A developmental perspective on research risk. *Child Development, 61,* 1–16.

5

Ethical Issues in Psychosocial Treatment Research With Children and Adolescents

Euthymia D. Hibbs
National Institute of Mental Health
Penelope Krener
University of California, Davis

Psychosocial treatment research of child and adolescent mental disorders is a relatively young field, but it presents long-standing and at times formidable challenges to investigators. Although participation in psychosocial treatment research might be thought of as presenting less of a risk than other forms of treatments, because such treatments are not physically invasive, the risks may, in fact, be substantial for children with mental disorders. The psychosocial researcher often must base his or her design on theories of development and of psychosocial functioning that are less well established than are medical principles of physiology or pathology. Research based on unsubstantiated theories may bias the investigator's assessment of the morality of research questions and experimental procedures and place the subjects at risk.

The challenges arise in part because the relationship between clinical responsibility for the well-being of clients and scientific objectivity present competing demands to the researcher. As is clear from the casebook in this volume, such tensions can be ethically resolved, but special precautions need to be taken to ensure that both clinical and scientific responsibilities can be met.

In this chapter, we discuss five specific ethical issues that confront investigators who study the efficacy or effectiveness of psychosocial treatments for children. These issues are competence, informed consent/assent, confidentiality, use of incentives, and selection and involvement of control subjects.

CLINICIAN/THERAPIST COMPETENCE

Investigators conducting psychosocial research need to ensure the competence of the professionals involved in both the scientific and intervention components. Limited research resources frequently lead to the practice of training graduate students to carry out the treatment in the intervention modality being tested. Objectivity and replicability are sought by manualizing the treatment procedure in a regimented treatment protocol. The training, as it is reported in the literature, is usually intensive. Supervision is done directly or through videotapes. Although standardized and focused, this approach to treatment raises issues of clinical competence. The clinician who deals with childhood psychopathology needs to be well experienced. Therapeutic difficulties or crises may arise during treatment sessions that must be understood and addressed immediately, not delayed until after consultation with the supervisor or discussion during a weekly supervisory session. For example, a clinician/therapist may be trained to follow a manual for the cognitive treatment of depression. One subject may have a comorbid secondary condition of anxiety disorder and, during a session, this child may exhibit distress, difficulty swallowing, breathing, and so on, due to an anxiety attack. The therapist needs to be able to diagnose and therapeutically intervene to relieve the child's anguish.

The implications of the issue of competence are that in all studies of psychosocial treatment where specific modalities are being assessed there should always be well-qualified clinical backup. It is important to use fully trained and certified clinicians, as subjects may be harmed if treated by inadequately trained clinicians.

INFORMED CONSENT/ASSENT

Informed voluntary consent is an ethical and legal requirement for any research study. The consent form is a written document that explains to an individual who volunteers to participate in a research protocol the goals, processes, and risks involved. The Department of Health and Human Services (DHHS) regulations require, as a condition for institutional review board (IRB) approval of any research, that the informed consent form include:

1. Description and purpose of the research.
2. Discussion of reasonably foreseeable research risks.
3. Expected benefits.
4. Availability of alternative treatments.

5. How and the extent to which confidentiality will be maintained.
6. Possible compensation if injury occurs from research involving more than minimal risk.
7. Disclosure about who to contact concerning pertinent questions and research-related injury.
8. A statement about the voluntary nature of beginning and continuing in the research (DHHS, 1991).

Consent procedures for children and adolescents recruited for psychosocial intervention research require special consideration because minors do not have the legal capacity to consent, have limited social power that makes them especially vulnerable to coercion, and may lack the cognitive maturity to comprehend risks and benefits of treatment and experimentation (Fisher, Hatashita-Wong, & Isman, in press; Fisher & Rosendahl, 1990; Keith-Spiegel, 1983; Melton, Koocher, & Saks, 1983; Thompson, 1990; Weithorn & Campbell, 1982). In light of these considerations, federal regulations require the informed consent of a legal guardian before a child can participate in research. In addition, the National Commission for the Protection of Subjects of Biomedical and Behavioral Research introduced the concept of assent procedures for children participating in research (Hershey & Miller, 1976). Assent means that the child has the right to be informed of and agree to the conditions of research participation without necessarily comprehending the information at the level required for legal informed consent, and the child's objection supersedes guardian consent unless the experimental treatment holds out the prospect of direct benefit that can only be achieved through the research (Campbell, 1987; Fisher, 1993; National Commission for the Protection of Human Subjects in Biomedical and Behavioral Research, 1977).

Consent and assent forms should be written in a language that can be understood by individuals unfamiliar with technical terminology, appropriate to the developmental level of the participant, and sensitive to the participant or guardian's familiarity with English. Children and families recruited for participation in psychosocial treatment research are especially vulnerable to confusion and potential exploitation during the recruitment phase of research because they are at risk for or have identifiable mental health problems. Accordingly, the investigator should verbally discuss the research issues and encourage questions to ensure that the children or their parents or guardians fully understand the significance of their participation prior to signing the written informed consent document.

As discussed in the casebook in this volume, in longitudinal treatment studies, informed consent needs to be conceptualized as an ongoing educational process between investigators and children and their guardians. Investigators should be particularly cautious when conducting studies in treatment contexts where guardians provide "blanket consent" for experimental assessments. Under these conditions, parents may not remember every procedure listed in the initial consent document and may be surprised or distressed to learn that their child has been taken out of class or away from a daily hospital routine to be given an extensive assessment battery. A recommended procedure is to review the study protocol with parents and children at specific points throughout the research process. An investigator can also provide parents (and children when appropriate) a written schedule or calendar of activities detailing the approximate dates of treatment, assessment, and parent meetings. Periodic parental review and renewed consent to research procedures may present some threat to the research design because some families will need more explanation or support than others. However, as the casebook and conclusion to this volume indicate, investigators have developed innovative ways to incorporate individual participant responses to consent and debriefing procedures into the experimental design. Psychosocial intervention studies with high-risk or disordered children and youth also raise ethical issues regarding what information and available treatments will be provided parents and children at the end of the study. In short-term treatment studies, it is standard practice to offer control groups the treatment found to be most effective. However, in longitudinal studies designed to evaluate the effect of an early intervention on later development, a treatment found to be effective may be developmentally inappropriate for the now older participants in the control group (Fisher, 1993). To address this problem, it has been suggested that in long-term psychosocial intervention studies for children, investigators design post intervention assessments and referral procedures that can be utilized to help parents whose children still need treatment find developmentally appropriate community services at the completion of the study (Fisher, 1993; Fisher, Higgins, et al., in press, chapter 8, this volume).

CONFIDENTIALITY

Protections Against Disclosing Personally Identifiable Information. Investigators conducting psychosocial interventions with children and youth need to set up procedures that can adequately protect participant confidentiality. This includes consideration of how to protect the confidentiality of assessment results, treatment outcomes, as well as information about a participant's family members. Protecting confidential information can be particularly difficult when working with minors because all states have some form of statutory reporting requirement regarding child abuse and neglect and in most states there is an absence of clear legal and professional parameters outlining parental access to treatment information (DeKraai & Sales, 1991; Fisher et al., in press; Liss, 1994; Putnam, Liss, & Landsverk, chapter 8, this volume; Schaefer & Call, 1994). Accordingly, both parents and prospective child participants must be fully informed about the procedures that will be used to ensure confidentiality (e.g., the use of subject codes, security measures for storing files) as well as the limits of confidentiality (e.g., what types of information will and will not be shared with parents, what information is required by law to be reported to outside authorities). Investigators conducting psychosocial treatment research with delinquent youth should also be sensitive to the possibility that data regarding legal offenses committed by a participant might be subpoenaed (Wolfgang, 1981). One way to provide research subjects and investigators immunity from subpoena of research records is to obtain a Certificate of Confidentiality issued by DHHS (Health Omnibus Programs Extension Act, 1988). The certificate provides legal protection for the investigator against being compelled to disclose personal, identifiable information about research subjects, and at the same time assures research participants that they are protected from such disclosure (Hoagwood, 1994).

The Use of Videotapes and Computer Technology. Investigators studying psychosocial interventions are increasingly using videotapes to perform complex behavioral analyses or to test hypotheses beyond those directly relevant to treatment efficacy (e.g., comparing the time of onset and strength of the therapeutic alliance between two treatment conditions). Videotaping promises an effective and economical way to ensure interrater reliability and to examine several hypotheses over a period of time extending beyond the completion of the treatment phase of the study. At the same time, videotaped sessions raise ethical concerns about confidentiality. For example, investigators need to consider the extent to which the original consent form adequately details which members of the treatment and research teams will have access to the videotapes (e.g., the child's psychotherapist, the head of the research team, research assistants), addresses secondary analysis procedures, or safeguards the privacy rights of the individuals videotaped during the treatment study.

Therapy material, especially videotapes gathered through research treatment protocols, can also be a helpful teaching tool to train students and other professionals or a means of disseminating information about research to the public. However, such exposure runs the risk of embarrassing or stigmatizing participants. For example, one student of psychology recognized her next door neighbors on a videotaped treatment study shown in class. As illustrated in Case 26 of the casebook, consent procedures can provide participants and their parents with several options for the use of their videotaped sessions, ranging from use by the primary investigator only to use by other investigators or for educational purposes. However, some participants may not have fully understood the consequences of educational or media exposure or may have forgotten they had granted permission for the release over an extended period of time. For example, one participant whose video interview was shown on television was enraged because he had forgotten that he had signed a consent, his life had changed, and he did not want to expose his past problems to the public. He threatened to sue the institution and the investigator conducting the study. Another alternative, therefore, is for investigators to draw up a new consent form, explaining in detail to the participants the meaning and consequences of being viewed in a classroom filming or on national television at the time when videotapes may be shown for educational or media purposes.

Investigators also need to give careful consideration as to how the videotapes will be secured both on site and when data may be sent to investigators at other sites. In one treatment study, concern for the inability to ensure confidentiality when videotaped data were transferred across sites led the investigators to limit the data to on site access (Imber et al., 1986).

A related threat to confidentiality is computer technology. For example, investigators need to consider the penetrability of data stored in computer banks. Because researchers cannot ensure against access by unauthorized individuals to computer stored data, they must ensure that the data are identifiable only to themselves through encryption or sophisticated subject codes.

Sharing Information With Parents. Because children and adolescents rarely refer themselves to treatment or intervention studies, parents are recognized as the "gatekeepers" with respect to referral and continued compliance in the research protocol (Melton & Wilcox, 1989). Consequently, parental involvement in the research process is critical to the ongoing participation of their offspring (Kovacs & Lohr, 1995). Usually love and concern as well as their legal and moral responsibility to protect the welfare of their children impels parents to want to be informed about the ongoing aspects of a treatment study. They may request to be updated concerning assessment results and therapy decisions. Investigators need to consider the extent to which sharing information with parents facilitates or compromises the child's treatment as well as the integrity of the research.

Children's privacy rights and their response to intervention strategies are dependent on a sense of trust in the service provider. This trust is not, however, limited to the child's faith in the therapist's and researcher's ability to keep information confidential, but also in the professional's responsibility and obligation to disclose information when it is necessary to ensure the child's welfare (Fisher, 1993; Fisher et al., in press; Taylor & Adelman, 1989). Methodological requirements of a psychosocial intervention study may, however, limit the type and amount of information that might be available to parents under nonresearch conditions. For example, time constraints, incomplete development of comparison norms, or the need for investigators to be blind to the treatment outcome of individual participants may mean that certain measures can be scored only at the end of the treatment. In addition, informing parents about certain aspects of the child's behavior revealed during the course of therapy may differentially impact their behavior toward the child or toward the research and compromise the validity of the study. Consequently, at the outset of the study, investigators need to consider the extent and limits of confidentiality with respect to therapeutic and methodological requirements, as well as the needs of family members, and work closely with parents to communicate the rationale for the procedures and thus gain their trust and cooperation.

Another issue related to sharing of information with parents concerns disclosure about comorbid conditions. Often the experimental hypothesis or limited resources make treatment of the comorbid disorder during the study period infeasible. Because comorbid conditions are the rule rather than the exception in children, the methodological integrity of a study might suffer by informing parents of this condition if this leads the parent to respond to the child differently or to refer the child out for additional treatment. Assuming the scientific validity of the experimental hypothesis and ruling out the possibility that failure to directly treat or provide a referral for the comorbid condition places the child at greater risk than if he or she had not entered the study, investigators should consider strategies for including parents as an integral part of the treatment project. Such strategies can include parent and community consultation in the design stages of the study regarding identification and communication of comorbid disorders, adequate informed consent procedures detailing the possibility that comorbid conditions may be identified during the course of the study, provision of a schedule for parent feedback during the study, parent training, and, when appropriate, parent treatment. More examples of ways to involve families in research are provided by Osher and Telesford (chapter 3).

INCENTIVES FOR PARTICIPATION

Psychosocial treatment research, like any other clinical research, will seek volunteer participants with particular mental disorders to participate in treatment studies. Investigators may advertise in newspapers, doctors' offices, schools, the media, and in other ways. Although subject participation is defined as voluntary, voluntariness is a relative term. The potential for incentives to be a coercive influence on children or their parents needs to be carefully considered by investigators. The question then becomes, at what level of reimbursement is remuneration potentially great enough to influence participants to consent to participate in a study? For individuals in great financial need, there may be little likelihood they will reject the offer to participate; does this, then, entail coercion? If the investigator appeals to an individual's altruism (e.g., "This study will help us understand how to treat this disorder and your participation will help people in the future") is he or she exerting moral coercion? If the study offers treatment that is otherwise unaffordable, will a potential subject feel compelled to participate? These are issues that should be considered in advance by the investigator.

Remuneration for participation in a study is permissible and is used extensively, not as an incentive but as a token to express the investigator's appreciation for the child's/parent's effort or to reimburse the subjects for travel or other expenses due to their participation in research (Small, Campbell, Shay, & Goodman, 1994). It is advisable to obtain advice from ethics consultants when developing recruitment strategies that include remuneration to participants.

In addition to ethical concerns, a threat to the research design may be posed by using incentives. Some participant volunteers may be desperate individuals who either could not find treatment elsewhere or who could not afford it. Others may be responding to an advertisement, but not be as symptomatic as they claim; some may merely be seeking novelty. It also happens that philanthropic organizations or churches encourage their constituents to volunteer and then donate the remuneration.

In all of these conditions, however, there is a risk of selective recruitment of subjects who read newspapers, attend church, or respond to advertisements. Selection bias may put the generalizability of the study at risk. To avoid such problems, a systematic outreach and effort to include a representative sample from all socioeconomic status and ethnic/cultural groups is crucial.

CONTROL SUBJECTS

The strongest designs in psychosocial treatment research include comparison or control groups. Depending on the hypothesis tested, control groups may include individuals without psychopathology, those with physical illness only, or subjects with a different diagnosis than the one under investigation. In the case of psychosocial treatment research, individuals falling within the same diagnostic category, but receiving a different treatment modality, are often used for the control condition. Ethical issues that arise in studies using some of the more common designs are described here.

No-Treatment Control.   No-treatment control groups help in discerning the extent to which subjects would improve without treatment. These groups are controlled for history, maturational level, the effects of repeated testing, and so on. The control and experimental groups are usually equivalent in all independent variables. The core issue here is that withholding treatment is unethical (Hibbs, 1993). For example, in the treatment of school phobia, it is unethical to allow a phobic child to remain in fear of and away from school for a prolonged period of time.

In addition, participation in a no treatment control group may lead to differential attrition. If, in order to alleviate their child's suffering, parents seek treatment elsewhere without informing the investigator, the results of the study will be diluted or muddled. If they drop out of the study, the remaining subjects will comprise a select group (Kazdin & Wilson, 1978) whose selection did not fit the study design.

Wait-List Control Group.   A wait-list control group has several advantages. An intake interview is usually performed prior to placement on the waiting list, and patients expect an appointment in the near future. Patient expectancy (the improvement that occurs in anticipation of treatment) provides important information on the natural history of the disorder (O'Leary & Borkovec, 1978). On the other hand, subjects may differ in characteristics such as severity of disorder and rate of attrition, as they are not often randomly assigned. Delaying treatment is unethical unless the subjects are assigned to the wait-list control group on the basis of their ability to wait for treatment. In this case, the research design is in trouble because of selection bias and the study's generalizability is thrown into question. Attrition may occur when treatment is readily available in the subject's locality. It is also unethical to delay treatment in situations when treatment is unavailable except through the research study.

Placebo Control Group.   Placebo control typically includes components of treatment that account for its effects, such as expectation of improvement, and attentional control. Both control and experimental subjects receive the same number of sessions. Process research, which attempts to investigate and isolate the active components of therapy, is best controlled for by using a placebo treatment group. Control group subjects should be equivalent in every way to the experimental group, except for the active components of therapy to be isolated and investigated. However, the placebo condition necessitates deception, which presents ethical problems (see the chapter on deception in the casebook in this volume). Unlike drug studies, where subjects are informed that they will receive an "inert pill," in psychosocial treatment, "placebo/inert" conditions are not usually explained. Hence, important information is withheld from the subject in the consent process (Hibbs, 1993). The Ethical Principles of Psychologists (1993) state that when methodological requirements make the use of deception necessary, the investigator has a special responsibility to determine whether the use of such techniques is justified by the study's prospective scientific, educational or applied value; to determine whether alternative procedures are available; and to ensure that the participants are provided with sufficient explanation as soon as possible.

CONCLUSION

Although biologically noninvasive, psychosocial interventions may be invasive psychologically, and may consequently have a powerful impact on patients. Therefore, minimal risk cannot be assumed. Five challenges to conducting ethical and high-quality psychosocial research with children and adolescents have been discussed in this chapter. These are summarized here.

First, funding constraints may compromise research design either by necessitating the employment of inexperienced assistants, or by limiting the accommodations available for addressing comorbid conditions or clinical crises. The clinician carrying out the treatment within the research protocol must employ well-trained staff, even if the cost of employing such individuals is higher. Therapeutic effectiveness is known to depend on therapist–patient factors, which are difficult to operationalize and quantify, and which potentially threaten the objectivity and interchangeability of treatment units. For example, treatment effectiveness increases if the therapist feels invested in the patient's well-being; however this may be seen as therapeutic bias, jeopardizing objectivity. Flexibility of therapist response to patients is a feature of clinical competence, as is the ability to perceive subtle behaviors and patterns which cannot be quantified in treatment manuals. Thus, there may be a negative trade-off of clinical information for quantifiable data, unless the investigators are able to apply both clinical mastery and rigor of research design.

A second challenge is posed by the problem of obtaining informed consent with proxy consenters (parents or other responsible adults) and determining children's assent to participate. Consent may need to be obtained at multiple points over the course of the study. In addition, developmental factors always must be taken into account in longitudinal studies involving children. These are examples of ethical problems in treatment research of children that have been explored elsewhere in the literature (Krener & Mancina, 1994).

A third challenge in conducting psychosocial research is that of ensuring patient confidentiality while collecting data which is intended for dissemination. Troubled individuals may find many ways to assist themselves with overcoming their symptoms and solving their problems in living. If participation in psychosocial research causes a patient to limit his or her search for assistance to one standardized intervention, then that patient may be walled off from other sorts of social assistance. Data from the treatment in the research project may be confounded by other therapeutic experiences which had been discovered outside the project. The increased use of videotaping in treatment research necessitates additional protections. Investigators need to create procedures for management of videotaped data, including obtaining additional consents from participants and developing policies for access to these data. A related threat to ethical treatment of subjects is presented by the question of preserving confidentiality while also meeting the scientific obligation to disseminate data and teach the next generation of researchers and clinicians. The power of the media to widely broadcast images—which are one person's personal experiences and another person's data points—magnifies this threat. The investigator must anticipate potential distortions and abuses, and both protect the patient from unwanted surprises by adequate informed consent, and protect the data from distortion in transmission by carefully controlling how it is exposed.

A fourth problem concerns the differential effects of incentives on participants. Clinical judgment, skill, and foresight should be brought to bear on the question as to whether the incentive structure will exert a differential effect upon selection or retention, and whether it constitutes undue inducement.

Finally, the selection of appropriate control groups, and the optimal design for their involvement, are often accompanied by a variety of ethical dilemmas. No-treatment control group designs are the most problematic, because withholding treatment from persons who, by definition, may require intervention, is clearly unacceptable. Such a design also risks loss of study participants. Wait-list control group designs do not pose the same problem as withholding treatment, but attrition of participants is a risk. Placebo control designs, while offering the advantage of rigor, generally involve deception, and this, of course, requires careful thought and justification.

Although these five ethical issues tend to arise in many studies of psychosocial treatments, there are creative ways to engage with the problems presented, and the casebook in this volume presents examples of such solutions. As the field of psychosocial treatment research with children continues to grow, one can expect the dilemmas likewise to reproduce. Several approaches will facilitate sound ethical decision making: strengthening the role of clinicians in such research; delineating the separate responsibilities for the clinical and scientific components of these studies; ensuring that new technology, which can strengthen scientific contributions, is accompanied by foresight and caution; and involving families in multiple aspects of the research process.

REFERENCES

Campbell, M. (1987). Consent issues with disturbed and/or retarded children. *Psychopharmacology Bulletin, 23*(3), 379–381.

DeKraai, M. B., & Sales, B. D. (1991). Liability in child therapy and research. *Journal of Consulting and Clinical Psychology, 59*, 853–860.

Department of Health and Human Services. (1988). *Health Omnibus Program Extension Act of 1988. paragr. 242a, 42 U.S.C. Paragr. 301(d).*

Department of Health and Human Services. (1991). Title 45 Public Welfare, Part 46, *Code of Federal Regulations, Protection of Human Subjects.*

Ethical principles of psychologists. (1993). *American Psychologist, 48*, 633–638.

Fisher, C. B. (1993). Integrating science and ethics in research with high-risk children and youth. *Society for Research in Child Development Social Policy Report, 7*(4), 1-27.

Fisher, C. B., Hatashita-Wong, M., & Isman, L. (in press). Ethical and legal issues in clinical child psychology. In W.K. Silverman & T.H. Ollendick (Eds.), *Developmental issues in the clinical treatment of children and adolescents.* Boston: Allyn & Bacon.

Fisher, C. B., & Rosendahl, S. A. (1990). Psychological risks and remedies of research participation. In C. B. Fisher & W. W. Tryon (Eds.), *Ethics in applied developmental psychology: Emerging: issues in an emerging field* (pp. 43-60). Norwood, NJ: Ablex.

Hershey, N., & Miller, R. D. (1976). *Human experimentation and the law.* Germantown, MD: Aspen.

Hibbs, E. D. (1993) Psychosocial treatment research with children and adolescents: Methodological issues. *Psychopharmacology Bulletin, 29*(1), 27–33.

Hoagwood, K. (1994). The Certificate of Confidentiality at the National Institute of Mental Health: Discretionary considerations in its applicability in research on child and adolescent mental disorders. *Ethics & Behavior, 4*, 123–131.

Imber, S. D., Glanz., L. M., Elkin, I., Sotsky, S. M., Boyer, J. L., & Leber, W. R. (1986). Ethical issues in psychotherapy research: Problems in a collaborative clinical trials study. *American Psychologist, 41*, 147-156.

Kazdin, A. E., & Wilson, G. T. (1978). *Evaluation of behavior therapy: Issues, evidence, and research strategies.* Cambridge, MA: Ballinger.

Keith-Spiegel, P. (1976). Children's rights as participants in research. In G. P. Koocher (Ed.), *Children's rights and the mental health professions* (pp. 383–431). New York: Wiley.

Keith-Spiegel, P. (1983). Children and consent to participate in research. In G. P. Melton, G. P. Koocher, & M. J. Saks (Eds.), *Children's competence to consent* (pp. 179-211). New York: Plenum.

Kovacs, M., & Lohr, W. D. (1995). Research on psychotherapy with children and adolescents: An overview of evolving trends and current issues. *Journal of Abnormal Psychology, 23*(1), 11–30.

Krener, P. K., & Mancina, R. A. (1994). Informed consent or informed coercion? Decision-making in pediatric psychopharmacology. *Journal of Child and Adolescent Psychopharmacology, 4*(3), 183–200.

Liss, M. B. (1994). Child abuse: Is there a mandate for researchers to report? *Ethics & Behavior, 4*, 133-146.

Melton, G. B. Koocher, G. P., & Saks, M. J. (Eds.). (1983). *Children's competence to consent.* New York: Plenum.

Melton, G. B., & Wilcox, B. L. (1989). Changes in family law and family life. *American Psychologist, 44*, 1213–1216.

National Commission for the Protection of Human Subjects of Biomedical and Behavioral Research. (1977). *Research involving children* (Pub. No. 0577–004). Washington, DC: Department of Health, Education and Welfare.

O'Leary, K. D., & Borkovec, T. D. (1978). Conceptual, methodological, and ethical problems in placebo groups in psychotherapy research. *American Psychologist, 9*, 821–830.

Schaefer, A. B., & Call, J. A. (1994). Legal and ethical issues. In R. A. Olson, L. L. Mullins, J. B. Gillman, & J. M. Chaney (Eds.), *The sourcebook of pediatric psychology* (pp. 405-413). Boston: Allyn & Bacon.

Small, A. M., Campbell, M., Shay, J., & Goodman, I. S. (1994). Ethical guidelines for psychopharmacological research in children. In J. Y. Hattab (Ed.), *Ethics and child mental health* (pp. 132–154). Hewlett, NY: Gefen.

Taylor, L., & Adelman, H. S. (1989). Reframing the confidentiality dilemma to work in children's best interests. *Professional Psychology Research and Practice, 20*, 79-83.

Thompson, R. A. (1990). Vulnerability in research: A developmental perspective on research risk. *Child Development, 61*, 1-16.

Weithorn, L. A., & Campbell, S. B. (1982). The competency of children and adolescents to make informed treatment decisions. *Child Development, 53*, 1589-1598.

Wolfgang, M. E. (1981). Confidentiality in criminological research and other ethical issues. *Journal of Criminal Law and Criminology, 72*, 345–361.

6

Ethical Issues in Psychopharmacological Treatment Research With Children and Adolescents

Henrietta Leonard
Brown University School of Medicine
Peter S. Jensen
Benedetto Vitiello
National Institute of Mental Health
Neal Ryan
Western Psychiatric Institute
John March
Duke University
Mark Riddle
Johns Hopkins University
Joseph Biederman
Massachusetts General Hospital

It has become increasingly clear that there is little, if any, safety and efficacy data in the pediatric age group for the majority of prescription medications. Indeed, most medications are not labeled for use in children by the Food and Drug Administration (FDA) because of the absence of sufficient studies. In a recent review, the Committee on Drugs of the American Academy of Pediatrics (AAP; 1995) cited data from an FDA report (Office of Drug Evaluation Statistical Report, FDA, 1989) that 80% of the new medications approved from 1984 to 1989 did not contain labeling for use in children. Additionally, the AAP noted that of the medications reviewed in the 1991 *Physician's Desk Reference* (*PDR*), 81% had descriptions that either disclaimed their use in children or restricted them to specific age groups (Gilman & Gal, 1992).

This paucity of safety and efficacy data in the pediatric age group raises immediate and important clinical concerns about pharmacologic treatment of this age group. Essentially, this absence results in children being left as "pharmacologic orphans." In order to make treatment recommendations for a child who might have a potentially medication-responsive illness, a physician must compare the risk of not treating, because of the lack of systematic information, with that of treatment based on limited data. The physician may be left to extrapolate from studies in adults, or to draw conclusions from anecdotal reports in children, either of which source may have significant limits. Children and adolescents, by virtue of their changing development, often have very different pharmacokinetics, clinical response (pharmacody-namics), and adverse reactions to medications than those seen in adults. Drug absorption, distribution, metabolism, and excretion vary through-out development, and these may have important clinical implications for prescribed dosage, clinical response, and toxicity (Branch, 1994). For example, the rate of absorption may be faster in children, and peak levels may be reached earlier (Bourin, Couetoux, & Tertre, 1992). The association between serum levels, clinical response, and side effects is not well studied for many medications; studies are needed to determine maturationally related changes of bioavailability, metabolism, and clearance (Wilens, Biederman, Baldessarini, Puopolo, & Flood, 1992).

Hepatic metabolism of some medications appears to vary with age, such that it is highest during infancy and childhood, approximately twice the adult rate in prepuberty, and equivalent to adult values by age 15 (Popper, 1993). Thus, younger children may require divided (instead of once a day) dosages and higher milligram/kilogram (mg/kg) daily dosages of hepatically metabolized medications to achieve a plasma concentration similar to that of adults. For example, Wilens and col-leagues (1992) reported that children had a lower serum concentration of desipramine than that of adolescents, and much lower than that of adults on equivalent weight-corrected (mg/kg) dosages. Interindi-vidual differences can be significant; a sixfold difference in nortriptyline drug levels, and a twentyfold difference in desipramine drug levels, have been reported in children who were administered a constant mg/kg daily drug dose (Wilens et al., 1992; Wilens, Biederman, Geist, Steingar, & Spencer, 1993). Thus, studies in adults may not predict the pharmacokinetics, therapeutic response, or adverse effects in children.

This lack of systematic study of the pharmacokinetics of medications in children poses a major problem for all of pediatric medicine, but perhaps an even more critical one for the field of pediatric psychophar-macology. Long-term effects of a medication on the developing systems, especially the central nervous system (CNS), need particular consideration in children, and this has received only very limited study. For example, metoclopramide, a dopamine antagonist, is indicated for the treatment of gastroesophageal reflux in adults. As with other dopamine antagonists, tardive dyskinesia, dystonic reactions, and other extrapyramidal symptoms have been reported in association with this medication (*PDR*, 1995). Metoclopramide is frequently prescribed for reflux in infants, yet it is unknown what its long-term effects on the developing brain are, nor whether there might be any increase in subsequent movement disorders.

The animal literature suggests that rats exposed to medications with CNS actions (i.e., haloperidol, apomorphine) before or shortly after birth have enduring changes in catecholamine levels and/or receptor cells (Haldeman & Quirion, 1983; Hill & Engblom, 1984; Rosengarten & Friedhoff, 1979). There is very limited literature on the long-term effect of exposure to CNS medications on the child during the prenatal or early childhood period, although it merits consideration (Farell, Lee, & Hirtz, 1990; Scolnik, Nulman, Rovet, & Gladstone, 1994). This remains one of the most compelling arguments for systematic study of the safety of medications that may be prescribed in children.

Another unique issue for the pediatric group is that since the mid-1980s there has been a dramatic increase in the prescribing of psychotropic medications in children and adolescents (Jensen, Vitiello, Leonard, & Laughren, 1994). This increase parallels changes in psychiatry, such as the recognition that many "adult" psychiatric disorders can now be diagnosed in childhood, and that many common psychiatric disorders have biological etiologies and may be amenable to psychotropic interventions. These changes, as well as the development of new medications with new indications and a different side effect profile, have resulted in the increased use of medications in adults, which may potentially have applications for children. The increased interest in pediatric pharmacology is indirectly evidenced by the twofold increase in numbers of psychopharmacology research articles in the *Journal of the American Academy of Child and Adolescent Psychiatry* and the development of a new journal (*Journal of Child and Adolescent Psychopharmacology*) devoted specifically to pediatric pharmacology (Jensen et al., 1994).

There is a dramatic discrepancy between actual clinical practice of prescribing medications in children and the FDA-approved indications and ages for those drugs. (Of note, an FDA-approved indication means that the pharmaceutical company can legally advertise that the medication is effective for a specific disorder in a specific age group based on research studies.) Other than the psychostimulants, only four neuroleptics (haloperidol, thioridazine, chlorpromazine, and pimozide) and two antidepressants (imipramine for enuresis and clomipramine for obsessive compulsive disorder [OCD]) have a specific indication and dose guidelines for children (Jensen et al., 1994). The neuroleptics have dosing guidelines starting at age 6 months for chlorpromazine, and ranging to 12 years for pimozide. Imipramine has guidelines for age 6 years and above, and clomipramine has them for age 12 years and above.

The discrepancy between clinical practice and FDA approval is apparent in the gap between perceptions of risk and actual prescription practices. For example, three neuroleptics are approved for use in children for "severe explosive behaviors" or "short-term management of attention deficit hyperactivity disorder (ADHD)." Yet, these medications would be seen by many as having more potential risks than other medications not approved for those uses but commonly prescribed for such symptoms (i.e., clonidine or imipramine).

Essentially, the FDA-approved indications bear little resemblance to common clinical practice. For example, the only FDA-approved indication for desipramine is for treatment of depression in adults. However, there is a controlled trial showing the efficacy of desipramine for ADHD in children (Biederman, Baldessarini, Wright, Knee, & Harmatz, 1989) and safety data from systematic treatment trials of depressed adolescents (Ambrosini, Bianchi, Rabinovich, & Elia, 1993). Moreover, it is often used to treat both of these disorders in the younger ages, and has become a second-line treatment for ADHD for children with tic disorders or those who are not responsive to stimulant medications (Biederman, Thisted, Greenhill, & Ryan, 1995). An estimated 140,000 prescriptions of desipramine were written for children from age 5 to 14 in 1992, and the number of prescriptions for desipramine increased more than sixfold from 1986 to 1992 (Biederman et al., 1995). Data on the actual number of children being treated with, or of prescriptions written for, desipramine are not available in this country; estimates were calculated from "drug mentions" (i.e., number of times a drug is prescribed, refilled, recommended, or administered by a physician; Biederman et al., 1995).

Additionally, there is a dramatic discrepancy between actual clinical practice and systematic research data that supports efficacy of most of the psychotropics. Psychotropics are quite widely prescribed, despite limited safety and efficacy data, as demonstrated by projected data calculated from a national drug marketing database (Jensen et al., 1994). The antidepressants are the most widely prescribed of all of the psychotropics (including CNS stimulants) in childhood and adolescence. In 1992, there were 2.8 million drug mentions for an antidepressant for children ages 5 through 12 in 1992 (Jensen et al., 1994).

Despite interest in pediatric pharmacotherapy, there are very few systematic trials for any of the childhood psychiatric disorders, other than perhaps for ADHD. Even though it has been estimated that depression is not uncommon in childhood, fewer than 250 children and adolescents have been studied in controlled pharmacologic treatment trials (Jensen, Ryan, & Prien, 1992). None of the systematic treatment trials for depression in adolescents have found an antidepressant to be significantly superior to placebo, despite anecdotal evidence suggesting otherwise. This speaks to the need for thoughtful consideration of methodological issues concerning the study of depression in the younger ages (Ambrossini et al., 1993).

Surprisingly, for all the anxiety disorders seen in children, only 13 controlled psychopharmacologic trials could be found (4 for separation anxiety, 4 for avoidant/overanxious/mixed disorders, and 5 for OCD) in the pediatric age group (Allen, Leonard, & Swedo, 1995). OCD is probably the best studied of the childhood anxiety disorders, and it is estimated that as many as 1% of adolescents may suffer from it (Flament et al., 1988). There are five systematic pharmacotherapy treatment trials for individuals with OCD under 18 years of age, and only clomipramine is approved for use in the younger ages (10 years and above; Allen et al., 1995).

Thus, there is a paucity of safety and efficacy data in the pediatric age group for medications that are commonly prescribed. Obstacles, current regulations, and ethical issues concerning studying medications in children are identified in this chapter.

OBSTACLES TO PSYCHOPHARMACOLOGIC RESEARCH IN CHILDREN

Acknowledging that there are many difficulties in developing new psychotropic medications for children, and in testing the safety and efficacy of those approved for use in adults, has led to a series of dialogues among members of the National Institute of Mental Health (NIMH), FDA, Office of Protection of Research Risks (OPRR), and other federal agencies and institutes, clinicians, researchers, pharmaceutical industry, and community and patient representatives (Jensen et al., 1994). Such interdisciplinary meetings have led to the identification of several key obstacles that currently delay or impede psychopharmacologic research in children (Jensen et al., 1994).

Although there is some uncertainty about the actual market size for pediatric indications, most patient and professional groups have not perceived the need as small (Jensen et al., 1994). Pharmaceutical development is a very expensive and time-consuming process, and there may be a perception that additional risks are posed by testing in the younger "more vulnerable" ages. Concerns have been raised that if significant adverse reactions were reported in children during the drug development stage, then this might potentially jeopardize the approval of the new drug application (NDA) process for adults, as well. Additionally, because children have an extended time period for the statue of limitations, concerns about long-term liability of drug manufacturers to lawsuits, even years after drug exposure, could constrain drug testing for children, despite the lack of cause and effect data. It is unclear whether these perceived vulnerabilities are actually likely (Jensen et al., 1994).

In addition to the practical issues of who would initiate and pay for clinical trials, there is an issue of who would carry them out. There are only a handful of specially trained pediatric psychopharmacologic clinical researchers who currently do the majority of the systematic research. With reductions in funding for training and research, and with academic institutions experiencing severe financial challenges, it is uncertain whether there will be enough "experts" or funding to deal with the complexity of developing psychopharmacologic studies.

RECENT REVISIONS IN THE FEDERAL GUIDELINES AND REGULATIONS FOR PEDIATRIC DRUG INFORMATION

Until recently, labeling for the majority of medications contained in the *PDR* was "not recommended for children below age 12." This typically represented the fact that a medication had not been studied in children during the NDA process, and that specific indications for its use in the pediatric age group were not sought. Examinations of the concerns that there were limited data available, and that labeling often did not contain adequate information about the use of drugs in the younger age group, led to the major revision of the pediatric use of prescription drugs subsection in the labeling in 1994 (Department of Health and Human Services, FDA, 1994a).

This new rule recognized several methods of establishing substantial evidence to support pediatric labeling claims, including studies carried out in adults that in certain cases could be extrapolated to children. Allowing data from adequate and well-controlled studies in adults, in combination with other information supporting pediatric use (e.g., pharmacokinetics, safety, and pharmacodynamic data), may allow for labeling for pediatric use. In response to concerns that direct pharmacokinetics data in children are often difficult to obtain, the regulation states that "additional information supporting pediatric use must ordinarily include data on the pharmacokinetics of the drug in the pediatric population for determination of pediatric dosage" (DHHS, FDA, 1994a, p. 64245). Some individuals have raised concerns that this rule will allow adult data to be extrapolated to children, and that treatments safe and effective in adults may not be such in the pediatric age group. For example, tetracycline was once used in pregnant women and in children, until it was discovered that permanent discoloration of children's teeth could result. Similarly, aspirin was used in children, until a possible association with Reye's syndrome was reported. Thus, some have argued that to allow adult data to be extrapolated to children may inhibit the development of pediatric studies, whereas the overall purpose is actually to generate more information about children and better access to information for prescribing physicians.

The regulatory constraints on psychopharmacologic studies have prevented this field from keeping pace with clinical practice. In addition, research in this field is beset by several ethical challenges; these are outlined here and are accompanied by recommendations.

DESIGN AND IMPLEMENTATION

The AAP (1995) described several ethical issues for clinical investigations of children, and emphasized the importance of the study design. First, the research should "be of value to children in general and, in most instances, to the individual child subject." Second, the research design should be appropriate for the stated purposes and scientifically valid. Third, the research design "must take into consideration the unique physiology, psychology, and pharmacology of children and their special needs and requirements as research subjects." Fourth, the design should "minimize risk while maximizing benefit." Additionally, the design should consider the "racial, ethnic, gender, and socioeconomic characteristics of the children and their parents" (p. 287). Several of these issues have immediate implications for psychopharmacologic trials and are developed in the following section.

Study Design. The study design must be scientifically sound in order for the results to be useful or valid, as well as to justify the risks for the subject. Although most would agree with this statement, the specifics of whether a study is developmentally sensitive and whether a certain design is merited can often be debated. For example, the issue of placebo-controlled trials for both children and adults has been met with controversy. Rothman and Michels (1994) argued that it is unethi-

cal to use a placebo given a proven treatment. The AAP (1995) concluded that "placebo or untreated observational control groups can be
used in pediatric studies if their use does not place children at increased
risk" (p. 294). They detailed four situations when a placebo trial is
ethical: (a) when there is no commonly accepted therapy for the condition, (b) when the commonly used therapy is of questionable efficacy or
carries significant undesirable side effects, (c) when the placebo is used
to study undesirable side effects of a new treatment added to an
established one, (d) or when the efficacy has not been demonstrated
because the disease process has frequent spontaneous exacerbations
and remissions.

This issue of placebo-controlled trials in children has been debated,
although the AAP recommendations have clarified the issues. There are
numerous examples of studies in which the investigator may need to
decide whether a placebo trial is appropriate. For example, is lithium
required for long-term maintenance in adolescents with bipolar disorder? Should one use a placebo discontinuation design? Should the
antidepressant trials for adolescents with major depressive disorder
have a placebo group or should psychotherapy be a comparison? If a
double-blind crossover design is used for two medications, how can the
carryover effect from the first drug be controlled? Would an A–B–A
design of a drug be considered methodologically sound? Although the
issues for specific protocols will merit debate, the guideline that the use
of placebo should not place a child at increased risk should be a key
factor for consideration.

Subject Enrollment and Recruitment.   The subjects should represent a cross-section of children with consideration of racial, ethnic,
gender, and socioeconomic characteristics (AAP, 1995). It is unethical
and unscientific to under or over include children from any specific
population. This is particularly true for pharmacokinetics or drug response trials, where there may be both age and ethnic differences in
metabolism. Thus, data from a limited population might not be able to
be extrapolated to others. This issue will become particularly important
with the expected increase in pharmacokinetic trials.

Participation in research must be voluntary for the child; there should
be no coercion, or perception of such, by either researchers or parents.
Thus, the issue of paying the child or parents for participation or for
costs incurred needs careful scrutiny. Recent recommendations by AAP
suggest that neither the child nor the parent should be paid for their
direct participation, other than a token gesture of appreciation (1995).
This is to avoid a situation in which a parent might be enrolling his or
her child in the study for financial gains. However, as Osher and
Telesford point out in chapter 3, reimbursement is often very appropri-

ate. Moreover, a child's participation in a study is more complex than an adult's. The child's participation depends on the parents and siblings; often babysitters need to be hired and parents need to miss work. Many investigators have suggested that reimbursement for time out of work, babysitting, and travel expenses might be appropriate. This area merits further consideration, as many investigators see reimbursement as appropriate and not as an inducement.

Long-Term Outcome.   A concern that is particularly relevant for psychopharmacologic trials is that of long-term outcomes after exposure to medications. As discussed earlier, one of the largest concerns is that there may be an untoward effect that would not become evident for years. This would suggest that for some medication studies, the possibility of long-term follow-up should at least be considered. Unfortunately, there is no generally accepted mechanism for such, and the feasibility of such is challenging. Nonetheless, investigators may want to consider the feasibility of follow-up for at least a subset of their sample.

Role of the Investigator and Conflicts of Interest.   The ethical imperative is that the investigator be qualified to conduct the studies planned and be able to address issues of potential bias. It is the investigator's responsibility to obtain as much information as is available about the safety and efficacy of the medications that are under study prior to enrolling children. The investigator should attempt to describe a balanced and factual view of the risks and benefits to the potential study child. The investigator must strive to prevent bias from affecting study design, execution of the study, deviation from the protocol, or interpretation of the data as it places other children at risk (AAP, 1995).

Any potential conflict of interest between those of the institution, the investigator, and the child needs to be assessed. Although true for nonpharmacologic studies, this may be more of an issue for pharmacologic studies, as often a product sponsor is involved. For example, if a pharmaceutical company funds the drug study, the salary of a research assistant, or the travel money to a meeting to present results from the study, this financial support could potentially represent a vested interest in the study, and present a biasing influence on the investigator. Although these situations would not likely be considered unethical, it is important to realize that any possible conflict requires consideration and disclosure. Recently, the FDA proposed a requirement to identify and consider financial arrangements between product sponsors and clinical investigators that might have the potential to bias the outcome of clinical trials (DHHS, FDA, 1994b). The sponsor of a drug for FDA approval would be asked to disclose any financial interests of the investigator in the study. Although the proposal is still under consideration, it will likely be approved in some form.

Steps can be taken to minimize bias; design factors (independent data monitoring, multiple investigators, blinding, and independent endpoint assessment) can render a potentially problematic financial interest unlikely to introduce bias (DHHS, FDA, 1994b). Any issues of potential bias must always be considered and dealt with directly, especially when financial support is provided from a specific source.

ASSESSING RISKS

In 1979, "The Belmont Report" (DHHS, 1979) set forth critical guidelines for research studies. The report emphasized three basic ethical principles: respect for person (autonomy), beneficence (informed consent and risk–benefit issues), and justice (fairness in access to research). That report specifically noted some of the ethical and practical difficulties of including children in research, such as having to balance benefits and risk. Additionally, the report noted that limiting research that does not benefit an individual child directly may rule out much research that might promise great benefit to other children in the future. The reader is directed to several excellent reviews of ethical issues by Levine (1989), Munir and Earls (1992), and Grodin and Alpert (1988).

Determination of Benefits and Risks.   Assignment of one of four risk–benefit ratio categories is necessary for children to participate in a research study (DHHS, 1983, 1991). This is an important difference between the regulations for children and those for adults. This requirement serves to protect the minor subjects but poses limitations on the research. Not only must a study meet the requirements for the risk–benefit ratio, but it should be scientifically sound and have potential benefit.

Research with "no greater than minimal risk" (Category 1) is limited by the definition of minimal risk ("the probability and magnitude of harm or discomfort . . . are not greater . . . than those ordinarily encountered in daily life or during the performance of routine physical or psychological examinations or tests" (DHHS, 1991, 46.102). Although open to an individual institutional review board's (IRB) interpretation for assignment of risk, most drug treatment trials would not fall under this risk category. However, a group of children who were taking a medication for a specific disorder could be studied to determine pharmacokinetics measures (i.e., plasma levels in relationship to age, gender, concomitant medications, dosage schedule). This type of study would not likely represent more than minimal risk to the child, because the issue would not be whether the child was choosing the medication or whether it was effective or not. With the recent revisions in the guidelines for pediatric labeling, there is likely to be increased interest in pediatric pharmacokinetics studies, and some would be subsumed under this category.

The majority of psychopharmacologic treatment protocols, however, would fall under the second category, "research that involves greater than minimal risk but presents the prospect of direct benefit to the individual subjects." This category requires that the "risk is justified by the anticipated benefit to the subjects," and that the "relation of the anticipated benefit to the risk is at least as favorable to the subjects as that presented by available alternative approaches." The premarketing controlled trials of clomipramine (vs. placebo) in children with OCD, ages 10 to 18, were likely to have been in this category. Initial safety and efficacy data in adults had suggested that clomipramine was effective for OCD and had the expected side effect profile of a tricyclic antidepressant. There was no specific reason to think that this response and side effect profile would be different in the younger age group. Children with OCD suffer from an incapacitating disorder, and there were no effective medications available at the time. Thus, there was reason to expect that clomipramine would be effective, and that the risk–benefit ratio would be at least as favorable (if not more so) than other interventions.

Category 3, "research involving greater than minimal risk and no prospect of direct benefit to the individual subjects, but likely to yield generalizable knowledge about the subject's disorder or condition" could be conducted if the risk represents a minor increase over minimal risk, if the intervention presents experiences that are "reasonably commensurate with those inherent in their actual or expected medical, dental, psychological, social, or educational situations," and if it will yield information which is of "vital importance for understanding or amelioration of the subjects' disorder." For example, a depressed child in a treatment protocol for a new antidepressant, might be asked to participate in a challenge study (which would involve a one-time exposure to a medication, such as clonidine, and measurement of peripheral neuroendocrine response via a phlebotomy) in order to better understand whether there is neuroendocrine dysregulation in depressed children.

Category 4, "research not otherwise approvable," must be approved by the secretary of Health and Human Services after consultation with experts. Rarely would psychopharmacologic studies fall in this category.

How do these federal regulations affect psychopharmacologic trials in children? The regulations necessitate attention to the following questions: What data would be necessary to conclude that the treatment "holds out the prospect of direct benefit"? Would effective open and/or closed treatment trials in adults be considered sufficient to justify a trial in the pediatric group? Would preliminary safety data in children be required? Would open treatment of the medication in children be required prior to controlled treatment trials? For example, although open to the individual IRB's interpretation, an experimental drug treatment might be approved if some data existed that suggested that there was prospect for direct benefit for the child from the investigational intervention. If the disorder were severe, and/or treatments were not available, such as was the situation with OCD in the late 1980s, presumably this would factor into the risk–benefit decision.

What difficulties are raised by research studies that do not have a direct prospect of benefit to the patient? For example, in the case of a challenge study that had been conducted in a specific (i.e., depressed or anxious) adult population, it might be difficult to obtain approval for a similar study in a pediatric population. If so, then information on the neurobiology of childhood psychiatric disorders has to be extrapolated from adults. Even normative neuroendocrine data would be difficult to obtain in normal pediatric controls, because this might be determined to represent more than a minor increase over minimal risk and without direct benefit to the individual.

IRB ISSUES

The large responsibility for determining whether a research study is ethical falls on the IRB. One of the principal issues is to determine whether the risk is justified by the anticipated benefit. For example, is the potentially successful treatment of ADHD symptoms in a child with Tourette syndrome by imipramine (or another antidepressant) justified by the risks of use of a tricyclic antidepressant? One would consider the treatment beneficial if a child who was previously unsuccessful in academic work and peer relationships (secondary to inattentiveness and impulsivity symptoms) were able to complete schoolwork, have academic success, and develop better social relationships. If the risks are those of anticholinergic side effects of medications, which are somewhat annoying but tolerable, then the risk–benefit ratio would appear to be at least as favorable as available alternatives. This is particularly true because stimulant medications (the approved medication for the treatment of ADHD) present the risk of exacerbating the tic disorder and this would be likely to present more problematic side effects than that of a tricyclic.

Additionally, it is up to the individual IRB to determine what is "minor increase over minimal risk." For example, a child participating in a fluoxetine treatment study of depression, might agree to several phlebotomies for the purpose of measuring plasma drug levels. This intervention would be reasonably commensurate with those inherent in their actual medical situations, and it would yield important information about the individual's pharmacokinetics that could be applied to others. This category would allow for normative data to be obtained on patient and control children. For example, neuroendocrine responses (i.e., growth hormone, cortisol, and prolactin) to challenge studies, in both control and patient groups, could be very important in elucidating underlying mechanisms involved in mental illness. In contrast, administering a psychotropic medication to normal controls to determine pharmacokinetics properties might represent more than minor increase over minimal risk, and therefore would not be approvable, even if it were to be likely to yield generalizable knowledge about childhood disorders.

In a general medical hospital IRB, there may be some unfamiliarity with childhood psychiatric disorders. Thus, for protocols to have appropriate consideration there should be members on or consultants to the IRB who can consider the relevant medical, psychological, and social needs of the child. Certainly, there are misperceptions that mental disorders aren't "real," and that it is "unethical to drug kids." Thus, it may become necessary to educate IRBs as to the nature of the psychiatric disorders and the necessity for the study of interventions. Additionally, risks for children of different ethnicities are not well studied and therefore difficult to determine. There is evidence that ethnicity may affect drug metabolism, both in normal and slow metabolizers (secondary to genetic polymorphism); thus consideration of their potential differential response to medications needs to addressed. Thus, the IRB has an important responsibility and may need to call on consultants to sensitize and educate members.

Informed Consent and Assent.   Informed consent is based on the premise that subjects "to the degree that they are capable, be given the opportunity to choose what shall or shall not happen to them" (DHHS, 1979). The consent process contains three key elements: information (purposes, procedures, risks, benefits, alternative treatments, ability to withdraw), comprehension, and voluntariness (without coercion or undue influence; DHHS, 1979). The process of consent (from parents or guardian) and assent (from the child) involves both a written consent/assent form with signature as well as a discussion in which there is a chance for the subject to ask questions (Munir & Earls, 1992). Failure for the child to object does not constitute assent. Assent to participate should not be obtained based on coercion, inducement, or reward (AAP, 1995).

It is the responsibility of the IRB to determine whether children are capable of assenting, taking into consideration their age, maturity, and psychological state. Specific judgments about the capacity for children at various ages are potentially problematic. (See Susman, Lorah, & Fletcher, 1993, for a detailed discussion.) These issues of judging a child's capacity to participate in agreeing to research treatment may arise particularly if the child is very young or if the psychiatric disorder interferes with cognitive capacity, and they may become quite complicated. Most researchers would agree that children should be actively involved in the agreement to participate in treatment trials, and that they should be presented information and explanations at their level of understanding.

CONCLUSION

The limited number of studies of medications in children presents ethical issues on many levels. Additionally, there is a dramatic discrepancy between actual clinical practice of prescribing medications in children and the FDA-approved indications and ages for those drugs. For children to avoid the status of "psychopharmacologic orphans," they must be granted equal access to medication studies. Scientifically sound and ethical studies are necessary to determine the safety and efficacy of psychotropic agents in children, and they can be conducted. Although many obstacles—both regulatory and ethical—exist, such studies are feasible. Establishment of a working coalition that includes representatives from clinical psychopharmacology, the research community, pharmaceutical industry, American Academy of Child and Adolescent Psychiatry, other professional organizations representing pediatrics, pediatric neurology, and family practitioners, clinicians, FDA, OPRR, NIMH, and others would be one way to facilitate and improve studies of the safety and efficacy of medications for children.

ACKNOWLEDGMENTS

The opinions and assertions contained in this chapter are the private views of the authors and are not to be construed as official or as reflecting the views of the Department of Health and Human Services or the National Institute of Mental Health. We thank Jean Frazier, Susan Swedo, Daniel Rosenberg, and Kimberly Hoagwood for their critical review.

REFERENCES

Allen, A. J., Leonard, H. L., & Swedo, S. E. (1995). In perspective: Current knowledge regarding medication for the treatment of childhood anxiety disorders. *Journal of the American Academy of Child and Adolescent Psychiatry, 34,* 976–986.

Ambrosini, P. J., Bianchi, M. D., Rabinovich, H., & Elia, J. (1993). Antidepressant treatments in children and adolescents: I. Affective Disorders. *Journal of the American Academy of Child and Adolescent Psychiatry, 32,* 1–6.

American Academy of Pediatrics, Committee on Drugs. (1995). Guidelines for the ethical conduct of studies to evaluate drugs in pediatric populations. *Pediatrics, 95,* 286–294.

Biederman, J., Baldessarini, R., Wright, V., Knee, D., & Harmatz, J. (1989). A double-blind placebo controlled study of desipramine in the treatment of attention deficit disorder. I. Efficacy. *Journal of the American Academy of Child and Adolescent Psychiatry, 28,* 777–784.

Biederman, J., Thisted, R., Greenhill, L., & Ryan, N. (1995). Estimation of the association between desipramine and the risk for sudden death in 5– to 14–year-old children. *Journal of Clinical Psychiatry, 56,* 87–93.

Bourin, M., Couetoux, D., & Tertre, A. (1992). Pharmacokinetics of psychotropic drugs in children. *Clinical Neuropharmacology, 15*(suppl), 114–225.

Branch, R. (1994). Characteristics of drug disposition during childhood. In D. Rosenberg, J. Holttum, & S. Gershon (Eds.), *Textbook on pharmacotherapy for child and adolescent psychiatric disorders* (pp. 7–16). New York: Brunner Mazel.

Department of Health and Human Services. (1979, April 18). The Belmont Report: Ethical principles and guidelines for the protection of human subjects of research. National Commission for the Protection of Human Subjects of Biomedical and Behavioral Research. *The Federal Register.*

Department of Health and Human Services. (1983). OPRR Reports: Protection of human subjects. *The Federal Register,* 48, 46 (revised March 8, 1983).

Department of Health and Human Services. (1991). OPRR Reports: Protection of human subjects. *The Federal Register,* 46 (revised June 18, 1991).

Department of Health and Human Services, FDA. (1994a). *The Federal Register* (21 CFR Part 201), 59:238, 64240–64250.

Department of Health and Human Services, FDA. (1994b). *The Federal Register,* 59, 48708.

Farell, J. R., Lee, Y. J, & Hirtz, D. G. (1990). Phenobarbital for febrile seizures–effects on intelligence and on seizure recurrence. *New England Journal of Medicine, 322,* 364–369.

Flament, M., Whitaker, A., Rapoport J., Davies, M., Berg, C., Kalikow, K., Sceery, W., & Shaffer, D. (1988). Obsessive compulsive disorder in adolescence: An epidemiological study. *Journal of the American Academy of Child and Adolescent Psychiatry, 276,* 764–771.

Gilman, J. T., & Gal, P. (1992). Pharmacokinetics and pharmacodynamic data collection in children and neonates. *Clinical Pharmacokinetics, 23,* 1–9.

Grodin, M. A., & Alpert, J. J. (1988). Children as participants in medical research. *Pediatric Clinics of North America, 35,* 1389–1401.

Haldeman, G. E., & Quirion, R. (1983). Neonatal exposure to morphine increases opiate binding in the adult forebrain. *European Journal of Pharmacology, 94,* 357.

Hill, H. F., & Engblom, J. (1984). Effects of pre- and postnatal haloperidol administration to pregnant and nursing rats on brain catecholamine levels in their offspring. *Developmental Pharmacological Therapy, 7,* 188–197.

Jensen, P. S., Ryan, N. D., & Prien, R. (1992). Psychopharmacology of child and adolescent major depression. *Journal of Child and Adolescent Psychopharmacology, 2,* 31–45.

Jensen, P. S., Vitiello, B., Leonard, H., & Laughren, T. P. (1994). Design and methodology issues for clinical treatment trials in children and adolescents. *Psychopharmacology Bulletin, 30,* 3–8.

Levine, R. J. (1989). Children as Research Subjects. In L. M. Kopelman & J. C. Moskop (Eds.), *Children and Health Are: Moral and Social Issues* (pp. 73–87). Dordrecht/Boston/London:Kluwer Academic.

Munir, K., & Earls, F. (1992). Ethical principles governing research in child and adolescent psychiatry. *Journal of the American Academy of Child and Adolescent Psychiatry, 31,* 408–414.

National Commission for the Protectioon of Human Subjects of Biomedical and Behavioral Research. (1977). *Research involving children: Report and recommendations* (DHEW Publication No. [OS] 77–0005). Washington, DC: Author.

Offices of Drug Evaluation Statistical Report. Center for Drug Evaluation and Research, Food and Drug Administration, Public Health Service. (1989). Rockville, MD: U.S. Department of Health and Human Services publication 89–233530.

Physician's Desk Reference (49th ed.). (1995). Montvale, NJ: Medical Economics.

Popper, C. W. (1993), Psychopharmacologic treatment of anxiety disorders in adolescents and children. *Journal of Clinical Psychiatry, 54,* 52–63.

Rosengarten, H., & Friedhoff, A. J. (1979). Enduring changes in dopamine receptor cells of pups from drug administration to pregnant and nursing rats. *Science, 203,* 1133.

Rothman, K. F., & Michels, K. B. (1994). The continuing unethical use of placebo controls. *New England Journal of Medicine, 331,* 394–398.

Scolnik, D., Nulman, I., Rovet, J., & Gladstone, D. (1994). Neurodevelopment of children exposed in utero to phenytoin and carbamazepine monotherapy. *Journal of the American Medical Association, 271,* 767–770.

Susman, E. J., Lorah, D., & Fletcher, J. C. (1993). Participation in biomedical research: The consent process as viewed by children, adolescents, young adults, and physicians. *Journal of Pediatrics, 121,* 547–552.

Wilens, T. E., Biederman, J., Baldessarini, R. J., Puopolo, P., & Flood, J. (1992). Developmental changes in serum concentration of desipramine and 2–hydroxydesipramine during treatment with desipramine. *Journal of the American Academy of Child and Adolescent Psychiatry, 31,* 691–698.

Wilens, T. E., Biederman, J., Geist, D. E., Steingar, R., & Spencer, T. (1993). Nortriptyline in the treatment of ADHD: A chart review of 58 cases. *Journal of the American Academy of Child and Adolescent Psychiatry, 32,* 343–349.

7

Biologic Procedures: Ethical Issues in Research With Children and Adolescents

L. Eugene Arnold
David M. Stoff
National Institute of Mental Health
Edwin Cook, Jr.
University of Chicago
Clinton Wright
Columbus Medical School
Donald J. Cohen
Yale Child Study Center
Markus Kruesi
Institute for Juvenile Research, Chicago
Jocelyn Hattab
Hadassah Medical School
Philip Graham
Private Practice, London
Alan Zametkin
F. Xavier Castellanos
National Institute of Mental Health
William McMahon
University of Utah Medical Center
James F. Leckman
Yale Child Study

Recent years have witnessed a burgeoning use of biological procedures in mental health research with children and adolescents. This encompasses both old and new technology, and is spurred by the increasing recognition of biological contributions to pathogenesis and treatment of major mental disorders. A literature survey of the research use of various such procedures reported in five major journals over a 5-year period ending in Spring 1994 revealed the following number of uses and relative proportions (in parentheses) of various procedures: noninvasive 46 (39%), venipuncture 30 (25%), challenges with multiple venipuncture or intravenous (IV) catheter, other IV catheter 4 (3%), spinal taps 5 (4%), brain imaging 18 (15%). In the brain imaging category, there were 9 uses (8%) of ionizing radiation. Obviously the most invasive biological procedures have been used far less frequently than the noninvasive and simple venipuncture, which together accounted for 64%. Generally, the more invasive procedures yield data more reflective of brain activity whereas the less invasive procedures reflect more peripheral systems.

Such research raises and is limited by ethical issues reviewed here. An additional concern is societal misinterpretation of research findings. For example, most experts now agree that genes influence behavior, but unfortunately, society (lay consumers of scientific information) may translate this fact into "neurogenetic determinism," in which genes unilaterally determine behavior rather than interacting with the environment. (A well-known example of interaction is phenylketonuria, in which genes interact with diet, and the genetic cognitive/behavioral disorder is preventable by specific nurture.) Fear by some that neurogenetic determinism will erode human dignity and the fact that some abuses have historically occurred in the treatment of research subjects form a counterpoint to enthusiasm for the benefit of scientific study. Nevertheless, the position taken by the authors is one of advocacy for children's and adolescents' access to research. We emphasize the need and means to find ethical ways to advance scientific mental health study that can benefit children and adolescents. Perhaps the first question to be addressed should be: Is there really a need for such research?

NEED FOR BIOLOGICAL MENTAL HEALTH RESEARCH IN CHILDREN AND ADOLESCENTS

It is now well recognized by clinical and scientific experts that many of the mental disorders of children and adolescents are early manifestations of serious, lifelong disorders that impair the quality of life and in some cases even threaten life itself. Major mood disorders, for example, are increasingly recognized at younger and younger ages, including an historic increase in youth suicide. Obsessive–compulsive disorder, often beginning in childhood, can impair victims of all ages. Posttraumatic stress disorder (PTSD), from abuse, community violence, or natural catastrophe, can have lifelong impairing sequelae. Pervasive developmental disorders (PDD) have, by definition, continued impact across the lifespan. For some children, disruptive behavior disorders have, in follow-up studies, shown a significant rate of serious adult psychopathology. Mounting effective prevention and treatment efforts require thorough biological as well as psychosocial understanding of the disorders and of the children they afflict. Modern technology has provided effective research tools to pursue such an understanding. However, invasive biological technology poses special ethical questions that must be resolved in the interest of allowing children to benefit from scientific advances.

A hope for many children and adolescents with neuropsychiatric and severe developmental disorders is rigorous, sustained investigation by groups able to use the most sophisticated methodology and technology. Klin and Cohen (1994) described how responsible clinical concern for the welfare of our patients imposes an ethical imperative to support, encourage, and conduct research—and of course, to make sure it is done in an ethical manner.

This chapter reviews, discusses, and makes recommendations about some salient issues in the use of biological procedures in mental health research with children and adolescents. This includes the issues of possible overprotection, the definition of minimal risk, assessment of risk–benefit ratio, risks of biological procedures, minimization of risk, normal controls, age-graded consent, "coercive" inducement, multiple institutional review boards (IRBs), unexpected or unwanted knowledge about individuals, cultural and ethnic issues, and special considerations about neuroimaging.

ARE WE BEING OVERPROTECTIVE
IN LOCO PARENTS?

Because of children's special vulnerabilities, society has established special legal and ethical protections for them, including protection from research risk. This generally adds to the safeguards afforded by parents' natural protection. In fact, society sometimes implies that parents' judgment cannot be trusted to be protective enough and, like a super-parent, limits parents' rights to decide for their children to ensure additional protection. In some settings, the legal concept of *in loco parentis* is invoked to justify societal authorities making decisions that ordinarily would fall to a parent. The special federal research safeguards for children (45 CFR, Subtitle A, Part 46, Subpart D, 10-1-91 Edition, detailed in chapter 2, this volume) provide that parents' or guardians' permission for research on their children may not be solicited or accepted for research with substantially greater than minimal risk unless there is direct benefit to the child with a risk–benefit ratio at least as good as available alternatives.

Technically, this restriction applies only to federally supported research, but the federal requirement for an IRB in order to receive federal funding, coupled with the application of IRB review to all research at respective institutions, essentially brings all research under the purview of such regulations. The practical effect is that parents and guardians cannot give permission for some kinds of research on children that competent adults could altruistically consent to on behalf of themselves (Kopelman, 1989a, 1989b; Laor, 1987). This issue is discussed further in the section on adolescent altruism. Further, some IRBs interpret the regulations even more restrictively, adding another layer of "protection." In some cases, IRBs have equated minimal risk with no risk for children.

An increasing suspicion has developed that children and adolescents may be overprotected by restrictive rules (or restrictive interpretations of rules) that deprive them of needed research. The tendency to abhor any research risk for children and adolescents (e.g., May, 1974; Ramsay, 1970, 1976, 1980, cited in Laor, 1987) may interfere with adequately addressing their needs (Kopelman, 1989a). The dearth of research directly with children has long threatened to make them research orphans, inappropriately dependent on work done with adults (Shirkey, 1968). When new treatments are introduced after clinical trials only on adults, clinicians are forced to extrapolate to children. They are faced with a dilemma: either deprive children of the new treatment or subject them to the risk of an untested treatment that may or may not work the same as in adults.

Animal models, although useful and desirable, also have limitations, perhaps more so for children and adolescents than adults. One might think that we could easily triangulate to knowledge about children by comparing findings in adult humans with findings in adult and juvenile animals. This strategy is often worth trying, but has many pitfalls. For example, although children metabolize drugs faster than adults, in some experimental animals, the adult animals metabolize faster than the young animals. Also, the relatively short juvenile stage of most animals may make them questionable analogies to humans for some mental disorders of children and adolescents. A problem shared with adult biological mental health research is that some receptors, such as $5HT_{1B}$ receptors, differ in key pharmacologic properties between rodents and humans (e.g., Metcalf, McGuffin, & Hamblin, 1992). Finally, a practical problem is the limited availability of animal models for many children's mental health disorders.

An historical analogy offers a relevant lesson. After the thalidomide scare, there was active discouragement of including women of childbearing age (whether pregnant or not) in clinical trials of new drugs for over a decade. However, when new drugs came on the market, they were used in women of childbearing age in a nonstudied fashion, posing a risk to more patients (or their fetuses) than if such patients had been included in controlled, well-monitored trials. And women were deprived of efficacy data to guide their treatment. This short-sighted policy has fortunately been reversed for women, who are now expected to be included in research generally from now on (Ellis, 1994; Varmus, 1994). May we hope that the lessons learned from this ethical detour will be applied to the benefit of children also? The consequences of not conducting research in children and adolescents might include the perpetuation or introduction of harmful practices, failure to discover etiology of illnesses, and failure to develop new treatments for psychiatric disorders of childhood and adolescence.

DEFINITION OF MINIMAL RISK

One problem mentioned earlier is the definition of *minimal risk,* which Kopelman (1989b) characterized as "pivotal." Unfortunately, some IRBs seem to interpret minimal risk as not any risk. A common sense definition is needed, and is suggested by 45 CFR, Subtitle A, Part 46, Subpart A, 46.102(g) 10-1-91 Edition: "'Minimal risk' means that the risks of harm anticipated in the proposed research are not greater, considering probability and magnitude, than those ordinarily encountered in daily life or during the performance of routine physical or psychological examinations or tests." This seems to imply taking into consideration the everyday risks that parents and society routinely approve for children, such as bike riding, riding in a car, and even seasonally limited but otherwise daily activities like swimming or sledding. However, authorities are not clear about this. For example, Kopelman (1989b) pointed out that the phrase "ordinarily encountered in daily life" can be interpreted three ways: "all the risks ordinary people encounter, or the risks all people ordinarily encounter, or the minimal risks all ordinary people ordinarily encounter." We should note that research is not itself an ordinary daily risk, but one added to the ordinary risk. Nicholson (1986) proposed a list of ordinary daily risks to which research risks can be compared in determining minimal risk. This may be a good idea as long as it is defined as a list of examples and not interpreted rigidly.

A question to be resolved is whether minimal risk should be defined the same for patients as for control subjects. Does the daily risk of a serious disorder by comparison change the estimation of minimal risk? It might be argued, for example, that patients who have daily exposure to electrolyte imbalance or malnutrition from an eating disorder, or clinically need daily administration of risky drugs, encounter more risk in daily life than normal controls. On the other hand, one could argue that their state of vulnerability from other risks makes them less able to tolerate an additional modicum of risk.

Risk and Aversiveness. Defining minimal risk also requires clarification of the relationship between aversiveness and risk. Both are negative outcomes and one may cause the other, but a procedure can be risky without being aversive or uncomfortable, or can be mildly aversive without being risky (at least physically). For example, finger stick or venipuncture, universally acknowledged to carry minimal risk under sterile conditions, may be considerably aversive to children (Fradet, MacGrath, Kay, Adams, & Luke, 1990; Humphrey, van Linden van den Heuvell, & van de Wiel, 1992; Turkeltaub & Gergen, 1989).

The aversiveness of a procedure is modified by a child's previous experience. A child who has learned to take clinically indicated spinal taps in stride through autohypnosis and recumbent games for a day may find little aversiveness in an additional spinal tap for research purposes. In fact, Kruesi et al. (1988) found spinal taps to be no more aversive to children than attending school. On the other hand, a child who has had a catastophic experience with a severe headache from a previous tap would be sensitized to fear and experience the procedure as even more aversive than a naive subject. Thus, the aversiveness of the same biological procedure can vary widely. The obvious need for some individual evaluation of aversiveness is partly met by the requirement for child assent as well as parent permission: If the procedure is extremely aversive, assent will presumably not be forthcoming. The same procedure may be less aversive as part of a research protocol than when done under routine clinical need because investigators typically invest time and effort in psychological preparation to maintain subject cooperation while the press of clinical emergencies and stringencies of cost containment often disallow the same degree of preparation for clinical patients. Several authors (e.g., Castellanos et al., 1994; Jay, Elliot, Ozolins, Olson, & Pruitt, 1982) documented that aversiveness can be minimized by preliminary rehearsal, role- playing, and so on.

REVIEW OF RISKS OF BIOLOGICAL RESEARCH PROCEDURES

A literature search yielded few systematic studies about the risks of biological research procedures. Smith (1985) carried out a 1-year follow-up of a group of 7-year-old children who had been venipunctured for research purposes, and found very few aftereffects. However, Turkel-taub and Gergen (1989), Fradet et al. (1990), and Humphrey et al. (1992) reported immediate (short-term) risk and discomfort from similar clinical tests. Kruesi et al. (1988) found a postlumbar headache prevalence of 22% in child and adolescent psychiatric patients age 6.5 to 19.8 years, comparable to that seen in adults. Similar results were found by Castellanos et al. (1994).

The relevant clinical literature about risks and side effects is somewhat richer. Table 7.1 displays the results of a literature review of reported adverse effects of some biological procedures used in psychiatric research, gleaned mainly from reports of clinical experience and nonpsychiatric research. This review is necessarily incomplete because the appropriate key words were not found in all computer literature services, and the review had to depend greatly on manual searching. Nevertheless, it probably samples fairly what has been reported. It can be used as a reference and literature guide by investigators wishing to research potential adverse effects of planned procedures.

ASSESSMENT OF RISK–BENEFIT RATIO
FOR INVASIVE BIOLOGICAL PROCEDURES

Assessment of the risk–benefit ratio should reflect consideration of the entire study, including any invasive procedures. An invasive procedure is no less ethical per se than any other procedure. The following considerations are recommended to potential investigators:

1. Evaluate risks broadly, considering known in vitro effects and in vivo effects in animals, adults, and other children, and the effect of the technician's or clinician's skill on the risk. For the database utilized for judgment about risk, include not only all available experimental findings, but also noncontrolled clinical and other observations.
2. Evaluate benefits broadly, considering the health and welfare of the individual subject and children in general, and advancement of medical knowledge that would benefit the subject in the long run.
3. Consider possibilities for improving the risk–benefit ratio by increasing benefits or decreasing risk or both. Potential benefits may be maximized by careful attention to protocol and design; the minimization of risk is discussed here.

TABLE 7.1

Published Adverse Effects Data on Procedures Used in Biological Mental Health Research

PROCEDURE Author (Type of Study)	Age Range (y)	N	Number of Complications	Patient Population	Reported complications	Expertise	Primary Purpose of Procedure	Suggestions for prophylaxis
Arterial Puncture								
Cole and Lumley, 1966 (prospective)	—	160	53	—	Bruising	MD	N	
Ena et al., 1992 (prospective)	—	26	—	Hospitalized	Phlebitis, catheter-related infection	N	N	
Marshall et al., 1984 (prospective)	1d–14.8y	70	0	Intensive care, operating room	Vascular insufficiency	—	N	—
Miyasaka et al., 1976 (prospective)	<2 - > 10 (n = 37 2–10)	53	18 27	Intensive care, operating room	Skin lesions, arterial obstruction	—	N	
Mortensen, 1967 (retrospective)	—	3,193	389	Hospitalized	—	—	N	
Saladino et al., 1990 (retrospective)	8mo–36y	41	10	Emergency room	Vascular changes, failure to draw blood	MD	N	
Sellden et al., 1987 (prospective)	1–20	78	0	Intensive care, operating room	NA	MD	N	
Smith-Wright et al., 1984 (prospective)	1wk–28y	330	—	Intensive care	Sepsis, embolism, bleeding	MD	N	
Lumbar Puncture								
Carbaat and Van Crevel, 1981 (prospective)	13+	100	41	Hospitalized	Headache, neck pain, neck stiffness, nausea, vomiting, giddiness, tinnitus, diplopia	MD	RP	—
Gupta, 1977 (case report)	17	1	1	Hospitalized	Pulmonary edema	—	N	—
Heide and Diener, 1990 (prospective)	16–58	90	29	—	Headache and posture-dependent complaints	—	RP	
Kruesi et al., 1988 (prospective)	6.5–19.8	60	13	Psychiatric, hospitalized	Headache, backache/local soreness	—	RS	
Richards and Towu-Aghantse, 1986 (case report)	17	1	1	Hospitalized	Respiratory arrest	—	N	

IM Injection

Study	Age	N	n	Setting	Outcome	Expertise	Purpose	
Babhulkar, 1985 (case report)	6–13	11	11	—	Triceps fibrosis	—	N	—
Bigos and Coleman, 1984 (case report)	16	1	1	—	Sciatic nerve injury	—	N	
Dhar et al., 1988 (case report)	1.5	1	1	Hospitalized	Gangrene	MD	N	
Hang and Miller, 1978 (case report)	9	1	1	Operating room	Deltoid fibrosis	—	N	—
Ling and Loong, 1976 (case report)	9	1	1	—	Radial nerve injury	—	N	
McCloskey and Chung, 1977 (case report)	2–6	7	1	Hospitalized	Quadriceps fibrosis	RN	N	
Mukherjee and Das, 1980 (case report)	≤14	37	37	Hospitalized	Quadriceps fibrosis	—	N	
Sarkar and Dasgupta, 1981 (case report)	4mo–5y	93	93	—	Abscess	RN, MD, Att.	N	
Shanmugasundaram, 1980 (case report)	1–20	169	169	Hospitalized	Quadriceps fibrosis	—	N	

Venipuncture

Study	Age	N	n	Setting	Outcome	Expertise	Purpose	
Fradet et al., 1990 (prospective)	3–17	196	37	Operating room	Pain	—	N	
Humphrey et al., 1992 (prospective)	2.5–18	223	10	Hospitalized	Panic	Att	N	
Turkeltaub and Gergen, 1989 (prospective)	6–19	4,121	14	—	Asthma, syncope, near syncope, malaise	—	RP	—

Expertise
MD = medical doctor
RN = registered nurse
N = nursing staff
Att = attendant

Primary Purpose of Procedure
N = normal diagnostic or therapeutic use
RS = research secondary, superimposed on routine clinical procedure
RP = research primary, main purpose of procedure

General
— = data not provided
+ = data provided
NA = not applicable to study

A problem in extrapolating reports of adverse effects from clinical samples is that the clinical experience is often confounded by complicating factors, including the illness for which the clinical procedure was done. For example, the informal review of clinical papers for lumbar puncture (LP) side effects summarized in Table 7.1 found the reports complicated by administration of cancer chemotherapy, spinal anesthesia, and contrast agents in the spinal canal, all of which could cause adverse effects that might be attributed to the LP. Further, because a research procedure is carried out on a voluntary basis rather than under clinical necessity, it is less likely to be done on those who anticipate the most distress from it; this probably reduces the psychological risk for the sample as a whole, although there still may be individuals who assent/consent despite negative anticipation. An interesting related question concerns the subsequent effect on the child's later psychological reaction to the same test if it is clinically indicated: Will the child weather it better because of success in the research administration or take it harder because of being sensitized to the risks? Systematic follow-up of child and adolescent research subjects regarding both physical and emotional consequences would be of great value for future formal risk estimation.

MINIMIZING RISK

Risks and fears should be minimized by limiting both the number and type of invasive tests. Responsible investigators have an obligation to do no more invasive tests than necessary to answer the central research questions and to devise designs that allow the minimum number of tests to suffice. A similar obligation pertains to the type and invasiveness of the test: Will a blood draw suffice rather than spinal tap? Will a buccal scraping suffice rather than a skin biopsy? Less invasive tests should be sought, and technology devised to make them yield the same information for which a more invasive test might have been needed. An example is development of polymerase chain reaction, which enables genetic analysis from saliva rather than blood. Because risk and discomfort may be inversely proportional to the skill of the technician or clinician doing the procedure, the most skilled should be recruited to do research procedures. Arranging the presence of parents, family, or peers during the procedure to encourage and comfort the subject may be useful in allaying the anxiety that can aggravate discomfort. Another strategy for minimizing risk is to "piggyback" invasive tests on routine clinically indicated procedures: for example, taking an extra milliliter of spinal fluid or an extra 5 ml of blood for research puposes during a clinically indicated spinal tap or blood draw. Of course, this lower risk still requires informed consent and is justified only if a sufficient increment of biological information can be obtained for an approved investigation. The frequency and number of invasive tests is complicated by the need for follow-up studies. Deciding the appropriate number and frequency of serial tests in a longitudinal study requires careful balancing of the value of incremental knowledge gained against the incremental risk for each repetition.

Another minimization of risk or at least discomfort involves carefully determining the value and hazards of preparatory procedures (e.g., fasting, special diets, resting) that are associated with the actual biological tests. Are these necessary for subject safety? Or are they merely necessary for quality of test results? If the latter, is the increment of knowledge worth the increment of subject discomfort?

Risk can be further minimized by implementation of procedures to prepare the subject and monitor consequences and aftereffects of biological tests (Castellanos et al., 1994; Jay et al., 1982; Kruesi et al., 1988). For example, Amiel (1985) devised a simple method of keeping children happily supine after a spinal tap: Show them videotape movies. This reduced the risk of spinal headache. Children may have a lower (or higher) threshold for aversive stimuli than adults, or the aftereffects of aversive stimuli may last a longer or shorter time. Studies of children's thresholds and perceptions of aversive procedures could be useful.

NEED FOR NORMAL CONTROLS

Biological assays, challenges, and other tests pose a special problem in the need for healthy, normal controls for comparison norms. Sometimes "cross controls" of subjects with contrasting disorders will suffice, but in many cases there is no substitute for healthy controls. Careful scrutiny of normal child volunteers, using a multistage screening process designed to detect psychopathology, is needed in biological psychiatric research to assure meaningful, truly normal, comparisons (Kruesi, Lenane, Hibbs, & Major, 1990). If the procedure poses more than minimal risk, current rules do not seem to allow child/adolescent normal controls to consent (i.e., to assent and have parents give permission for them). Children and adolescents are essentially disenfranchised from being altruistic by a regulatory double bind: They are considered incapable of consenting for themselves, and their parents are not allowed to be altruistic on their behalf (i.e., permit altruistic participation). The question arises as to why adolescents should not be allowed to be altruistic (i.e., voluntarily undertake risk or discomfort for the common good), because this would reflect a developmental tendency detectable as early as preschool (Sroufe & Cooper, 1987) and reaching full flower in adolescence. Does denying them the opportunity for altruistic consent deprive them of a developmental right?

Of course, not all motivations for normal controls are altruistic. Aside from subject compensation, discussed later, a child may find getting out of school for a day rewarding enough. Another may cherish the opportunity to impress peers. Yet another may be trying to feel special. There may even be neurotic motivation, such as guilt-motivated punishment (e.g., healthy siblings might feel guilty about not sharing the patient's problems). The investigator needs to be alert to the motivation of the normal control subject during the process of informed assent.

DEVELOPMENTALLY SENSITIVE CONSENT

The current system does not adequately recognize the gradual maturation of ability in children and adolescents. Why should the ability to consent altruistically activate abruptly at 18? Laor (1987) and Leikin (1993) suggested a continuous process of empowerment for consent paralleling the maturational process. One possibility might be increments of consent ability at the natural ages of cognitive ability increment. A considerable amount is now known about minors' understanding of the consent process, in addition to Piaget and Inhelder's (1958) basic work suggesting increments of ability at about 7 years and about puberty, when adult-like formal operations are attained. Lewis, Lewis, and Ifekwunigue (1978) found significant increases by grade level in awareness of risk, future consequences, wariness of individuals with vested interests, and need for independent professional advice. Keith-Spiegel and Maas (1981) found that the reasoning of 9-year-olds about research risk is similar to adults. Weithorn and Campbell (1982) found that 14-year-olds show the same risk–benefit reasoning as 21-year-olds, and that 9-year-olds reach the same conclusions through a different reasoning strategy. Lewis et al. (1978) found that 7- to 9-year-olds (but not 6-year-olds) asked all the relevant questions needed for an informed consent. Leikin (1993), after reviewing the literature, concluded that by age 9 children have enough cognitive capacity to participate in the decision. Weithorn and Scherer (1994) concluded that school-age children have the capacity to assent and that 14-year-olds on average have the capacity to consent in the same manner as adults. Thus, enough seems known about children's understanding and judgment to justify more empowerment in the consent process, including the right to make some altruistic decisions.

Laor (1987), in fact, resolves the situation thus: "every individual can achieve, and exercise, different levels of autonomy at different times. . . . The question as to who is or is not autonomous should be replaced by the questions of how much autonomy can/should be ascribed to/required of the individual in different circumstances, be the individual a child or an adult" (pp. 131–132). He proposed that children age 12 and above should be able to consent to research on their own (like adults); that between age 7 and 12 they can consent but parents' assent is also needed (the reverse of the current rules); and below age 7 parental consent is needed, whenever possible coupled with the child's assent. This recommendation was not adopted in 1977 by the U.S. National Committee for the Protection of Human Subjects of Biomedical and Behavioral Research because of a lack of public consensus at the time (Grisso & Vierling, 1978; Laor, 1987; Melton, 1980). Is it time to reconsider the recommendation, perhaps with some modification? For example, one expert who reviewed this manuscript felt that 14 would be a better age than 12 for adult-like consent, but otherwise endorsed Laor's proposal.

Neutral Clinician to Ensure Understanding. As Porter pointed out and the casebook demonstrates, ensuring thorough understanding of all information presented during consent can be achieved in various ways. Consent auditors or monitors can be used, for example, to validate that comprehension is complete. When the investigator is the child's regular clinician, Weithorn and Scherer (1994) suggest that consent be obtained by another clinician. The participation of a neutral clinician can act as a counterbalance to the investigator's bias. Cost and effort considerations would suggest that involvement of an additional clinician in day-to-day consent with individual child subjects is necessary and advisable only for research deemed more than minimal risk by the IRB.

Another important aspect of ensuring children's understanding is to make sure they actually realize they have a choice. Weithorn and Scherer (1994) reviewed the development of locus of control (external in 40% of prepubertal children, 80+% of late adolescents) and other relevant psychological dimensions. They listed several ways to help the child feel more autonomous (e.g., ask them to choose which chair to sit in; ask assent or consent neutrally, not leading). They noted that this not only promotes valid consent/assent, but also improves compliance with the research procedures and treatments.

SPECIAL RISKS ASSOCIATED
WITH NEUROIMAGING TECHNOLOGY

Many severe child and adolescent mental disorders are believed to arise from abnormal development and function of the brain; thus tools that directly measure brain structure and function are essential to understanding the pathogenesis and pathophysiology of these disorders. In addition, the effects in the brain of psychopharmacological agents used in treating children and adolescents should be studied to learn how to maximize treatment effects and to guide development of new therapeutic agents. Because of the importance of this growing area of biological mental health research, the special risks involved deserve specific attention.

Techniques for studying the brain have evolved rapidly during the past several decades, beginning with x-ray computed tomography (CT). Each type of imaging carries its own special risks. Although now almost obsolete, the history of CT scan use illustrates an interesting point about the concept of minimal risk and the impact of research on clinical risk. Before systematic research, many clinicians routinely obtained such scans when diagnosing developmental disorders such as autism. Research results and the careful thinking about risk and benefit associated with the informed consent process in research have led to a reduction in the number of clinical neuroimaging tests. Although magnetic resonance imaging (MRI) does not have the ionizing radiation risk that CT scans have, the potential risk of exposure to a high magnetic field cannot be measured accurately. In MRI studies, the greatest risk is probably sedation for those who require it. Still, many IRBs have not allowed minors to participate in studies at the high magnetic field strengths (3–4 tesla) required to reduce large vessel noise in functional MRIs. Although functional MRI allows studying brain physiology without the ionizing radiation associated with positron emission tomography (PET) or single photon emission computed tomography (SPECT), it is not a currently viable method of studying neurochemistry or the receptors that are important in development and in pharmacological mechanisms of action.

There seems no doubt that with adequately informed assent from the subjects and informed permission of parents, PET studies of children and adolescents with severe mental disorders pose an acceptable level of risk if designed to provide information that may benefit the affected children themselves. However, is it ever acceptable for normal controls? The International Commission on Radiological Protection (ICRP) sets general public involuntary risk guidelines at 1 mSv per year (approximately 100 mrem), which is slightly above most background levels due to soil radioactivity and cosmic radiation at sea level. The ICRP sets occupational limits for whole body exposure at 50 mSv (5 rem) per year.

In addition, a 30 mSv (3 rem) limit for exposure to any individual organ or tissue has been established by 21 CFR Ch. 1 Part 361.1.

Considering even 17-year-old subjects less capable of consent, the ICRP and FDA have limited the exposure of normal children and adolescents as subjects to one-tenth the dose equivalent limit for adult research subjects. Under this guideline, with current detector systems for positron emission tomography and longer acquisition times, some studies are feasible. Normal control minors have been studied with PET. To appreciate the stringency of this guideline, the risk from exposure to 3 mSv (one-tenth the adult limit of 30mSv) is equivalent to the risk of dying in 900 miles of highway driving (Huda & Scrimger, 1989).

Effectively Utilizing Radiation Safety Expertise.   Studies with human subjects using ionizing radiation must be reviewed by both the local Radioactive Drug Review Committee (RDRC) and the IRB throughout the research. RDRC committees are composed of members with the expertise in radiation biology to assess the risk of exposure. This degree of expertise is often lacking on the IRB. It may be helpful to the IRB process for the RDRC to provide an estimate of risk of studies based on current knowledge of radiation biology for use by the IRB in considering the risk–benefit ratio of a study. A process of careful collaboration and consultation among researchers, RDRC, and IRB members is essential for a logical, unfragmented review, with each party contributing their specific expertise and taking the appropriate responsibility.

Sedation or Anesthesia for Imaging.   Sedation of minors for imaging is a routine part of pediatric practice, associated with very low risk. For patients (not normal controls) the use of sedation in situations of no direct or immediate benefit requires careful justification but should not be categorically rejected, given the low risk. In view of the catastrophic nature of PDD, childhood-onset schizophrenia, and similarly crippling disorders, this adjunct to imaging should not stand as a rigid impediment to brain imaging. Although anesthesiologists often argue that general anesthesia with intubation is safer than deep sedation, the added psychological impact will probably be unacceptable to most IRBs. In some instances sedation may be obviated or reduced by such preparation as a preliminary visit to the lab and touching the machine.

INDUCEMENT

The possibility of "coercive inducement" requires a determination of how much is too large a compensation for the risk, discomfort, inconvenience, and lost time of subjects and their parents. Paradoxically, the greater the risk, the harder it is to justify a large subject compensation.

This in itself raises some ironic issues of fairness and justice: It seems that in fairness those who undergo greater risk should be rewarded with more compensation, but it is precisely in the high-risk situations that subjects need to be protected from undue inducement.

Another difficulty in determining appropriate compensation is the varying economic status of the families. The same payment may be much more of an inducement for a poor subject than a wealthy one, but the inducement is not easily equalized because it does not seem right to pay a poor subject less. The child's view of dollar amounts needs to be considered in any amount given directly to the child. For example, Keith-Spiegel and Maas (1981) found that minors age 9 to 15 were more interested than adults in the compensation at the lower amounts. However, parents also need to be compensated for lost time from work and transportation costs. How generously parents are compensated may be an issue: Would a poor parent be tempted to coerce the child into research for the compensation? Such exploitation would run counter to the usual expectation that the parent's judgment about the best interests of the child would protect the child from undue inducement. This presents a dilemma: Working middle-class parents should be reimbursed fairly for lost time from work, but this rate may verge on coerciveness for some poor families and it does not seem right to pay poor or unemployed parents less.

It is understandable why some IRBs and even some ethics experts are tempted to dispose of such thorny decisions by banning compensation in child research, at least for the children themselves. This does not seem fair to the subjects and their parents. It is the practice in some places to reimburse only transportation for the child and one parent. In fact, Graham endorses that restriction. However, the majority of us propose that fair compensation at middle-class levels be offered when the study budget can afford it, and in high-risk studies where there is a concern about this being too tempting for the poorer subjects in the expected sample, some provision could be made for monitoring the consent process by a neutral clinician.

Other suggested solutions have not elicited enthusiasm or general acceptance. For example, some ethicists suggest that there be no discussion about compensation until after consent in order to preclude any inducement. However, others feel that this raises new ethical issues of autonomy and may lead to false expectation for large remuneration, or might unfairly exclude some families who could not afford to take time off from work and pay transportation without some reimbursement. In practice, most IRBs take the position that knowledge about compensation is part of fully informed consent and many even require it to be in the consent form, at least for parents. (Some IRBs prohibit the child being told about compensation given the parents.) Another controversial recommendation not commonly followed is that none of the funding come from pharmaceutical companies or other interested parties (Small, Campbell, Shay, & Goodman, 1994).

Paradoxically, insurance for injury during research, to which no one would object ethically, is an inducement not universally used despite general agreement about its desirability. This particular inducement, in fact, would make any research more ethical by reducing economic risk to the subject.

A nonmonetary inducement may occur when the sibling of a patient is used as normal control. Is the sibling psychologically coerced by guilt and by the expectation of taking responsibility to help the ill family member? A partial answer can come from observations such as those reported by Amiel (1985), who found that siblings of patients were enthusiastic about volunteering for a procedure involving two indwelling venous lines for a day, because it allowed them to share in the attention the sick sibling had been getting and to satisfy their curiosity about what the patient had been going through.

MULTIPLE IRBS

Multiple IRBs are sometimes required for the same protocol because of cross-institutional links of research teams. Because IRBs may have conflicting requirements, this can put the investigator in a position of being unable to satisfy both. Better coordination among IRBs is needed, with education of IRB members as to how other IRBs operate.

UNEXPECTED OR UNWANTED
KNOWLEDGE ABOUT INDIVIDUALS

Another special problem for biological procedures is disposition of unexpected or unwanted knowledge gained in the course of research, especially with normal controls. This can actually be two problems: an internal one for the investigator and an external problem for the family. For example, what should the investigator do with the discovery of an untreatable disorder in a normal control, or the discovery of misattributed paternity in a genetic study? What if the misattributed paternity means that the subject has not really inherited the high risk of a catastrophic dominant-gene disease that he or she thinks he or she has? This dilemma poses twin risks of paternalism (protecting subjects and/or families from something they don't want or need protection from) and irresponsibility (placing a burden on the subject or family by a policy of telling all). Several authors have pointed out the subject's "right not to know" in genetic testing of nonpatients (Knoppers & Chadwick, 1994; Wertz, Fanos, & Reilly, 1994).

The preceding quandary is framed in terms of the personal conflict for the investigator. However, even when an investigator has resolved the internal conflict, there may be external ethical considerations. What if parents don't want the child to know something that the investigator believes he or she should know. Age considerations will obviously impact the solution of both types of problem. For example, the case of misattributed paternity might be handled quite differently with a 6-year-old who might not understand the biological facts of parenthood than with a 16-year-old.

It appears advisable to discuss with the child and parents their wishes about possible contingencies before the results are known. Wertz et al. (1994) suggested that the child or adolescent should be the primary decision maker about being provided information with no direct health benefits (i.e., no treatment or prevention possible) but useful to the minor in making reproductive decisions. Such a pretest discussion carries its own risks of arousing anxiety and curiosity unnecessarily, and needs to be handled skillfully and reassuringly. There is also need for general policy guidance from self-help groups for the respective disorders, and from other nonresearch sources. Such groups could help formulate general guidelines about when and what subjects in various scenarios would like to be told.

A risk of unwanted knowledge increasingly noted by IRBs is an economic one: If a previously undiagnosed chronic disease or genetic propensity to it is found in the course of research, it could prevent the subject from getting medical insurance (and possibly life insurance) in the future. Reportedly, some IRBs have interpreted this economic risk as more than minimal and have disapproved genetic protocols on this basis even though the other risks were acceptable. This particular risk is a cultural artifact and peculiarly American. It is not such a problem where universal health coverage obtains or where discriminatory coverage is prohibited. Provision by the study budget of insurance against this risk would make all research more ethical and acceptable, and it could be part of a more general insurance against injury as a research subject.

CULTURAL, ETHNIC, AND SOCIOECONOMIC ISSUES

In recruiting a sample, generalizability is an important consideration. Norms should reflect the general population, and a clinical sample should reflect the clinical population. This requires some attention to the socioeconomic status (SES) and ethnic composition of the sample.

Cultural and socioeconomic preferences, biases, opportunities, and confounds with exclusion criteria may skew a sample.

A special cultural/ethnic/SES problem for biological research arises from the consideration that some lower SES and single-parent families may be less able to support the subject before, during, and after invasive procedures, which may put such subjects at higher risk. If subjects are chosen on the basis of minimizing risk, it may result in underrepresentation of some ethnic minorities, and certainly of the lower SES. This is an example of the protection versus equal opportunity dilemma. Is exclusion protection or paternalism? Is inclusion equal opportunity or exploitation? This issue relates to the principle of "equity" in access to research mentioned by Knoppers and Chadwick (1994).

Some children in the lowest socioeconomic classes are already exposed to such a high degree of risk that some observers might consider it unacceptable to increase that degree of risk by adding to it the physical and emotional risks of being a research subject. For instance, the Working Group on Inequalities in Health (1980) found that British children in lower social classes are already exposed to between five and seven times the risk of accidental death of children in higher social classes. Barber, Lally, Makarushka, and Sullivan (1979), in a U.S. survey, noted that research subjects of lower social classes tended to be in research projects of greater risk than subjects from higher social classes. He found that research projects with the possibility of considerable therapeutic benefit to the subject were most likely to be carried out on private patients, whereas projects of little or no therapeutic benefit were most likely to be carried out on welfare recipients. Analyzing for both risk and benefit, he found that projects in which the risks were relatively high compared to the possible benefits were twice as likely to be carried out on welfare recipients as projects with a more favorable risk–benefit analysis. It is not clear whether these general findings represent the specific situation of biological mental health research in children and adolescents 15 years later.

The inclusion of appropriate ethnic representation is important for biological research because of possible biological differences between ethnic groups on such things as drug response, toxicity, and so on. If major ethnic groups are not represented in the sample, important findings could be missed that might be useful to the absent or underrepresented ethnic groups and to the advancement of clinical science. There has been official recognition of the need to ensure equal access to research and its fruits (Ellis, 1994; Varmus, 1994). This is another instance where family support groups may be useful in evaluating the benefit–risk ratio for particular populations and providing the extra support to allow full representation of minorities and lower SES subjects, and assist with the longer preparation that might be necessary.

CONCLUSION

Our literature review and collective experience in clinical biomedical research suggests that the degree of actual risk implicit in many biologic procedures used in mental health research (including the aversiveness of these procedures to children) is sometimes overstated. The available data suggest that the degree of discomfort assosciated with most biomedical procedures may not exceed that assosciated with children's everyday experiences. Likewise, the degree of physical risk as a result of many biologic procedures appears to be less than commonly assumed. As we described, many of these risks can be minimized by appropriate sensitivity and planning.

Despite popular notions to the contrary, evidence suggests that adolescents can meaningfully evaluate risks and benefits in a fashion similar to adults. Younger children, although cognitively less able, nonetheless reach sensible conclusions concerning risks and benefits, albeit through rationales somewhat different from those used by adolescents and adults. We suggest that current regulations excessively limit children's opportunities both to contribute altruistic service and to benefit as a group from research. Developmentally enlightened revisions of current regulations and research practices may be advisable to ensure that children and adolescents can reap full benefits of medical research for mental illnesses afflicting this entire class of citizens. The risks of biomedical research with children and adolescents should be carefully balanced against the risks of depriving children of state-of-the-art knowledge concerning the severe mental illnesses that afflict too many of them.

ACKNOWLEDGMENT

This chapter is adapted from an article previously published in the *Journal of the American Academy of Child and Adolescent Psychiatry*. The authors are grateful for permission to republish it.

REFERENCES

Amiel, S. A. (1985). Pediatric research on diabetes: the problem of hospitalizing youthful subjects. *IRB: A Review of Human Subjects Research, 7*(1), 4–5.

Babhulkar, S. S. (1985). Triceps contracture caused by injections. *Journal of Bone Joint Surgery, 67B*, 94–96.

Barber, B., Lally, J. J., Makarushka, J. L., & Sullivan, D. (1979). *Research on human subjects: Problems of social control in medical experimentation.* New Brunswick, NJ: Transaction Books.

Bigos, S. J., & Coleman, S. S. (1984). Foot deformities secondary to gluteal injection in infancy. *Journal of Pediatric Ortrhopedics, 4*, 560–563.

Carbaat, P., & Van Crevel, H. (1981). Lumbar puncture headache: Controlled effect of 24 hours' bed rest. *Lancet, 2,* 1133–1135.

Castellanos, F. X., Elia, J., Kruesi, M. J. P., Gulotta, C. S., Mefford, I. N., Potter, W. Z., Ritchie, G. F., & Rapoport, J. L. (1994). Cerebrospinal fluid monoamine metabolites in ADHD boys. *Psychiatry Research, 52,* 305–316.

Cole, P., & Lumley, J. (1966). Arterial Puncture. *British Medical Journal, 1,* 1277–1278.

Dhar, A., Baga, D., Taneja, S. B. (1988). Extremity gangrene following intramuscular injection. *Indian Pediatrics, 25,* 1209–1215.

Douglas, J. W. B. (1975). Early hospital admissions and later disturbances of behaviour and learning. *Developmental Medicine and Child Neurology, 17,* 456–480.

Ellis, G. B. (1994). *Inclusion of women and minorities in research* (OPRR Reports #94–01). Bethesda, MD: NIH Office of Protection from Research Risks.

Ena, J., Cercenado, E., Martinez, D., & Bouza, E. (1992). Cross-sectional epidemiology of phlebitis and catheter-related infections. *Control Hospital Epidemiology, 13,* 15–20.

Fradet, C., MacGrath, P.J., Kay, J., Adams, S., & Luke, B. (1990). A prospective survey of reaction to blood tests by children and adolescents. *Pain, 40,* 53–60.

Grisso, T., & Vierling, L. (1978). Minors' consent to treatment: A developmental perspective. *Professional Psychology, 9,* 412–427.

Gupta, D. K. (1977). Pulmonary edema following lumbar puncture. *Postgraduate Medical Journal, 23,* 127–129.

Hang, Y. S., & Miller, J. W. (1978). Abduction contracture of the shoulder. *Acta Orthopedics Scandinavia, 49,* 154–157.

Heide, W., & Diener, H. C. (1990). Epidural bloodpatch reduces the incidence of post lumbar puncture headache. *Headache, 30,* 280–281.

Huda, W., & Scrimger, J. W. (1989). Irradiation of normal volunteers in nuclear medicine. *The Journal of Nuclear Medicine, 30,* 260–264.

Humphrey, G. B., Boon, C. M. J., van Linden van den Heuvell, G. F. E. C., & van de Wiel, H. B. M. (1992). The occurrence of high levels of behavioral distress in children and adolescents undergoing routine venipunctures. *Pediatric, 90*(1), 87–91.

Hyde, C., Bentovim, A., & Monck, E. (in press). Clinical implications of a treatment outcome study of children who have been sexually abused. *Child Abuse and Neglect.*

Jay, S. M., Elliot, C. H., Ozolins, M., Olson, R. A., & Pruitt, S. D. (1982). Behavioral management of children's distress during painful medical procedures. *Behavior Research and Therapy, 23*(5), 513–520.

Keith-Spiegel, P., & Maas, T. (1981). Consent to research: Are there developmental differences? *Proceedings of American Psychological Association.*

Klin, A., Cohen, D. J. (1994). The immorality of not knowing: The ethical imperative to conduct research in child and adolescent psychiatry. In J. Hattab (Ed.), *Ethics in Child Psychiatry* (pp. 1–17). Jerusalem, Israel: Gelfen.

Knoppers, B. M. & Chadwick, R. (1994). The human genome project: under an international ethical microscope. *Science, 265,* 2035–2036.

Kopelman, L. M. (1989a). Children as research subjects. In L. M. Kopelman & J. C. Moskop (Eds.), *Children and Health Care: Moral and Social Issues* (pp. 73–87). Boston, MA: Kluwer Academic.

Kopelman, L. M. (1989b). When is the risk minimal enough for children to be research subjects? In L. M. Kopelman & J. C. Moskop (Eds.), *Children and health care: Moral and social issues* (pp. 89–99). Boston, MA: Kluwer Academic.

Kruesi, M. J. P., Lenane, M. C., Hibbs, E. D., & Major, J. (1990). Normal controls and biological reference values in child psychiatry: defining normal. *Journal of the American Academy of Child and Adolescent Psychiatry, 29*(3), 449–452.

Kruesi, M. J. P., Swedo, S. E., Coffey, M. L., Hamburger, S. D., Leonard, H., & Rapoport, J. L. (1988). Objective and subjective side effects of research lumbar punctures in children and adolescents. *Psychiatry Research, 25,* 59–63.

Laor, N. (1987). Toward liberal guidelines for clinical research with children. *Medicine & Law, 6,* 127–137.

Leikin, S. (1993). Minors' assent, consent, or dissent to medical research. *IRB: A Review of Human Subjects Research, 15,* 1–7.

Lewis, C., Lewis, M., & Ifekwunigue, M. (1978). Informed consent by children and participation in an influenza vaccine trial. *American Journal of Public Health, 68,* 1079–82.

Ling, C. M., & Loong, S. C. (1976). Injection injury of the radial nerve. *Injury, 8,* 60–62.

Mann, C. C. (1994). Behavioral genetics in transition. *Science, 264,* 1687–1689.

Marshall, A. G., Erwin, D. C., Wyse, R. K. H., & Hatch, D. J. (1984). Percutaneous arterial cannulation in children. *Anaesthesia, 39,* 27–31.

May, W. E. (1974). Experimenting on human subjects. *Linacre Quarterly, 41,* 238–252.

McCloskey, J. R., & Chung, M. K. (1977). Quadriceps contracture as a result of multiple intramuscular injections. *American Journal of Diseases of Children, 131,* 416–417.

Melton, G. (1980). Children's concepts of their rights. *Journal of Clinical Child Psychology, 9*(3), 186–190.

Metcalf, M. A., McGuffin, R. W., & Hamblin, M. W. (1992). Conversion of the human 5–HT1D beta serotonin receptor to the rat 5–HT1B ligand-binding phenotype by Thr355Asn site directed mutagenesis. *Biochemical Pharmacology, 44,* 1917–1920.

Miyasaka, K., Edmonds, J. F., & Conn, A. W. (1976). Complications of radial artery lines in the pediatric patient. *Canadian Anaesthesiology Society Journal, 23*(1), 9–13.

Mortensen, J. D. (1967). Clinical sequelae from arterial needle puncture, cannulation, and incision. *Circulation, 35,* 1118–1123.

Mukherjee, P. K., & Das, A. K. (1980). Injection fibrosis in the quadriceps femoris muscle in children. *Journal of Bone Joint Surgery, 62A,* 453–456.

Nicholson, R. (1986). *Medical research with children: Ethics, law, and practice.* Oxford, UK: Oxford University Press.

Piaget, J., & Inhelder, B. (1958). *The growth of logical thinking from childhood to adolescence.* New York: Basic Books.

Quinton, D., & Rutter, M. (1976). Early hospital admissions and later disturbances of behaviour: An attempted replication of Douglas' findings. *Developmental Medicine and Child Neurology, 18,* 447–459.

Ramsay, P. (1970). *The patient as person.* New Haven, CT: Yale University Press.

Ramsay, P. (1976). The enforcement of morals: Non-therapeutic research on children. *Hastings Center Report, 6,* 21–30.

Ramsay, P. (1980). Unconsented touching and the autonomy absolute. *IRB: A Review of Human Subjects Research, 2,* 9–10.

Richards, P. G., & Towu-Aghantse, E. (1986). Dangers of lumbar puncture. *British Medical Journal, 292,* 605–606.

Saladino, R., Bachman, D., & Fleisher, G. (1990). Arterial access in the pediatric emergency department. *Annals of Emergency Medicine, 19*(4), 382–285.

Sarkar, P., & Dasgupta, S. (1981). Complications of intramuscular injections in children. *Journal of Indian Medical Association, 77,* 145–147.

Sellden, H., Nilsson, K., Larsson, L. E., & Ekstrom-Jodal, B. (1987). Radial arterial catheters in children and neonates. *Critical Care Medicine, 15,* 1106.

Shanmugasundaram, T. K. (1980). Post injection fibrosis of skeletal muscle: A clinical problem. *International Orthopedics, 4,* 31–37.

Shirkey, H. C. (1968). Therapeutic orphans. *Journal of Pediatrics, 72,* 119–120.

Small, A. M., Campbell, M., Shay, J., & Goodman, I. S. (1994). Ethical guidelines for psychopharmacological research in children. In J. Hattab (Ed.), *Ethics and child mental health* (pp. 244–253). Jerusalem, Israel: Gefen.

Smith, M. (1985). Taking blood from children causes no more than minimal harm. *Journal of Medical Ethics, 11,* 127–131.

Smith-Wright, D. L., Green, T. P., Lock, J. E., Egar, M. I., & Fuhrman, B. P. (1984). Complications of vascular catheterization in critically ill children. *Critical Care Medicine, 12,* 1015–1017.

Sroufe, L. A. & Cooper, R. G. (1987). *Child development: Its nature and course.* New York: Knopf.

Turkeltaub, P. C., & Gergen, P. J. (1989). The risk of adverse reactions from percutaneous prick-puncture allergen skin testing, venipuncture, and body measurements: Data from the second National Health and Nutrition Examination Survey 1976–80 (NHANES II). *Journal of Allergy and Clinical Immunology, 84,* 886–890.

Varmus, H. (1994). NIH guidelines on the inclusion of women and minorities as subjects in clinical research. *Federal Register, 59*(59), 14508–14513.

Weithorn, L., & Campbell, S. (1982). The competency of children and adolescents to make informed decisions. *Child Development, 53,* 1589–1598.

Weithorn, L., & Scherer, D. G. (1994). Children's involvement in research participation decisions: Psychological considerations. In M. A. Grodin & L. H. Glantz (Eds.), *Children as research subjects: Science, ethics, and law* (pp. 133–179). Cary, NC: Oxford University Press.

Wertz, D. C., Fanos, J. H., & Reilly, P. R. (1994). Genetic testing for children and adolescents. *Journal of the American Medical Association, 272,* 875–881.

Working Group on Inequalities in Health. (1980). Sir D. Black (Chair.), *Inequalities in health.* London: DHHS.

8

Ethical Issues in Maltreatment Research With Children and Adolescents

Frank W. Putnam
National Institute of Mental Health
Marsha B. Liss
U.S. Department of Justice
John Landsverk
San Diego State University

Recent national studies document high rates of familial and extrafamilial victimization in children and adolescents (Finkelhor & Dziuba-Leatherman, 1994). There is considerable evidence that experiences of childhood victimization and maltreatment significantly contribute to a range of negative psychological, social, and medical outcomes (National Research Council, 1993). Victimization of children is now recognized as a major public health problem in the United States and is attracting the interest of mental health, medical, social, and criminal justice researchers.

This chapter addresses some of the complex ethical and legal dilemmas raised in research with maltreated and victimized children. Our goal is to articulate a set of ethical issues, particularly as they pertain to informed consent and the potential disclosure of maltreatment by participating children. There are no simple or universal answers for these dilemmas; each researcher must determine the appropriate balance of conflicting ethical and legal duties raised by the specifics of his or her research study.

We begin by considering why it is important to directly question children about possible victimization. Next, we consider the general legal and ethical principles for informed consent/assent with minors and the role of parents in consenting for their children to participate in research studies. We enumerate common concerns raised by researchers and institutional review boards (IRBs) considering research protocols with maltreated children. One of the most difficult dilemmas is raised by the conflict between the usual guarantees of confidentiality explicit in research and the legal and ethical requirements to report suspected maltreatment. Another dilemma is the issue of consent for children in out-of-home placements. Many children are placed in foster care because of suspected or confirmed maltreatment. Foster care children are often in legal limbo with respect to the informed consent/assent process. We use the experience of one author to elucidate the issues and potential solutions to this problem. Finally, we discuss the range of mechanisms available for clarification of this array of problems. The appendix contains a synopsis of all recommendations discussed in the text.

DISCLOSURE OF MALTREATMENT

It should be noted that many researchers who are not specifically interested in or looking for disclosures of maltreatment are none-the-less faced with this eventuality at some point in the course of their research. Research with children and adolescents that focuses on their behaviors, feelings, social life, or their health is likely to elicit disclosure of maltreatment by some participants. As a matter of principle, every researcher studying children and adolescents should be aware of the legal and ethical issues activated by unsolicited disclosures of maltreatment in the course of data collection on other questions.

There are numerous reasons why researchers need to know if children and adolescent subjects were maltreated. A history of maltreatment is a significant risk factor for a range of psychiatric, medical, and behavioral outcomes of interest (e.g., psychiatric symptoms, HIV infection, early pregnancy, low educational attainment, aggression; National Research Council, 1993). Correct classification of maltreatment status is necessary to test theory-driven models and to calibrate screening and diagnostic instruments. Researchers must know the details of specific maltreatment parameters (e.g., age of onset for sexual abuse, types of abuse, relationship to the perpetrator, etc.) to investigate the contribution of these variables to different outcomes. Evaluation of the effectiveness of child abuse prevention programs is dependent on accurate assessment of maltreatment status in target populations.

Currently, most research studies rely on secondary sources of information for the documentation of maltreatment experiences. Common secondary sources include Child Protective Services (CPS)/Department of Social Services (DSS) records, criminal justice system records, use of group consensus as to abuse status by researchers or CPS/DSS workers, and retrospective reports by adults about childhood maltreatment experiences. Studies comparing direct and indirect sources of information demonstrate that relying on CPS/DSS and court records significantly underreports the true incidence and prevalence of maltreatment. For example, Russell (1984) and Saunders, Kilpatrick, Resnick, Hanson, and Lipovsky (1992) found that only 6% to 12% of child sexual abuse cases were reported to authorities. Finkelhor, Hotaling, Lewis, and Smith (1990) found that at the time of the abuse only 40% of sexual abuse victims told anyone. Direct inquiry about abuse appears to significantly increase the rate of reporting of maltreatment by children (Lanktree, Briere, & Zaidi, 1991). However, even when abuse may be inferred from medical evidence, there are still high direct inquiry nondisclosure rates (Lawson & Chaffin, 1992).

It appears that few studies directly ask children about maltreatment experiences. A recent literature review and informal survey by Amaya-Jackson, Socolar, and Runyan (1994) identified 11 clinical/research instruments that directly ask children and adolescents about maltreatment experiences. However, they were only able to find ten studies actually collecting such data. The reluctance of researchers to ask children directly about maltreatment experiences arises in large part from a host of thorny ethical, legal, and methodological questions and dilemmas.

INFORMED CONSENT AND CONFIDENTIALITY IN MALTREATMENT RESEARCH

Principles of Informed Consent

One of the three moral principles that has guided behavioral research since the publication of the Belmont Report (Department of Health, Education and Welfare, 1978) is "respect," the ethical guideline "to respect participant autonomy and privacy" (Fisher, 1993). As Fisher stated:

> The principle of respect reflects a moral concern that individuals be treated as autonomous agents and that more vulnerable persons with diminished autonomy have these rights protected. This principle is reflected in professional codes and federal regulations that require that potential subjects be fully informed about the nature of the research, what will be required of them, the potential risks and benefits of participation, and their right to withdraw or withhold consent without penalty. (p. 3)

All current IRB approaches to children and adolescents classify them as vulnerable persons with diminished autonomy. In this section, we argue that consent procedures for adequately addressing the moral principle of respect are even more complex with minor participants in child maltreatment research than in other research involving children and adolescents. We review the issues of consent with minors in research, indicate the special issues when child maltreatment phenomena are involved in the study aims, and suggest some approaches to consent in child maltreatment research that may be helpful in both honoring the moral principle of respect and permitting child maltreatment research to be carried out robustly.

Three special considerations dominate ethical requirements for consent procedures for minors to participate in research. First, the legal capacity to consent is not granted to children and adolescents (Melton, Koocher, & Saks, 1983). Second, children and adolescents, and young children in particular, may have difficulty understanding the research process "because of their more limited cognitive competencies and experiential background" (Thompson, 1990, p. 4). Third, minors "may perceive they lack power to refuse participation" (Fisher, 1993, p. 3; Keith-Spiegel, 1983; Koocher & Keith-Spiegel, 1990; Levine, 1986).

In all research with children and adolescents, these three considerations have led to regulations that mandate the consent of one or both parents prior to their children participating in a research study. In addition, current IRB regulations stipulate that minors reaching a certain age (usually 7 or 8 although federal regulations do not stipulate an age) must formally "assent" to participation in research even in the context of parental consent (see Protecting Human Research Subjects: Institutional Review Board Guidebook, U.S. Government Printing Office, 1993). The use of an assent procedure addresses the principle of respect in the context of minors' lacking a "legal capacity to consent." Requirements for both parental consent and minor assent carry the clear intent that the agreement to participate must be an informed one, even within the potentially lowered capacity of the minor to understand the complexities of the proposed research participation.

It is important to note that children and adolescents should be afforded the opportunity to assent to their involvement in research regardless of parental motivations and involvement. Children and adolescents in child maltreatment research may provide new disclosures, identification of perpetrators, and additional information about their welfare. In so doing, they present situations wherein the investigators face the dilemma of reporting (see discussion later). Informed consent procedures therefore need to take account of these consequences that present greater than minimal risk to the prospective participant and involve child and adolescent participation in a responsible and sensitive manner. Moreover, these considerations raise questions about the age at which youth may consent to participate in research. Interestingly, adolescents are allowed by law to independently obtain some medical treatments, but not to independently consent to participate in research except in very special circumstances (Grisso, 1992; Weithorn & Scherer, 1994). Reconsideration of these age constraints for research may be of assistance for abused and maltreated children.

We would argue, as have others (e.g., Fisher, 1993; Kinard, 1985), that research involving child maltreatment is particularly complex in regard to these special considerations about consent for minor participation. IRB requirements for prior parental consent assume an intact family with a loving relationship between parent and child in which the best interests of the child will certainly be considered when the parents decide on the issue of their child's participation. However, in the area of child maltreatment, none of these conditions can be assumed. The parent, in fact, may be the agent of the maltreatment. If the maltreatment becomes visible to the community, the parent is likely to be reported to child protective services and/or the police and the parent may face criminal charges for child maltreatment and a dependency hearing in juvenile court. Finally, in cases where the court decides that the level of risk from maltreatment may not be reduced without removal of the child from the home of the parent, the child will come under the legal custody of the court with future legal procedures to determine whether the child will remain under the rights of the natural parent or whether those rights will be severed. In many cases of child maltreatment, an adversarial relationship will develop between the parent(s) and the community at large (as represented by the courts) where research data collection may be perceived as relevant to the outcome of the court decisions. These situations drive the complexity of the consent regulations in research about child maltreatment.

Consequences of Disclosure of Maltreatment

Potential consequences for the child of disclosing maltreatment that may be identified by researchers and IRBs include emotional distress, risk of provoking further abuse as punishment for disclosure, intrusive CPS/DSS/police investigations, and separation from parents (e.g., out-of-home placement, removal, or imprisonment of parent). CPS/DSS/police investigations can be intrusive and stigmatizing for children and their families, even when the maltreatment report is not substantiated or dismissed. In the event that a report is substantiated, legal action may run the gamut from no response to imprisonment of the parents. For example, only 38% of the sexual abuse cases in the Tufts' Maltreatment Study were investigated by the police, only 24% went to prosecution and only 10% resulted in imprisonment of the offender (Sauzier, 1989).

The question of potential emotional distress is often raised by IRBs concerned about a number of possibilities: (a) that telling the researcher the details of the abuse will cause the individual to abreact or "relive" the experiences and produce a psychiatric decompensation; (b) that asking a child about maltreatment may induce confusion about whether or not he or she has been abused (e.g., difficulty in making a distinction between conventional corporal punishment and physical abuse); and (c) that the child may be placed in a "double-bind" forced-choice situation between the researcher and parents (Berliner & Conte, 1994).

In general, researchers asking adults about a range of traumatic experiences have found that even tearful retellings of traumatic experiences do not seem to produce overwhelming emotional responses. To date, no research has been conducted to determine the subjects' perceptions of the effects, positive or negative, of such discussions. Nor is anything known about parental responses to disclosures of maltreatment during research.

We know very little about the process and effects of different types of disclosure experiences (Browne & Finkelhor, 1986; Campis, Hebden-Curtis, & Demaso, 1993; Greenberg & Stone, 1992; Sauzier, 1989; Sorenson & Snow, 1991). Limited data suggest that disclosure is easiest for children experiencing a one time maltreatment act by someone to whom the child does not feel close or loyal (Sauzier, 1989). Volitional disclosure appears most difficult for children involved in long-standing incestuous relationships with a biologic parent, where the sexual involvement has been associated with special attention, affection, and favors and where disclosure will produce significant turmoil in the family (Sauzier, 1989). Preliminary data suggest that some children (~25%) appear more symptomatic weeks to months after disclosure than at the time of disclosure. There may be complex reasons for this apparent worsening of symptoms in a subset of children, but some investigators have suggested that negative parental (usually maternal) responses to the disclosure may be contributory (Browne & Finkelhor, 1986; Sauzier, 1989). Virtually nothing is known about longer term effects of disclosure.

A researcher asking children about experiences of maltreatment is not a priori likely to know about the kind of abuse, the relationship with the perpetrator, or the family supports or psychopathology that may affect the postdisclosure process for a given child. However, given these preliminary data, some regard for the possibility that research-generated disclosures of maltreatment may negatively impact a subset of children should be part of the ethical questions considered in the design of the study.

Informed Consent for Parents

Federal regulation 46.408 requires that investigators must obtain permission from the parents before obtaining assent from their children (Department of Health and Human Services, 1988). Unlike many other research questions, asking children about possible maltreatment places their parents at risk for CPS/DSS investigation and criminal prosecution as well as serious marital and parent–child problems. It is unclear how to best inform parents of the range and likelihood of such consequences. Currently, many research studies include a simple statement to the effect that guarantees of confidentiality by the researcher will be superseded by the reporting of any information required by law. It is likely that many parents do not understand the nature of such cryptic references to mandated reporting or its potential consequences.

However, it is unclear what a researcher should include in the consent document that would adequately inform a parent about the possible risks and benefits to the parent and the child, should the child disclose maltreatment that is then reported by the researcher. In most instances, it is impossible for a researcher to do more than to broadly sketch out a possible course of events that could occur following a hypothetical disclosure of abuse or neglect. Especially without knowing the details of a specific case, a researcher is unable to provide an informed discussion of all of the possible consequences that might occur for parent and child if maltreatment should be disclosed. Many of the uncertainties reflect the variety of ways in which a maltreatment report may be processed by the CPS/DSS system (e.g., a large percentage of reports are not actively investigated in some jurisdictions).

MANDATED REPORTING

With the advent of mandated child abuse reporting laws under the Child Abuse Prevention and Treatment Act (CAPTA), its revisions and amendments (P.L. 102-295 CAPTA, 1992), increasing numbers of medical, social science, and mental health professionals have become obligated to report suspected cases of child abuse or neglect (Kalichman, 1993; Myers, 1992). Each state is required to have legislation defining mandated reporters of child abuse and neglect in the state; however, CAPTA does not endorse any particular definition of mandated reporter and thus states have wide discretion in defining the mandate. As a result, the breadth of the category of mandated reporters varies considerably. In some states, mandated reporters are restricted to a narrow enumerated list usually including medical and school personnel; in other states mandated reporters include all mental health professionals, whereas in still other states all citizens are mandated reporters (Liss, 1994). In addition, most states include provisions for the voluntary or discretionary reporting of suspicions of child abuse and neglect by a wide range of individuals.

The obligation to report suspected cases of child abuse and neglect is commendable for moral reasons in securing the safety of children and indeed has been critical in identifying children at risk for abuse and neglect. However, at the same time, it raises conflicting issues and circumstances for the researcher. These issues include but are not limited to: (a) conflicts between confidentiality as promised in the informed consent and the obligation to report, (b) multi-site studies across states with varying reporting requirements, (c) cases where the natural parents are not available to provide consent for child participation, and (d) adult participants' reports of past incidence of child abuse. There are no easy answers to these conflicts as researchers are reminded to balance the welfare of child participants and their families against the promises of confidentiality and trust inherent, as well as explicitly stated, in the research process. Commentators have questioned the limits of the ethic of the welfare and safety of the participants and the extent to which the researcher can foresee consequences to participation (Williams, 1994). No one method or formulaic language addressing all these issues will suffice for all studies and researchers; however, careful case-by-case consideration of the issues will assist researchers in developing scientifically rigorous, societally responsible, ethically sound informed consent procedures, protocols and sampling techniques that will satisfy state and federally mandated child abuse reporting statutes.

General Considerations

Prior to determining if the researcher will face any of the aforementioned questions, the investigator must review the state legislation and examine whether he or she is indeed a mandated reporter generally and in the research setting specifically (Liss, 1994). Several factors will be critical in reaching a decision: (a) which individuals are mandated to report, (b) what categories of professions are so obligated, and (c) whether the professionals' activities fall within the state statute's definition of the profession. For example, in some states a clinical psychologist would be mandated to report suspicions of child abuse uncovered during the provision of clinical services. However, depending on the state's definition of a psychologist, the same clinical psychologist interviewing a child in a research setting might not be a mandated reporter. In some states, however, all individuals in the state comprise the class of mandated reporters. In such states, the types of activities in which the psychologist engages would be immaterial and all disclosures would presumably be reportable. Furthermore, if only medical or school personnel are mandated reporters, then the same clinical psychologist might never be a mandated reporter in that state.

Even in states where a particular researcher is not included in the enumerated lists of mandated reporters, the researcher may nevertheless have the option of reporting under discretionary reporting statutes. These options usually occur as a general condition for all citizens and clearly include all researchers as well. As is discussed later, considerations of reporting, breaching confidentiality, and the structure of the informed consent face both mandated and discretionary reporters who struggle with the balance between confidentiality and the welfare of the children.

Conflicts With Confidentiality

Both mandated and discretionary reporting suggest problems, albeit different ones, for the researcher. The mandated reporting statutes present a direct conflict between the duty to report and the promise of confidentiality in the informed consent (Myers, 1992). Participants agree to be included in a research project with the understanding that what they say will remain anonymous and undisclosed to anyone not directly involved in the project. The dilemma is the mandated requirement to report versus maintenance of confidentiality.

The dilemma for researchers who fall within the classification statutory of discretionary reporters is the conflict between the maintenance of confidentiality and their ethical responsibilities as professionals. The ethical codes of several professional organizations specifically direct the researcher to be respectful of the welfare of their participants and to avoid bringing harm to the participants directly or indirectly (American Psychological Association, 1992; Society for Research on Child Development, 1990). This directive may be interpreted as implying that it is in the best interest of the children if the abuse or neglect were reported and the child receive proper attention and social services. Alternatively, if the researcher reports the abuse and an investigation ensues in which the child is removed from the home but the allegations are later not substantiated, the researcher may have caused a chain of events which resulted in parent–child separation, lack of trust, and psychological harm to the child.

To address these concerns, some researchers have developed strategies to avoid reporting themselves. For instance, some investigators go to elaborate lengths to encourage a discloser of child abuse to report to an authority, perhaps a teacher, police officer, or social service agency. Others have taken the strategy of not knowing any participants' names, thereby avoiding the possibility of identifying the victim or perpetrator. Researchers working with populations recruited from clinical or social service agency rosters of those already identified as abused or abuser differ on the extent to which they report new allegations of abuse. Some would mention all allegations, while others would only mention allegations regarding new victims or perpetrators. Many of these researchers apply for Certificates of Confidentiality, as discussed later, creating an option not to report suspicions of child abuse and neglect . Still other investigators eliminate high-risk participants from their research or avoid questions that would elicit responses of abuse or neglect.

Although interesting bypasses, these strategies compromise the level of scientific inquiry as well as the utility and generalizability of the findings. Each is an attempt to avoid confronting answers to these difficult issues. Serious inquiry and research should be undertaken by investigators to clarify their obligations.

Reporting Requirements and Informed Consent. Another factor for the researcher to consider is how to phrase the reporting requirements during the informed consent process. In child maltreatment research, reporting families to child protection services is a risk that needs to be explained during informed consent. Researchers not examining child maltreatment issues are divided regarding whether to inform participants and their families that disclosures about abuse or neglect may be reported. These investigators are often concerned that informing parents that they plan to inquire about maltreatment as part of the larger study will discourage participation and introduce a sampling bias (Egeland, 1991; Lynch, Stern, Oates, & O'Toole, 1993). These concerns have curtailed inquiry about maltreatment in epidemiological studies of child and adolescent mental disorders, depriving the field of crucial data on the role of maltreatment as a risk factor. Other researchers believe that not making such statements about abuse should it be discovered violates the nature of informed consent itself. These commentators note the conflict between mandates and options to report versus the content of the consent that should outline the responsibilities of the researchers toward the participants. Anecdotal reports from researchers indicate that when investigators present families with the possibility of reporting their suspicions to the authorities, the families usually opt to voluntarily report the behaviors and seek treatment themselves (Putnam, personal communication, 1994; National Institute of Mental Health, 1993).

There is very little data, anecdotal or empirical, to support either position. The limited extant data suggest that detailed informed consent statements do not deter participation (Singer, 1984). However, Singer's (1984) work did not involve high-risk participants for abuse, nor did she consider the full nature of the participants' understanding of the breadth of what researchers might report as abuse. Moreover, in child maltreatment research, the investigator must consider not only whether to tell the participants and their families that disclosures may be reported, but also potentially what the consequences of reporting might be for the family as a whole. Thus, there is little guidance in providing an answer to how extensively the informed consent should outline consequences of disclosures.

Unfortunately, there are also no legal decisions to guide the discussion. No published cases on appeal have dealt with the researchers' conflict between mandate to report and breaches of the promise of confidentiality. No researcher has yet been sued for reporting child abuse or neglect while breaching confidentiality in research, and there is no literature reviewing instances in which researchers have faced difficulties in reporting child abuse and neglect (Williams, 1994). Thus, this conflict is more apparent than real; those individuals who are reported for child abuse may not hold the researcher responsible. In fact, in a recent survey of urban adolescents, a majority of middle and high school students believed that investigators should break confidentiality and report incidents of physical and sexual abuse to parents or other concerned adults if a respondent revealed this information during the course of abuse (Fisher, Higgins, Rau, Kuther, & Belanger, in press). As more research is done on child maltreatment, it will be important to track the case decisions and to disseminate such results and their implications for research.

Multisite Studies. Recent major collaborative studies, such as the National Institute of Mental Health Cooperative Agreement for a Multisite Study of Mental Health Service Use, Needs, Outcomes and Costs in Child and Adolescent Populations (UNOCCAP), have brought an additional aspect to the discussion. Maltreatment researchers have begun studies involving multiple sites in several states thereby increasing the size of the sample, the diversity of programs and treatments, and range of issues (e.g., the LONGSCAN study funded by the National Center on Child Abuse and Neglect). It is clearly desirable that each of these sites be able to use comparable methodologies, interviews, access to records, informed consent procedures, and debriefing strategies. However, each of these sites and each of the researchers involved in these programs may be subject to different state mandated child abuse and neglect reporting laws. As a result, it may be difficult for the sites to develop jointly protocols to deal with suspicions of child abuse and neglect that arise during the course of the research.

In addition, many multisite studies also include longitudinal or treatment components in their design. These studies follow children who have been abused, are at risk for abuse, or comprise a comparison group, over a number of years with a battery of tests performed at several points in time. In order to follow the changes in development, implications of interventions, and family dynamics, it is critical to compare individual children's and families' responses at each point in time. Thus, some form of identification of participants is needed. In addition, the trust and cooperation of these families is required to maintain their participation in work that will have benefits for them and many other children as well as the formation of policies. However, clearly these individuals cannot be anonymous to the researcher and the more information collected and followed on a family, the more likely it is that suspicions of child abuse and neglect will be found or sustained. Thus, the longitudinal nature of important research creates further issues regarding the reporting of child abuse and neglect by researchers. The process of developing multisite and longitudinal studies of the magnitude needed to answer the significant questions in child abuse and neglect calls for a coordinated approach to guide researchers' responses to suspicions of child abuse and neglect, including a national definition of *child abuse* and designation of mandated reporters with reference to the role of researchers' obligations to report (National Research Council, 1993).

Certificates of Confidentiality

One means for dealing with these issues comes from the U.S. Department of Health and Human Services Health Omnibus Program Extensions Act of 1988, Section 242a, 42 U.S.C., Section 301[d] (1988). This act provides a mechanism whereby investigators doing sensitive research may secure a Certificate of Confidentiality that serves as a shield against discovery by subpoena in court cases (Hoagwood, 1994). Although not unanimous, most ethics opinions indicate that the certificate does not completely negate the obligation to report (National Institute of Mental Health, 1993). Indeed, the certificate merely indicates that the researcher cannot be compelled to report child abuse allegations or suspicions; however, it does allow the researcher to report allegations or suspicions voluntarily. As previously noted, many researchers are concerned with the welfare of child participants and wish to report suspicions of child abuse and neglect. As with the reporting of child abuse by researchers in general, there are no legal opinions upholding the shield of confidentiality in cases of abuse or neglect. Whether a Certificate of Confidentiality is secured or not, researchers should state the limits of confidentiality in the informed consent.

CONSENT ISSUES IN FOSTER CARE
AND SPECIAL POPULATIONS

Current IRB regulations provide some guidance for situations where functional parent–child relationships cannot be assumed. Guardians may be appointed for the child in the absence of a parent to give consent and advocates may be used when the best interests of the child and the best interests of the parent (in the case of criminal prosecution) may be in conflict. However, it has been our research experience that the conditions under which alternative procedures may be instituted are neither well codified nor well known by IRBs in the complex area of child maltreatment. Therefore, it is useful to review some of our experience and suggest some procedures for addressing consent issues in this research area. We use Landsverk's experience in research on the mental health of foster children to illustrate difficulties involved in this type of research and some approaches that can be used to carry out the research while honoring the principle of respect (Landsverk, 1994; Landsverk, Madsen, Litrownik, Ganger, & Newton, 1995).

Provision of Consent for Children in Foster Care

Almost all children currently entering foster care do so because of suspicion of child maltreatment. A court petition must be filed showing cause why the child should remain in out-of-home care and a legal disposition must be made for the child to remain in foster care. The National Institute of Mental Health (NIMH) funded study in San Diego County, California was designed to test the impact of behavioral problem feedback to social workers on referral patterns and use of mental health services. Because physical custody of the foster child by the court after disposition into out-of-home care does not sever the basic parental rights, the question of who can provide for consent in a study of foster children is ambiguous. Although the courts had legally placed the child under the care of the foster care system, judges were hesitant to assign full parental rights in regard to consent for research participation either directly to the court or to the social worker and foster parent who were temporarily providing for care. The situation, in fact, was identical to the problematic issue of who can sign for a foster child to receive medical treatment.

The consent protocol was developed in consultation and negotiation with the juvenile court, the Department of Social Services (DSS), and the governing university IRB. The juvenile court required that no child in out-of-home care would be considered for consent and assent procedures prior to the court's disposition that the child remain in out-of-home placement because of the level of risk to the child. This was done in order to formally establish what is essentially a temporary joint custody arrangement. On average, this disposition was recorded between 30 and 45 days after removal of the child from the home of his or her parents. However, in some child sexual abuse cases, legal disposition was in contention for more than 1 year while the child remained in foster care, resulting in the loss of that child for possible participation in the study.

The research team proposed and the IRB concurred that consent for the child's research participation would be sought from both the natural parent and the substitute parent in foster care. If the natural parent could not be found, the protocol allowed for obtaining consent from the substitute parent only. Only a very small proportion of natural parents chose not to provide consent for their child's participation (less than 5%), less than the percent of substitute parents who withheld consent (10%). It should be noted that the high proportion of natural parents providing consent was likely due to the disposition of the case and the lack of questions in the protocol for the minor about the maltreatment experience.

In addition, the consent protocol included notification to the case worker that a foster child under their supervision was being considered for study participation. Caseworkers, with their supervisor's approval, could request that the child not be approached. In very few cases, all of which involved either custody disputes between the parents or co-occurring spouse abuse with a threat of disclosure and kidnapping, did the caseworker request that a child be kept from participation in the study. This example illustrates the complexity of consent procedures in child maltreatment cases when custody of a child is in "limbo," which is the case in foster care. Multiple adults may need to provide consent in a legitimate process to fully protect these especially vulnerable children.

A further issue arose in the foster care study that illustrates the complexity of appropriate child assent procedures. Children tested, on average, a full standard deviation below norms on the Peabody Picture

Vocabulary Test (PPVT), which is a measure of language functioning, and on the Vineland Adaptive Behavior Scales (VABS), a general assessment of adaptive behavior across the four domains of communication, daily living skills, socialization, and motor skills. Consequently, both developmental level as well as chronological age had to be considered in determining how much information to provide to the children in order to constitute truly "informed" assent. Minors involved in child maltreatment may have diminished capacity for comprehending the "rationale or nature of the experimental procedures" (Fisher, 1993, p. 3).

Our experience with children who have been maltreated would also suggest the increased likelihood that they may perceive they lack power to refuse participation. If children have been involved with the experience of maltreatment and then with the experience of involvement with court procedures and even removal from their natural homes, they are even less likely to perceive themselves as individuals with much power to choose or not choose to participate in an activity defined by adults.

Use of Advocates for Consent Procedures

A creative approach to the use of an advocate in a juvenile detainee study has been reported in the casebook in this volume (Case 28). Due to the problem of contacting parents within the very few days that the juvenile detainee could be approached for study participation, the investigators and IRB concurred on the use of an advocate in the consenting process. This was the only practical way that the research could have been carried out. It should be noted that parental consent was sought if the parent appeared at the jail location. The participant advocate "was a psychologist who regularly met with the juvenile detainees, who had no formal or informal connection with the research project." In the event of noncontact with the parent or guardian, "the participant advocate interviewed the youth, evaluated the juvenile's comprehension of procedures, determined if he or she wished to consent, and that consent was voluntary." If the juvenile was "judged capable of informed, rational, and voluntary consent" a member of the research team was allowed to approach the juvenile and initiate the assent procedure (Fisher, Hoagwood, & Jensen, this volume). The use of a participant advocate in child maltreatment and other types of research with complex consenting situations holds promise for greater use by research teams and IRBs. It would have been an excellent addition to the foster care study mentioned earlier.

Although this section does not exhaust the coverage of consent issues in child maltreatment research, we hope it has provided both insight into the complexity of the circumstances surrounding consent procedures as well as concrete examples of realistic protocol elements that honor the moral principle of respect.

MECHANISMS FOR CLARIFICATION
OF ETHICAL AND LEGAL ISSUES

It is apparent that very little is known about the effects, positive and negative, of disclosure of maltreatment. In the absence of empirical research on the effects of disclosure in research settings and lack of case law on Certificates of Confidentiality and mandated reporting obligations by researchers, any guidelines or suggestions must be adapted to each researcher's methodologies and interpretations of their ethical and legal mandates. At the present time, rather than avoiding questions that may result in child maltreatment disclosures, there are some strategies that researchers may use to address ethical concerns in child maltreatment research and to deal with unanticipated disclosures of child maltreatment in a variety of research programs.

One prevailing option is to encourage the child/adolescent or the family to seek assistance and report the maltreatment themselves. The advantage to this approach is that it empowers the family to move forward in treatment, while at the same time preserving the research protocol and data collection but in most states it must be reported in 24 to 48 hours. In this way, the researcher does not violate the confidentiality and contract with the participants. However, this option does not obviate legal responsibility for mandated reporters to report abuse. In some instances, the family may waive their rights and make some relevant data available to a treatment therapist. There is little or no evidence to date about the relative outcomes of voluntary versus enforced reporting to social service and child protection authorities.

One straightforward response is to report families where there are suspicions of child abuse and neglect. This option may be exercised both when the informed consent has included a statement about the effects of disclosures and when there are no such statements. To date, there are few if any instances anecdotally discussed by researchers when a family has objected to the reporting or refused participation in the study because of the disclosure. As discussed earlier, many researchers firmly believe that telling the prospective participant that they may be reported for disclosures decreases the likelihood of their participation; future research on this issue is critical to guide the development of informed consent procedures in a knowledgeable rather than a conjectural manner. The remaining concern is the researcher's abrogation of the confidentiality indicated in the informed consent; dealing with this promise and the reporting mandates as they apply to the researcher may need to be an issue not for the courts but for the individual researcher. In addition, it will be important to disseminate any case law that develops guiding researchers in balancing the need to report with confidentiality issues. In general, the courts are likely to use a case-by-case balancing approach and to determine whether the breach of confidentiality is necessary.

Under the present CAPTA, states continue to be able to set different mandated and discretionary reporting statutes. This is likely to continue as an issue of state determination of family welfare. Researchers working in multisite situations should remember that one can always afford greater protections and that legal issues only determine the minimum standards to be set. Researchers should therefore consider providing the participants with the greatest amount of leeway in making decisions. As noted previously, the mandate to report under CAPTA and its state variations, seems to be at odds with the Certificates of Confidentiality. It would be helpful to researchers if these two statutes could be reconciled providing for the balancing of interests. In order to continue serving families and minimizing abuse it is necessary for researchers to be unhampered in their efforts to identify maltreatment victims, and to study family dynamics, treatment effects, effects of disclosures, and court and welfare system interventions. Some have argued that efforts to reconcile CAPTA and the Certificate of Confidentiality should incorporate legislation specifically including child maltreatment under the Certificate of Confidentiality (Runyan, 1994). Others argue that failing to report instances of abuse relayed by a child or adolescent research participant may inadvertently communicate to the child that the abuse is unimportant or that adults in authority will be of no assistance (Fisher et al., in press).

Child abuse and neglect is a critical public health problem that is poorly understood from a scientific and social perspective. Researchers studying child maltreatment and its effects face numerous daunting methodological problems and ethical dilemmas. Progress can only be made by clearly articulating and confronting these problems as they arise in the course of a given study. To inform the field, research reports should include descriptions of ethical issues and their resolution. Results sections should describe beneficial and negative effects of the methodological approaches adopted by the investigators. Increased dissemination of researchers' experiences with ethical and methodological problems is crucial to advancing knowledge and to improving future research designs.

APPENDIX: RECOMMENDATIONS

1. All child and adolescent researchers should be familiar with their state laws requiring mandated reporting of child abuse and neglect.
2. Researchers working in the field of childhood maltreatment should apply for a Certificate of Confidentiality.
3. Researchers should include a clause in their informed consent documents describing their response to a disclosure of maltreatment during the course of research.
4. If disclosure of maltreatment occurs during the research process, the child/adolescent and/or family should be encouraged to initiate a report to the appropriate agency.
5. In research with children in out-of-home placements, consent should be obtained from both the natural parents and the foster parents. If the natural parents cannot be located, provisions should be made for consent from the foster parents.
6. In research with juvenile detainees, consent may be obtained from an advocate not connected (directly or indirectly) with the research, when a natural parent cannot be located.
7. Researchers should discuss ethical and methodological issues in their published reports and include information on the beneficial and negative effects of their approaches to these issues.

REFERENCES

Amaya-Jackson, L., Socolar, R. S., & Runyan, D. K. (1994). Directly questioning children and adolescents about maltreatment: A review. In D. Runyan (Ed.), *The North Carolina Conference on the Ethical, Legal and Methodological Implications of Directly Asking Children about Histories of Maltreatment (The Siena Group Report).* Chapel Hill, NC.

American Psychological Association. (1982). *Ethical Principles in the conduct of research with human participants.* Washington, DC: Author.

Berliner, L., & Conte, J. (1994). Clinical issues in asking child subjects about abuse experiences. In D. Runyan (Ed.), *The North Carolina Conference on the Ethical, Legal and Methodological Implications of Directly Asking Children about Histories of Maltreatment (The Siena Group Report).* Chapel Hill, NC.

Browne, A., & Finkelhor, D. (1986). Impact of child sexual abuse: a review of the research. *Psychological Bulletin, 99*, 66–77.

Campis, L. B., Hebden-Curtis, J., & Demaso, D. R. (1993). Developmental differences in detection and disclosure of sexual abuse. *Journal of the American Academy of Child and Adolescent Psychiatry, 32*, 920–924.

Child Abuse Prevention and Treatment and Adoption Reform Act of 1992, Pub. L. No. 102–295, 42 U.S.C.A. 5101 *et seq* (1992).

Department of Health, Education and Welfare. (1978). *The Belmont report: Ethical principles and guidelines for the protection of human subjects of research.* Washington, DC: U.S. Government Printing Office.

Department of Health and Human Services. (1988). *Protection of human subjects, 45 CRF* (Vol. 46). Washington, DC: Author.

Egeland, B. (1991). A longitudinal study of high-risk families. In R. Starr & D. Wolfe (Eds.), *The effects of child abuse and neglect: Issues and research* (pp. 43–46). New York: Guilford.

Finkelhor, D., & Dziuba-Leatherman, J. (1994). Children as victims of violence: A national survey. *Pediatrics, 84,* 413–420.

Finkelhor, D., Hotaling, J., Lewis, I. A., & Smith, C. (1990). Sexual abuse in a national survey of adult men and women: Prevalence, characteristics and risk factors. *Child Abuse and Neglect, 14,* 19–28.

Fisher, C. B. (1993). Integrating science and ethics in research with high-risk children and youth. *Social Policy Report: Society for Research in Child Development, 7,* 1–27.

Fisher, C. B., Higgins, A., Rau, J. M., Kuther, T., & Belanger, S. (in press). Referring and reporting research participants at risk: Views from urban adolescents. *Child Development.*

Greenberg, M. A., & Stone, A. A. (1992). Emotional disclosure about traumas and its relation to health: Effects of previous disclosure and trauma severity. *Journal of Personality and Social Psychology, 63,* 75–84.

Grisso, T. (1992). Minors' assent to behavioral research without parental consent. In B. Stanley & J. E. Sieber (Eds.), *Social research in children and adolescents: Ethical issues* (pp. 109–127). Newbury Park, CA: Sage.

Hoagwood, K. (1994). The Certificate of Confidentiality at the National Institute of Mental Health: Discretionary considerations in its applicability in research on child and adolescent mental disorders. *Ethics and Behavior, 4,* 123–31.

Kalichman, S. C. (1993). *Mandated reporting of suspected child abuse: Ethics, law and policy.* Washington, DC: American Psychological Association.

Keith-Spiegel, P. C. (1983). Children and consent to participate in research. In G. P. Melton, G. P. Koocher, & M. J. Saks (Eds.), *Children's competence to consent* (pp. 179–211). New York: Plenum.

Kinard, E. M. (1985). Ethical issues in research with abused children. *Child Abuse and Neglect, 9,* 301–311.

Koocher, G. P., & Keith-Spiegel, P. C. (1990). *Children, ethics and the law.* Lincoln: University of Nebraska Press.

Landsverk, J. (1994). *Barriers to effective mental health services for children in foster care: Implications from research.* Paper presented at the annual conference of the American Public Health Association, Washington, DC.

Landsverk, J., Madsen, J., Litrownik, A., Ganger, W., & Newton, R. (1995). *Mental health problems of foster children in three California counties.* Manuscript submitted for review.

Lanktree, C., Briere, J., & Zaidi, L. (1991). Incidence and impact of sexual abuse in a child outpatient sample: The role of direct inquiry. *Child Abuse and Neglect, 15,* 447–453.

Lawson, L., & Chaffin, M. (1992). False negatives in sexual abuse disclosure interviews: Incidence and influence of caretaker's belief in abuse in cases of accidental abuse discovery by diagnosis of STD. *Journal of Interpersonal Violence, 7,* 532–542.

Levine, R. (1986). *Ethics and regulation of clinical research* (2nd ed.). Baltimore-Munich: Urban & Schwarzenberg.

Liss, M. B. (1994). Child abuse: Is there a mandate for researchers to report? *Ethics and Behavior, 4,* 133–146.

Lynch, D. L., Stern, A. E., Oates, R. K., & O'Toole, B. I. (1993). Who participates in child sexual abuse research? *Journal of Child Psychology and Psychiatry, 34,* 935–944.

Melton, G. B., Koocher, G. P., & Saks, M. J. (1983). *Children's competence to consent.* New York: Plenum.

Myers, J. E. (1992). *Legal issues in child abuse and neglect.* Newbury Park, CA: Sage.

National Institute of Mental Health. (1993, May). *Ethical and human subjects issues in mental health research with children and adolescents.* Conference proceedings, NIMH, Rockville, MD.

National Research Council. (1993). *Understanding child abuse and neglect.* Washington, DC: National Academy Press.

Runyan, D. (1994). Recommendations for federal policy and legal changes. In D. Runyan (Ed.), *The North Carolina Conference on the Ethical, Legal and Methodological Implications of Directly Asking Children about Histories of Maltreatment (The Siena Group Report).* Chapel Hill, NC.

Russell, D. E. H. (1984). *Sexual exploitation: Rape, child sexual abuse and workplace harassment.* Newbury Park, CA: Sage.

Saunders, B. E., Kilpatrick, D. G., Resnick, H. S., Hanson, R. A., & Lipovsky, J. A. (1992). *Epidemiological characteristics of child sexual abuse: Results from Wave II of the National Women's Study.* Paper presented at the San Diego Conference on Responding to Child Maltreatment, San Diego, CA.

Sauzier, M. (1989). Disclosure of child sexual abuse: For better or for worse. *Psychiatric Clinics of North America, 12,* 455–469.

Singer, E. (1984). Public reactions to some ethical issues of social research: Attitudes and behavior. *Journal of consumer research, 11,* 501–509.

Society for Research on Child Development. (1990, Winter). Ethical standards for research with children. *SRCD Newsletter.*

Sorenson, T., & Snow, B. (1991). How children tell: The process of disclosure in child sexual abuse. *Child Welfare League of America, LXX,* 3–15.

Thompson, R. A. (1990). Vulnerability in research: A developmental perspective on research risk. *Child Development, 61,* 1–16.

Weithorn, L. A., & Scherer, D. G. (1994). Children's involvement in research participation decisions: Psychological considerations. In M. A. Grodin & L. H. Glantz (Eds.), *Children as research subjects: Science, ethics and law* (pp. 133–180). New York: Oxford University Press.

Williams, L. (1994). Asking about abuse and the limits of confidentiality: A discussion of ethical issues facing child abuse researchers. In D. Runyan (Ed.), *The North Carolina Conference on the Ethical, Legal and Methodological Implications of Directly Asking Children about Histories of Maltreatment (The Siena Group Report).* Chapel Hill, NC.

Part III

Casebook

Casebook Contents

WITHHOLDING TREATMENT: THE USE OF CONTROL GROUPS, PLACEBOS, AND RANDOMIZED CLINICAL TRIALS

IDENTIFICATION AND RECRUITMENT OF SUBJECTS

INFORMED CONSENT PROCEDURES

CHILD ASSENT IN THE ABSENCE
OF PARENTAL CONSENT

DECEPTIVE RESEARCH PROCEDURES

CONFIDENTIALITY

MODIFYING PROCEDURES DURING
THE COURSE OF CLINICAL TRIALS

OFFERING SERVICES BEYOND THOSE
REQUIRED BY THE RESEARCH PROTOCOL

DEBRIEFING AND DISSEMINATION

9

Casebook on Ethical Issues in Research With Children and Adolescents With Mental Disorders

Celia B. Fisher
Fordham University
Kimberly Hoagwood
Peter S. Jensen
National Institute of Mental Health

Researchers applying the scientific method to describe, explain, and enhance the status of children and youth at risk for or suffering from mental disorders are encountering ethical dilemmas to which current federal and institutional guidelines offer incomplete answers. The scientific and ethical dimensions of such work often appear to have contradictory goals. Scientific responsibility requires validation of knowledge through experimental controls, whereas ethical responsibility requires the protection of participant welfare and rights that may appear to jeopardize controls (Fisher, 1993). Researchers must confront such questions as:

"How is an appropriate balance between research risks and benefits achieved?"
"How are members of high-risk and vulnerable populations identified and recruited without violating their privacy or coercing their participation?"
"How are the autonomy rights of children and adolescents protected when parental consent may or may not be in the child's best interest?"
"How is researcher–participant confidentiality maintained when one learns that a child's welfare may be in jeopardy?"

The development of this casebook arose in response to such questions repeatedly asked by investigators seeking guidance from staff and administrators at the National Institute of Mental Health (NIMH). At their monthly meetings, members of the NIMH Child Consortium discussed possible activities that might assist investigators who were confronting ethical dilemmas. They concluded that NIMH might best assist mental health researchers by bringing leaders in the field together to surface issues and share with other scientists how they were responding to their ethical responsibilities.

The first step in this initiative was to bring together members from professional organizations dedicated to promoting the mental health of children and adolescents to discuss the strengths and limitations of current professional and federal guidelines for advancing science and protecting the welfare of human research subjects. This was followed by the NIMH Conference on Ethical and Human Subject Issues in Research on Child and Adolescent Mental Disorders held in May 1993. At this conference, representatives from professional and scientific organizations, family groups, and the federal government identified issues of import to investigators and research participants. The most frequently mentioned recommendation was for the creation of a casebook of examples of ethical dilemmas and solutions encountered by investigators conducting research on mental disorders of childhood and adolescence

This casebook was written in response to that recommendation. It includes specific examples of dilemmas that have arisen during the design or conduct of research projects, and how those dilemmas were resolved by the investigator. It also provides concrete examples of specific research risks to child and adolescent subjects and ways to define, identify, and minimize risks without forfeiting the integrity of the studies. Cases were developed through a national survey of researchers working with children and adolescents with or at risk for mental disorders. Of the approximately 300 research scientists who were mailed requests for participation, approximately 100 responded by phone interview or provided cases, articles, and informed consent protocols by mail describing their ethical practices and challenges. The development of the casebook also benefited from the wisdom of those scholars and scientists whose works are cited in the references and suggested readings section.

Sixty-one ethics cases emerged from this process. Many of the cases follow in close detail and writing style specific incidents described by contributors; others are composites of issues presented by several contributors or highlighted in the research ethics literature. The cases are organized within 10 sections representing broad ethical concerns:

- Balancing research risks and benefits.
- Protecting participant welfare in research designs requiring the withholding of treatment.
- Protecting participant rights during identification and recruitment of subjects.
- Developing adequate informed consent procedures.
- DevelopIng adequate child assent procedures when guardian consent is unavailable or inappropriate.
- Protecting participant rights when designing and conducting deceptive research.
- Protecting participant confidentiality.
- Modifying research procedures in response to participant needs.
- Offering services beyond those required by the research protocol.
- Debriefing participants and disseminating research findings.

Ethical decision making in research with children and youth with mental disorders is enhanced by empirical data on participant and guardian responses to recruitment practices, random assignment, informed consent procedures, experimental methods, and debriefing procedures. For the readers benefit, the references and suggested readings section highlights articles that provide empirically derived information on ethical decision making or that incorporate into a research article detailed description of actual ethical practices.

At the heart of all the incidents represented in this casebook is the struggle to design and conduct research that attains both the highest scientific standards of human subjects research and the highest standards of humanitarian concern for participant welfare, autonomy, and justice. Although relevant federal guidelines are highlighted in the introductions to each section, the cases themselves are not meant to provide definitive rules or guidelines for ethical practice. The ethical demands of a situation are best understood when seen within the context or the culture of a given study. As such, ethical decision making is a process of constructing the best procedures possible within a given situation rather than discovering rules that can be universally applied across situations. Thus, the value of the cases lies in providing models of ethical decision making that focus on the scientist as a moral agent rather than a moral judge.

It is not always easy to share the deliberations that are involved in one's ethical decision making. It requires self-reflection and the courage to analyze and reveal one's values. We are fortunate that our case contributors and consultants have so generously shared their experiences and concerns with us. Their dedication to promoting the science and ethics of research on child and adolescent mental disorders has and continues to help investigators achieve the highest standards of scientific integrity and humanitarian concern.

As illustrated by the cases presented here, researchers dedicated to explaining and developing empirically sound treatments for children and adolescents with mental disorders are no longer looking at scientific rigor and ethical treatment of individuals as either–or positions. They are constructing new and innovative empirical approaches that are integrating scientific responsibility with participant care. There are no easy or universal solutions to ethical dilemmas facing researchers in the field of child and adolescent disorders. It is hoped that the approaches described in this casebook will help guide others in the continuing dialogue on ethical practice.

The following is a list of case contributors and consultants.

CASE CONTRIBUTORS AND CONSULTANTS

Howard Abikoff, *Schneider Children's Hospital & Albert Einstein College of Medicine*
Howard S. Adelman, *School Mental Health Project, UCLA*
Jean Adnopoz, *Yale Child Study Center*
Mutya San Agustin, *North Central Bronx Hospital and Albert Einstein College of Medicine*
Janet K. Allen, *Phoenix House Foundation*
Heidelise Als, *Enders Pediatric Research Laboratories, Harvard Medical School*
Michael Aman, *Massey University*
Arthur D. Anastopoulox, *University of Massachussetts Medical Center*
Adrian Angold, *Duke University Medical Center*
L. Eugene Arnold, *Child & Adolescent Disorders Research Branch, NIMH*
Marc S. Atkins, *Institute for Juvenile Research, University of Illinois at Chicago*
Gerald J. August, *University of Minnesota*
David E. Balk, *Kansas State University*
Manuel Barrera, Jr., *Arizona State University*
Ellen L, Bassuk, *The Better Homes Fund and Hawood Medical School*
Herbert Bauer, *University of California at Davis, School of Medicine*
Jay Belsky, *College of Health & Human Development, The Pennsylvania State University*
Gail Bernstein, *University of Minnesota Medical School*
Leonard Bickman, *Vanderbilt University Center for Mental Health Policy*
Boris Birmaher, *Western Psychiatric Institute & Clinic*
Jack Block, *University of California at Berkeley*

James Breiling, *National Institute of Mental Health*
David A. Brent, *Western Psychiatric Institute & Clinic*
Daniel J. Burbach, *Riverhill Psychological Associates*
Nancy Busch-Rossnagel, *Fordham University*
Magda Campbell, *New York University Medical Center*
Glorisa Canino, *Behavioral Sciences Research Institute, University of Puerto Rico*
Emily H. Canning, *University of Pittsburgh, Western Pyschiatric Institute and Clinic*
Deborah M. Capaldi, *Oregon Social Learning Center*
F. Xavier Castellanos, *Child Psychiatry Branch, NIMH*
Stephen J. Ceci, *Cornell University*
Laurie Chassin, *Arizona State University*
Edward R. Christophersen, *Children's Mercy Hospital*
Dante Cicchetti, *Mount Hope Family Center, University of Rochester*
Donald J. Cohen, *Yale Child Study Center*
John F. Curry, *Duke University Medical Center*
Geraldine Dawson, *University of Washington*
Harold E. Dent, *Center for Minority Special Education, Hampton University*
Norin Dollard, *New York State Office of Mental Health*
Ralph Mason Dreyer, *Louisiana State University*
Byron Egeland, *University of Minnesota*
Leona L. Eggert, *Reconnecting At-Risk Youth Research Program, University of Washington*
Josephine Elia, *St. Christopher's Hospital for Children*
Mary Evans, *New York State Office of Mental Health*
Joseph Fagen, *Saint John's University*
James Garbarino, *Erikson Institute for Advanced Study in Child Development*
Barbara Geller, *Washington University School of Medicine*
Susan Goldberg, *The Hospital for Sick Children, Toronto*
Gail Goodman, *University of California, Davis*
Irving I. Gottesman, *University of Virginia*
Madelyn S. Gould, *Columbia University College of Physicians & Surgeons, Public Health*
Katheryn E. Gustafson, *Duke University Medical Center*
Christoph M. Heinicke, *University of California Los Angeles*
Lily Hechtman, *Montreal Children's Hospital*
Sylvia Herz, *New Jersey Public Health Administration*
Stephen P. Hinshaw, *University of California, Berkeley*
Jacquelyne Jackson, *Institute of Human Development, University of California, Berkeley*

Katurah Jenkins-Hall, *The Florida Mental Health Institute, University of South Florida*
Jeannette L. Johnson, *University of Maryland at Baltimore, School of Medicine*
Jerome Kagan, *Harvard University*
Sandra Kaplan, *Cornell University*
Joan Kaufman, *University of Pittsburgh Medical Center, Western Psychiatric Institute/Clinic*
Philip C. Kendall, *Temple University*
Meg Kerrigan, *University of Michigan*
E. Milling Kinard, *Family Research Laboratory, University of New Hampshire*
Kathleen Kostelny, *Erikson Institute for Advanced Study in Child Development*
Markus Kruesi, *Institute for Juvenile Research, University of Illinois at Chicago*
John V. Lavigne, *Children's Memorial Hospital, Northwestern University*
Lewis P. Lipsitt, *Brown University*
Catherine Lord, *University of Chicago*
Raymond P. Lorion, *University of Maryland*
Ellen D. Nannis, *Henry M. Jackson Foundation*
Charles Oberg, *University of Minnesota Medical School*
Roberta Ann Olson, *Health Psychology Associates*
Joy Osofsky, *Louisiana State University Medical Center*
Deborah A. Pearson, *University of Texas Medical School at Houston*
William E. Pelham, Jr., *University of Pittsburgh, Western Psychiatric Institute & Clinic*
Amy Perwien, *University of Minnesota Medical Center*
Cynthia R. Pfeffer, *Cornell University Medical College*
Marion Radke-Yarrow, *Laboratory of Developmental Psychology, NIMH*
Helen Reinherz, *Simmons College School of Social Work*
John E. Richters, *Child and Adolescent Disorders Research Branch, NIMH*
Mark Riddle, *Johns Hopkins University Hospital*
Arthur Rifkin, *Albert Einstein College of Medicine*
Anne W. Riley, *School of Hygiene & Public Health, Johns Hopkins University Hospital*
Abram Rosenblatt, *University of California, San Francisco*
Mary Jane Rotheram-Borus, *University of California Los Angeles*
M. David Rudd, *Scott & White Clinic & Hospital, Texas A&M University*
Mary Carmel Ruffolo, *School of Social Work, Syracuse University*
Deborah Rugs, *Florida Mental Health Institute*
Laura Schreibman, *University of California, San Diego*
David Shaffer, *New York State Psychiatric Institute*

Wendy K. Silverman, *Florida International University*
Magda Southamer-Loeber, *University of Pittsburgh, Western Psychiatric Institute/Clinic*
Robert L. Sprague, *University of Illinois at Urbana-Champaign*
Scott Spreat, *Woods Services Incorporated*
Aubyn C. Stahmer, *University of California, San Diego*
David Stoff, *National Institute of Mental Health*
Teresa Sweeney, *Duke University Medical Center*
Peter E. Tanquay, *University of Louisville*
C. Barr Taylor, *Stanford Medical School*
Linda A. Teplin, *Psycho-Legal Studies Program, Northwestern University Medical School*
Edward Tronick, *Children's Hospital Harvard Medical School*
Maribel Vargas, *Fordham University*
Norman F. Watt, *University of Denver*
Jeanne Rodier Weber, *Edinboro University of Pennsylvania*
Merrill Weiner, *Cornell University Medical College*
Roger Weissberg, *University of Illinois at Chicago*
Alan J. Zametkin, *Section on Clinical Brain Imaging, NIMH*

* * *

Casebook

Balancing Research Risks and Benefits

Research designed to describe, explain, and evaluate treatments for mental disorders in childhood and adolescence presents both the probability of benefits and the probability of risks for research participants. For example, research designed to assess a new biomedical or behavioral treatment can have remedial as well as iatrogenic effects on participant welfare. Studies examining the developmental correlates of violent and illegal adolescent behaviors can contribute to preventive strategies for ameliorating these problems, or if sensitive information is revealed, can result in punitive actions against research participants. Ethical justification for the conduct of research, therefore, rests on demonstrating a favorable balance of risks to benefits. This balance, embodied in the dual moral principles of beneficence (to do good) and nonmaleficence (to do no harm), is reflected in federal guidelines requiring that research risks are justified by and reasonable with respect to the anticipated benefits to the research participants or to society (OPRR, 1993).

RESEARCH BENEFITS

That a study holds out the possibility of doing good is a minimal requirement for the ethical justification for conducting the research (Veatch, 1987). In research with children and adolescents with mental disorders, no risk is acceptable if the research does not have the potential to directly benefit the participant or enhance our knowledge of the child or adolescent's disorder or condition.

Scientific Validity and Value. A critical factor in determining the benefit of a research design is whether the study has scientific merit (Fisher & Fyrberg, 1994; Freedman, 1987). To be scientifically valid, research must be designed to produce reliable information according to accepted principles of research. For example, experiments must have a sufficient number of subjects to produce reliable findings and adequate experimental control against the influence of extraneous variables. However, a study may be well designed but may be of no value because the hypothesis itself will not meaningfully enhance the understanding of a specific disorder or help to ameliorate a mental health problem. To be of benefit, an "experiment should be such as to yield fruitful results for the good of society" (Nuremberg Code, 1946, Principle 2). Scientific validity and value are thus at the heart of evaluating the risk–benefit balance of mental health research. If the scientific integrity or societal contribution of a study can not be ensured (i.e., because of institutional regulations), methodologically sound research with the potential to improve existing knowledge or treatments may not be conducted because the probability of benefit does not outweigh the probability of research risk (see Case 1).

Direct and Indirect Benefits. Beneficial outcomes in research with children and youth can be achieved directly or indirectly (Fisher, 1993). On the one hand, research designed to evaluate the efficacy of a medication to treat a disorder of childhood has the potential to benefit directly the child or adolescent assigned to the "treatment" group. On the other hand, research designed to identify the natural developmental course of a childhood disorder has the potential to benefit indirectly other minors who share the participant's disorder through future application of research findings by practitioners.

Maximizing Benefits. The benefits of participation in therapeutic research can be maximized by helping participants receive the empirically effective treatment once the study is completed. In studies with no expected direct benefit, such as some descriptive or explanatory studies, benefits can be maximized by providing research participants with information about mental health services that they might not otherwise receive. When evaluating the benefits of mental health research, investigators need to be mindful that the assessment of doing good may be subject to cultural norms and professional bias. Thus, some have suggested that the perspectives of potential research participants should be considered in all ethical decision making (Fisher & Fyrberg, 1994; Fisher, Higgins, Rau, Kuther, & Belanger, in press; Veatch, 1987).

RESEARCH RISKS

Risks that may result from research should be distinguished from those associated with therapies children would undergo even if they were not participating in the research (OPRR, 1993). Thus, although some pharmacological agents used in standardized treatment may have potentially negative side effects, the responsibility of the investigator examining the efficacy of this clinically established procedure (and his or her institutional review board [IRB]) is to assess the risks of the research design and procedures themselves (e.g., a placebo washout period, randomization to a no-treatment or alternative treatment condition, the biomedical or psychosocial measures used to assess outcome) rather than the treatment per se.

Direct and Indirect Risks.   Research with children and youth can also expose participants directly or indirectly to experiences that result in harm that is minor or serious, transient or permanent (Fisher, 1993). For example, both biomedical and psychosocial procedures can directly contribute to transient and minimal discomfort (e.g., the immediate discomfort and potential minor bruising from venipuncture; dizziness or dry mouth from a medication; negative feelings associated with questions about personally distressing events) or less transient more severe discomfort (e.g., headaches sometimes associated with a spinal tap procedure; medication induced memory loss or cognitive impairments; guilt or "inflicted insight" from recognizing through the research experience negatively perceived self-attributes). Other risk factors that need to be considered include withholding of treatment, invasion of privacy, failure to protect confidentiality, and dissemination of misinformation that can have negative personal or societal consequences for children and youth suffering from a disorder under investigation.

ADDITIONAL PROTECTIONS FOR CHILDREN INVOLVED AS SUBJECTS IN RESEARCH

Federal guidelines, in recognizing the special vulnerability of child participants in human subjects research, have developed added protections to ensure that their rights and welfare are protected. In general, all research risks can be minimized by avoiding dual role relationships, ensuring the competence of all research personnel, determining that consent and assent are adequately informed, maintaining confidentiality, using the least invasive technologies, and whenever possible using procedures already being performed on subjects for diagnostic or treatment purposes.

Minimal Risk Research.   The Department of Health and Human Services (DHHS) regulations 45 CFR 46 Subpart D strictly limits research with children presenting more than minimal risk. Research is considered minimal risk when "the probability and magnitude of harm or discomfort anticipated in the research are not greater in and of themselves than those ordinarily encountered in daily life or during the performance of routine physical or psychological examinations or tests" (DHHS 46.102[i]). Research involving venipunctures and most psychological assessments routinely fit under this category . As illustrated in Cases 2 and 3, in minimal risk research, one can minimize risk even further by piggybacking research procedures onto regularly scheduled medical procedures or by selecting the minimum levels of experimental manipulation necessary.

Research Involving Greater Than Minimal Risk, But Presenting the Prospect of Direct Benefit to an Individual Subject. When research involves greater than minimal risk, investigators must justify probable risks and associated discomforts in terms of the expected benefits to the child or to society as a whole. For example, in research involving greater than minimal risk (side effects of an experimental drug or lumbar puncture; see Kruesi et al., 1988), DHHS 46.405 requires that the investigator demonstrate that any risks are justified by the anticipated direct benefits to the participants, that the relation of these benefits to the risk is at least as favorable to the participants as that presented by available alternative approaches, and that adequate provisions are made for soliciting both guardian consent and the child's assent. Case 4 illustrates how an investigator can assess the risk–benefit ratio and minimize harm in a study testing the effects of a new medication for a childhood disorder.

Research Involving Greater Than Minimal Risk With No Prospect of Direct Benefit to Individual Subjects, But Likely to Yield Generalizable Knowledge About the Subject's Disorder or Condition. When research involving greater than minimal risk holds out no prospect of direct benefit to the child participants, an acceptable balance of risk to benefits must include the likelihood that the research will yield generalizable knowledge that is of vital importance for the understanding or amelioration of the subject's disorder or condition. In addition, the increased risk must represent only a minor increment over minimal risk and the research experiences must be reasonably commensurate with those inherent in situations the child would be expected to experience. Finally, adequate provisions must be made for soliciting both guardian consent and child assent (DHHS 46.406). Case 5 provides an example of how such risk–benefit judgments are made and the additional procedures used to further reduce the possibility of risk.

Research Not Otherwise Approvable. Under exceptional circumstances, when research may provide an understanding, prevention, or alleviation of a serious problem affecting the health or welfare of children, the secretary of DHHS may approve research not otherwise considered acceptable under the above regulations.

JUSTICE AND RESEARCH RISKS

Estimations of the balance of risks and benefits must also include a consideration of the special life circumstances of potential research participants. When planning to recruit impoverished, disenfranchised, or institutionalized children and adolescents, investigators must consider whether the selection of participants is equitable (Federal Regulation 46.111[3]). At issue is whether it is fair to add to these children's lives the additional burden of research participation (Veatch, 1987). The principle of justice, the equitable distribution of research risks and benefits, requires that especially vulnerable classes of children not be involved as research subjects merely because they present a sample of convenience. For example, from this moral perspective a study of physiological correlates of anxiety, targeting indigent or institutionalized children rather than members of the general population, would be considered an unfair distribution of burden on those whose lives are already burdened with substantial problems. On the other hand, recruiting institutionalized children for research designed to study the consequences of the debilitating illness responsible for their institutionalization might be considered morally just if it held out the possibility of directly improving the participant's condition or providing important knowledge that might help members of the participant's class (see Case 6).

CASE 1: COGNITIVE CORRELATES
OF DEPRESSION IN HOSPITALIZED
ADOLESCENT PATIENTS

Research Goals

The experimenters were conducting research on the assessment of cognitive and coping factors related to depression in inpatient adolescents. One purpose of the study was to validate a new diagnostic interview against routine standardized hospital evaluations of depression. The research personnel were also clinical staff members.

Reevaluating the Scientific Validity of Research
Under Changing Hospital Conditions

An ethical dilemma emerged when hospital regulations shifted from allowing children to be hospitalized for 60 days to a maximum of only 14 days. Under the former regulations, a clinical team meeting to formerly diagnose the child's condition and identify his or her treatment needs was conducted 3 weeks following admission. This had allowed the research team 3 weeks in which to assess independently the child's behavior before sharing information with the clinical team. Thus, the 60-day hospitalization and delayed team meeting had enabled conclusions to be drawn from the experimental interview to be independent of other clinical data on the patient and conducted in a way that did not interfere with the patients' diagnostic and treatment schedules.

With the new regulations, a formal diagnosis had to be developed and a team meeting held a few days following admission. The investigators were also part of the treatment team; thus the shortened regulations made it difficult to separate their research activities from their clinical activities. The investigators also believed that performing routine hospital evaluations and the experimental assessment procedures within a 3-day period would place an undue burden on the patients. As a consequence, they concluded that they could not protect patient welfare and scientific integrity simultaneously under the new regulations. They decided to modify the study (with IRB approval) to compare the clinical interview against information (e.g., biological markers) not needed for treatment decisions.

CASE 2: PHYSIOLOGICAL INDICATORS OF DEPRESSION AND ANXIETY IN DIABETIC CHILDREN

Research Design

The purpose of this study was to measure biological indicators of depression and anxiety in diabetic children (6–11 years of age). Children were admitted into the hospital for a 5-day program to teach patients and their families how to regulate their medication and diet. As part of the medical regimen, blood tests to monitor sugar and insulin levels were routinely administered on an average of four times a day. The researchers needed to measure platelet serotonin and cortisol levels three times a day for 2 days at regular intervals to obtain information on physiological indicators of depression and anxiety, respectively.

Evaluating Research Risks and Benefits

Venipuncture is considered a safe procedure that produces only minimum discomfort. In addition, drawing blood is a standard part of the diabetic child's experience while in the hospital and injections are a routine event in the diabetic child's life. The researchers believed that any additional blood tests required for this study did not pose a risk of harm or discomfort greater in and of themselves than those ordinarily encountered in the children's daily life and during the performance of routine physical examinations. Moreover, the assessment of biological correlates of anxiety and depression in diabetic children has the potential for significant benefits for enhancing knowledge about psychological sequelae of diabetes because these physiological factors may interact with variations in insulin levels. The investigators and their IRB thus concluded that the research presented a favorable balance of probable research benefits to probable research risks.

Minimizing Research Risks

Measurements of platelet serotonin and cortisol levels could be derived from samples drawn during the child's routine blood tests to monitor sugar and insulin. However, because the timing of these routine venipunctures was based on children's behaviors, self-reports, and diet, blood was not drawn at the same time each day. Such inconsistency in the timing of the venipunctures would jeopardize important scientific controls. As a consequence, to ensure regularity over the course of 2 days the researchers might have to administer additional blood tests.

The research team decided to use the routine blood samples whenever possible. They also decided to schedule the testing intervals at times that medical venipunctures would most likely be conducted (e.g., just before or after meals) and at times that did not interfere with the child's educational activities. Parental consent and child assent forms explained that additional venipunctures might be required if the child participated in the study. (See Case 33 for a discussion of confidentiality issues raised by this research.)

CASE 3: ASSESSING BRAIN METABOLISM IN SCHIZOPHRENIC ADOLESCENTS AND NORMAL CONTROLS USING RADIOACTIVE GLUCOSE

Research Goals

The purpose of this research was to study biochemical brain functions related to schizophrenia. Specifically, brain metabolism would be studied using Positron Emission Tomography (PET), a procedure that required the use of radioactive glucose. The hypothesis to be tested was that low metabolism rates are associated with a biological predisposition to schizophrenia.

Evaluating the Adequacy of Alternative Methodologies

Federal guidelines allow minor research participants to be exposed to radioactive tracers if the radiation is one tenth that of the radioactivity level allowed for adult participants. At these adult levels, there is no known or documented risk of physical harm for humans. The first ethical challenge for the investigators was to determine whether the benefits of using the PET methodology were sufficient to outweigh the possibility of any unknown risks. The research team first examined whether alternative nonradioactive methods could yield empirical evidence on neurochemical functions. For example, the advantages and disadvantages of using magnetic resonance imaging (MRI) data were explored. Although the MRI could provide information on the size and shape of brain structures (and possibly patterns of blood flow) it could not provide information on chemical processes.

The research team also considered whether information on brain processes underlying schizophrenia could be adequately determined using only adult subjects. Previous theoretical and empirical work suggested that some neurochemical processes in adult schizophrenics might be affected by years of pharmacological treatments and/or institutionalization. In addition, some brain functions in schizophrenics that were indistinguishable from normals in adult samples, might have arisen from different and distinguishable developmental trajectories in childhood and adolescence. Thus, studying adult schizophrenics would not necessarily reveal information about the biochemical processes underlying childhood schizophrenia.

Identifying Potential Benefits and Minimizing Risk

Once the investigators decided that the PET procedure had critical advantages over alternative methodologies, they went about further identifying the potential benefits of the study and determining how to minimize the risk. They accomplished this by conducting several studies with adults to further demonstrate that there was empirical reason to study brain metabolism in adolescent schizophrenics; and that the study could be accomplished at very low levels of radioactivity. This first phase of the research did indicate lower metabolism levels in schizophrenic as compared to normal adult controls and demonstrated that metabolism could be studied at levels lower than the recommended federal guidelines for radioactive research with minors.

Assessing the Risk–Benefit Balance

After concluding that alternative methods could not provide sufficient information on brain chemistry potentially underlying schizophrenia, providing further empirical support for the scientific value of the research, and empirically determining the minimal level of radiation that could be used, the investigative team turned to weighing the risk–benefit balance of the study. In evaluating this balance they considered the devastating effects of schizophrenia on affected individuals and their families and the potentially negative side effects of current pharmacological treatments. This led the investigators to conclude that although the experimental procedure did not hold out direct benefits to participants it was likely to yield generalizable knowledge about the schizophrenic subject's disorder and provide normal participants with an opportunity to contribute to an understanding of a serious problem affecting the mental health of children.

The investigators provided their IRB with their data on adult schizophrenics and normal controls, a summary of the extant literature on the absence of known risk associated with the low levels of radiation to be used in the study, literature pointing to the scientific value of the hypothesis, and a copy of the proposed informed consent procedures for fully detailing the radiation levels and possibility of unknown risk to participants and families. The IRB agreed that the minimal and unknown risk factors of low-level radiation research were outweighed by the potential benefits for understanding childhood schizophrenia.

CASE 4: PHARMACOLOGICAL TREATMENT OF HYPERACTIVE CHILDREN WITH MENTAL RETARDATION

Research Goals

The purpose of this study was to assess the behavioral, cognitive, and physiological side effects of fenfluramine (Pondimin) as an alternative to methylphenidate (Ritalin) in hyperactive children (5–13 years) with mental retardation. Five drug conditions were to be compared: a placebo, three different doses of fenfluramine, and one dose of methylphenidate. Each drug condition was to be given for 2 weeks with order determined by a complex Latin square assignment. All parties having contact with the children, including their parents, teachers, and study personnel, were blind to the medication sequence. Prior to starting the protocol, each child would also take a known placebo for 1 week (see

Cases 40 and 56 for discussions on managing side effects and debriefing parents, respectively).

Evaluating Research Risks and Benefits: The Neurotoxicity Issue

Fenfluramine is controversial in some circles because of animal studies that suggest that doses given over a brief period can cause long-lasting depletion to serotonin content in certain midbrain structures. Some animal researchers argue that this suggests that the drug could have an irreversible effect on serotonin function in human beings.

When the investigators were designing their study they drew this issue to the attention of the university IRB and provided copies of much of the relevant research suggesting fenfluramine may have neurotoxic effects in certain laboratory animals. They also provided the following reasons, grounded in logic and the research literature, why they thought that fenfluramine would not pose unacceptable risks in human beings:

1. Doses have typically been much higher in animal studies than are used in people.
2. There appear to be marked interspecies differences in physiological response to fenfluramine.
3. Not all researchers have been able to replicate the phenomenon in animals.
4. To the investigators knowledge, no one has shown functional losses to be associated with these changes.
5. No one has been able to show long-lasting serotonergic changes or functional changes in human beings treated with the drug (although it may not be possible with current technologies to thoroughly examine serotonergic status in people taking fenfluramine).
6. Most importantly, the drug has been used with adults for at least two decades without reports of adverse consequences related to CNS functioning.

The IRB in accepting these arguments agreed with the investigators that the potential benefits of determining whether fenfluramine could help hyperactive children who respond poorly to Ritalin outweighed the probability that the drug would cause participant harm. To further protect the children from potential risks, parents were fully informed about the fenfluramine controversy. Parent informed consent indicated that animal research exists suggesting that fenfluramine may cause permanent changes to serotonergic structures and that there is some

unknown risk that the drug could cause permanent neurological damage in the children taking part in the study (see Case 21 for a description
of the informed consent procedures).

CASE 5: AN ANALYSIS OF CEREBRAL
FLUID DOPAMINE METABOLITES
IN CHILDREN WITH ADHD

Research Goals

The purpose of this research was to evaluate whether different levels of
dopamine production are associated with individual variation in the
symptomology of 6- to 12-year-old children with attention deficit hyperactivity disorder (ADHD). A test of this hypothesis required analysis
of dopamine metabolites acquired through extraction of cerebral spinal
fluid. The spinal fluid is extracted through a needle inserted into the
spinal cord.

Evaluating Research Risks and Benefits

The use of the spinal tap procedure involves a minor increase over
minimal risk to children because studies have indicated that 20% to 25%
of research participants may experience headaches for several hours (up
to 1 week) and/or experience some soreness at the site of needle
insertion (Kruesi et al., 1988). The ethical decision regarding whether to
use this procedure rests on the extent to which the potential benefits of
research outweigh these risks. Although ADHD affects at least 3% of
children, biological markers of this disorder have yet to be discovered.
Furthermore, the neurochemical reactions underlying the effect of
standard pharmacological treatments for ADHD (e.g., Ritalin) have not
been determined. Moreover, not all children successfully respond to
these treatments. Therefore, although participants would not directly
benefit from this research, the investigators believed that the study of
biological correlates of ADHD provided an important opportunity to
understand the nature of the child's disorder.

Considering the Use of Normal Controls.   As in any experimental
investigation, comparing data from a clinical sample and a sample of
normal controls strengthens conclusions drawn about the biological
correlates of a psychological disorder. However, the investigators concluded that, at this point in time, the research benefits did not outweigh
the risks for normal children because the study would not lead to
increased understanding of neurochemical correlates of normal func-

tioning and the vast majority of nonaffected children are not at risk for developing ADHD.

Minimizing Research Risks

Having determined that the balance of risks and benefits favored conducting the study, the investigators turned their attention to optimally minimizing the risks of the spinal tap procedure. The investigators wanted to reduce the child's anxiety about the spinal tap and the possibility of a spinal headache.

Minimizing Anxiety. The investigators used role playing to reduce potential anxiety about the procedure. On the day before the spinal tap, children attended a "practice" session in which all facets of the procedure (except for the needle) were rehearsed. The child practiced the positions he or she would take in the bed, staff enacted their roles, and the child was familiarized with the equipment used for the spinal tap and the sounds that would be associated with the procedures. Most importantly for hyperactive children who find it difficult to remain inactive, was a practice period in which they were taught how to lie on their sides in a still position for 5 minutes. In addition to the practice session, potential participants were also encouraged to speak with children who had undergone the procedure.

To allay children's anxiety during the procedure, parents were invited to stay with the child. In addition, at each new step in the procedure, children were asked if they were uncomfortable and constantly reminded that they could stop the procedure at any time. The investigators believed that it was most important that the child be given a sense of control over the procedure and would leave with a sense of trust that his or wishes had been respected.

Minimizing Physical Discomfort. Several steps were taken to minimize the possibility of physical discomfort. First, the investigators added a second local anesthetic to the traditional procedure of injecting the lumbar area with Lidocaine—a fluid that can sometimes cause a burning sensation. A numbing cream (approved by the FDA for use with infants) was applied 1 hour before the local anesthetic was to be injected. In addition, the Lidocaine was injected very slowly so that the child could signal if there was any discomfort. If the child did indicate discomfort, the investigator waited for the site to further numb before any more Lidocaine was released.

The second concern following the spinal tap was to minimize the possibility that children would get a spinal headache. Research on adults suggested that lying flat in bed could prevent such headaches.

Accordingly, the researchers made great efforts to ensure that the children did not lift their heads from the pillow for 3 hours—while allowing the children to move other parts of their bodies. These precautions proved to be very successful. To date, none of the children have experienced spinal headaches, they describe their experiences positively to other children, and some participants have volunteered for a second spinal tap.

CASE 6: NEUROLOGICAL CORRELATES OF AIDS IN INFECTED INSTITUTIONALIZED CHILDREN

Research Goals

The purpose of this study was to examine the neurological correlates of AIDS in infected children whose mothers had transmitted the HIV virus during pregnancy. The children (8–12 years of age) were in a state hospital being treated for the last stages of AIDS. The mothers of most of the children were deceased and many were wards of the state. The research procedures included neuropsychological testing and MRI.

Evaluating Research Risks and Benefits

The procedures presented no more than minimal risk and held out no direct benefits for the terminally ill child participants. The investigators believed that the research was likely to yield generalizable knowledge about the child participants' disorder that could be applied to the diagnosis and treatment of other children with AIDS contracted through maternal transmission. They concluded that the benefits of research outweighed the minimal risk to the participants (see Case 29 for a discussion of informed assent for this population).

Applying Principles of Justice to the Risk–Benefit Evaluation

Demonstrating significant research benefits was not sufficient to determine whether this study should be conducted. Because these children, as poor and institutionalized wards of the state, were especially vulnerable, the question of justice in subject selection had to be addressed. Was the selection of these children as subjects equitable in terms of the

distribution of research risks and benefits? To evaluate equitable distribution of research burdens to institutionalized patients, one must demonstrate either that noninstitutionalized children will also be the focus
of study or that the research has special applicability to the child's
institutionalized status. In this regard, the investigators noted that the
majority of HIV infections currently found in children are contracted
either through maternal transmission or blood transfusions. In the latter
cases, the children usually suffer from hemophilia and therefore possess
a physiology and medical history significantly different from children
who contracted HIV during pregnancy. In addition, many children
infected through maternal transmission are likely to become wards of
the state because their infected mothers may have died, become severely
ill, or indigent. On this basis, the research risks to these institutionalized
children were not considered an unfair burden, because the research
would directly address the special circumstances of this population.

* * *

Casebook

Withholding Treatment: The Use of Control Groups, Placebos, and Randomized Clinical Trials

In some forms of research, the investigator's responsibility to conduct a scientifically valid study in itself creates participant risks. This is especially true in research on treatment efficacy where the necessity for experimental control in the form of placebos, control groups, and randomized assignment often intentionally denies treatment to children and youth with identified mental disorders. In many instances where no effective treatments have been established, the use of such techniques may pose few risks and hold out the potential of direct benefit to both experimental and control participants (because those who do not receive the experimental treatment during the research should be routinely offered the treatment if it is found to be effective).

NO-TREATMENT AND ALTERNATIVE TREATMENT CONTROL GROUPS

Ethical concerns are raised about the use of a no-treatment control group in situations where there is a persuasive literature that certain basic services are at least minimally effective. In addition, it is not ethically responsible to assign minor participants to an alternative treatment control condition that has been shown to produce poor developmental outcomes when the effectiveness of one of the experimental conditions is well documented. This holds in situations where the experimental therapy is known to be superior to a comparison therapy as well as situations where a third treatment is known to be superior to either or both treatments being compared in a study (OPRR, 1993). In such

156

situations, while providing control groups with standard treatment can jeopardize conclusions that the treatment per se is significantly better than no treatment at all, comparing the new intervention to an established therapeutic regimen may be the more honest intellectual question, especially in times of limited economic resources (Fisher, 1991, 1993). Case 7 describes a situation where use of a *positive (or standard) treatment control* condition provides sufficient experimental control and participant protection. In other circumstances, a standard treatment may not have strong empirical support, but the risk to patients of no treatment (e.g., in the case of suicide risk) may require a treatment-as-usual control (see Case 8).

Placebos. In the absence of strong empirical support for the effectiveness of a clinically established treatment, the scientific validity, and thus benefits of the research, may require the use of a placebo control (see Case 9). Placebos, for example, may be used in drug studies when there is no known or available alternative medications that can be tolerated by the subjects or when available treatments have known serious side effects (Levine, 1986; OPRR 1993). Under other circumstances there may be ethical justification for including a *placebo washout* period in which any drugs taken prior to the experimental intervention are terminated to eliminate any contaminating effects. The placebo washout condition, although providing necessary experimental controls, can also have beneficial effects, because it can identify children who are "placebo responders" and who therefore may not be in need of drug therapy.

A third context under which the use of placebos is ethically justified is when empirically validated treatments are not effective for all children or youth diagnosed with the same disorder. Under these circumstances, investigators may choose to use a cross-over design in which an individual child's response to the new treatment, the established treatment, and a placebo condition are compared. This method can often provide a more accurate assessment of the utility of the new treatment for different children (see Case 4 for a discussion on how to minimize harm in a cross-over study).

Wait-List Control Groups. The use of wait-list control groups has received a great deal of ethical attention, especially in situations where participants may be deprived of standard services that might be immediately available to them. Under these conditions, the *only* ethical approach may be to limit this type of research to situations in which services are unavailable outside the research context (see Case 10). At the same time, evaluating the efficacy of an intervention against the natural course of a disorder may be an important source of information, especially in situations in which an adverse condition may attenuate without intervention. Under these circumstances both wait-list and treatment participants can be offered emergency assistance if needed, and requests for such assistance included as a variable in the statistical analysis (see Case 11).

WITHHOLDING OF COLLATERAL TREATMENTS

When testing the effects of a new treatment, investigators typically require that patients stop all collateral treatments to ensure the internal validity of the study. However, such procedures may simultaneously interfere with the clinical validity of an intervention and jeopardize participant welfare. For example, the generalizability of research to practice may be seriously limited, if the experiment fails to study the efficacy of the treatment within the context of routine collateral treatments. This is especially true in the treatment of patients with dual diagnoses. Under these conditions, a more ethically defensible study might include a phase that examines the efficacy of the treatment within the context of other biomedical or psychosocial interventions (see Case 10).

RANDOM ASSIGNMENT

Once an investigator has determined that the risk–benefit balance justifies the use of either a placebo or control condition, the participant and his or her guardian are informed that if they agree to participate, they will be randomly assigned to either a control or treatment condition. Random assignment enhances scientific validity by minimizing the possibility of bias in the selection of experimental and control subjects. When a child or family declines to participate because of a preference for one arm of clinical trials research, the generalizability of the research to other such families is jeopardized (Fisher, 1991; Veatch, 1987). For example, if an investigator is comparing the efficacy of family therapy to individualized child therapy, those families who refuse random assignment because they prefer the family intervention condition may be just those individuals who would benefit most from this therapy. Offering random assignment under conditions in which no effective treatment is available may also be potentially coercive to parents who are desperate to help their children (Carroll, Schneider, & Wesley, 1985; Fisher & Tryon, 1990; Veatch, 1987).

Veatch (1987) developed a unique approach to address these concerns. In the semi-randomized clinical trial, participants are assigned to one of four conditions: two randomized groups for participants who have agreed to be randomly assigned to the treatment or control group and two nonrandomized groups for participants who have a preference for one arm of the research. As Case 12 illustrates, this approach (when feasible) can decrease the possibility of participant coercion and increase the population generalizability of intervention research.

CASE 7: ASSESSING THE EFFICACY OF A PSYCHOEDUCATIONAL INTERVENTION FOR PARENTS OF CHILDREN WITH SED

Research Goals

The purpose of this research was to develop and assess a multiple group psychoeducational intervention for parents of children with serious emotional disturbance (SED). The principal investigator (PI) was the director of an agency serving as primary provider of social and mental health services to children with SED and families in the area. The psychoeducational intervention would consist of 15 sessions followed by a 6-month follow-up period.

Designing a Positive-Control Randomized Study

The PI was aware that by the time children with SED and their families enter the mental health service system any delay in treatment access might result in more negative consequences for the child and his or her family. The PI held meetings with parents and other mental health professionals to discuss the risks and benefits of a wait-list control group. Based on this input, the PI decided that because there were no other agencies serving SED children in the area, families would be unduly burdened by assignment to a wait-list control. Thus, a positive-control randomized design was implemented. All families were enrolled into an intensive case management program designed specifically for this study. The experimental group received an additional multiple family group psychoeducational intervention program. By using two treatment groups, the children with SED and their families received services immediately regardless of the random assignment. In addition, the use of a case management control group added to the clinical validity of the study, since the value of the experimental intervention could be weighed against standard nontherapeutic services.

CASE 8: ASSESSING THE EFFICACY
OF A PROBLEM-SOLVING INTERVENTION
TARGETING SUICIDAL ADOLESCENTS
AND YOUNG ADULTS

Research Goals

This study evaluated the effectiveness of a time-limited, outpatient problem-solving intervention targeting suicidal adolescents and young adults. Participants were randomly assigned to either the experimental treatment or the control condition. Patients engaged in the experimental treatment attended 14 days of intensive group meetings at the treatment facility. The treatment was structured on a problem-solving and social competence paradigm. A comprehensive intake assessment and bian-nual follow-up was conducted over a 2-year period. It was predicted that both groups would improve over time, but that those in the experimental group would gain significantly better problem-solving skills immediately after the intervention and during the follow-up period, whereas controls would evidence degradation of any initial problem-solving gains (see Case 45 for discussion of responses to staff requests for specific patient assignments).

Designing a Treatment-as-Usual Control Condition

Given the clinical and ethical concerns apparent when working with high-risk suicidal patients, randomization to a no-treatment control was neither appropriate nor possible. The investigators decided to provide control patients with treatment-as-usual that included a combination of short-or long-term hospitalization employing milieu therapy and indi-vidual or group outpatient care. The experimental approach differed from standard care in that it was an intensive, time-limited outpatient intervention that required participants to remain in the very circum-stances that precipitated the initial suicidal crisis.

Protecting the Welfare of Experimental Subjects
Waiting for Treatment

Because the treatment groups required a minimum number of eight patients, some patients assigned to the experimental group would have to wait for the critical mass for a new rotation. To protect the welfare of these patients, they were enrolled in a weekly monitoring group: an unstructured weekly support group with a problem-solving focus.

CASE 9: THE EFFECT OF LITHIUM
ON AGGRESSIVE BEHAVIORS IN
ADOLESCENTS WITH MENTAL RETARDATION

Research Goals

The investigators wanted to conduct a 4-month investigation of the effect of lithium in the treatment of aggressive adolescents with mental retardation. Although the effect of lithium on aggressive behaviors has long been recognized in the nonhandicapped population, quality research addressing this question for persons who have mental retardation was lacking. All subjects lived in a residential treatment center for persons with mental retardation. The study was to be a parallel group study with one group on lithium and the other on a placebo.

Placebo Trials in Research on Clinically Established, But Scientifically Untested, Treatments

Despite the absence of strong empirical support, many of the staff at the hospital had adopted lithium as one of their tools for treating the aggressive and self-injurious behavior of persons with mental retardation. As a result, the staff believed that using a placebo control would in fact be depriving the patients of an established treatment. The investigators believed that although the "logical" extension of research on other populations is quite common in the field of mental retardation, it cannot substitute for direct validational research. They therefore decided to use a non-lithium control group in the study. Although this decision was supported by their IRB, they had difficulty with individual staff members during patient recruitment and during drug trials. To address this difficulty, the investigators met weekly with staff to discuss procedures for monitoring children's reactions to experimental conditions as well as potential risk factors that would indicate a child should be excluded from the study. (See the section on modifying procedures for further discussion of managing risk in clinical trials research. Also note that 45 CFR 46 contains regulations on special protections required for wards of the state.)

Withholding Collateral Treatments During Clinical Trials

A second dilemma that arose was that in order to study the efficacy of lithium alone, it was necessary to withdraw individuals from all other psychotropic medications. For example, a child who was being treated with Serentil was withdrawn from it and then treated with either lithium or placebo. As might be expected, this created some behavioral difficulties that exposed subjects, peers, and staff to increased risk due to assaultive behavior. Although withdrawing the subjects from all other medications would allow the researchers to assess the validity of lithium alone in the treatment of aggression and self-injurious behavior, they were concerned that these results would have little generalizability to actual treatment. For example, in clinical practice lithium is typically used in consort with other medications (usually a tranquilizer). To study lithium in isolation was to study something other than the typical treatment practice. The investigators weighed the risks to subjects and staff against the scientific validity and value of a medication-free lithium trial and decided that a more clinically defensible study would be a two-phase design. During the first phase, the efficacy of lithium was tested alone. During the second phase, the effect of lithium was studied against a background of other medications. This two-phased design received greater support from the hospital staff.

CASE 10: THE IMPACT OF A HOME-BASED INTERVENTION FOR PARENTS WITH CHRONIC MENTAL ILLNESS ON CHILD OUT-OF-HOME PLACEMENT

Research Goals

The director of a family support service wanted to conduct an outcome evaluation on a short-term, home-based intervention for families in which children are at high risk for out-of-home placement because of parental chronic mental illness. The investigator wanted to compare the parenting skills of parents enrolled in this program to those of parents whose children were placed out of the home.

Staff Resistance to an Out-of-Home Placement Control Group

The director faced a dilemma involving the ability to utilize a scientifically rigorous research design. Despite the absence of empirical evidence, the mental health providers affiliated with the service believed that home-based programs developed to maintain children with their families are successful. In addition, because there are few alternative resources available to these families, there was deep reluctance on the part of social service agency staff to deny home-based service to eligible children in order to develop a randomized trial. As a result, in the past, evaluations of these programs relied largely on data gathered without matched controls.

Utilizing Overflow Referrals as a Control Condition

As both a reseacher and head of a family support service, the PI recognized the need to evaluate the efficacy of the agency's work and to better understand both the intended and unintended effects of the agency's home-based interventions. As a result, the PI chose to create a comparison group by maintaining a record of overflow referrals to the service. These were cases that would meet all the criteria for service, but that could not be accepted because there were no family support treatment teams available at the time of the referral. The agency was not able to maintain a wait list; thus these families typically did not receive services. Because all referrals for this intensive family preservation program came from a single source, the state child protection agency, placement data were available for long-term follow-up. This allowed the research team to assess differences in utilization of primary care resources and differences in frequency and severity of additional abuse or neglect for children within the treatment group as compared to children in the group for which family-based services were not available.

CASE 11: ASSESSMENT OF AN OUTPATIENT COGNITIVE BEHAVIORAL TREATMENT FOR DEPRESSED ADOLESCENTS

Research Goals

The purpose of this research was to assess the efficacy of cognitive behavioral treatment for moderately depressed adolescents receiving outpatient treatment. Previously nonreferred adolescents were recruited from the community. The intervention was to last 12 weeks and would be evaluated by comparing the mental health status of participants to those in a wait-list control group.

Protecting the Welfare of Adolescents in a Wait-List Control Group: A Treatment on Demand Design

The investigators were concerned that even though the study focused on adolescents with moderate levels of depression, some members of the wait-list control group might be at risk for suicide. They decided to use a treatment-on-demand strategy. During recruitment, patients were informed that if they participated in the study they would be randomly assigned to a treatment or wait-list control group that would last 12 weeks. Those who did not wish to be randomly assigned were excluded from the study and offered standard outpatient treatment.

Individuals who were assigned to either the wait-list or treatment groups were told they could call their research team whenever they felt they were in crisis. If, following the call, the research staff or patient felt the crisis had not abated, a meeting would be set up to formally assess the adolescent. If the assessment indicated a high risk of suicide, treatment (for an adolescent in the wait-list group) or additional treatment (for an adolescent in the experimental group) would be recommended and the subject would be withdrawn from study. If the assessment did not indicate suicidal risk, the subject would be asked if he or she would like to continue participating in the study. At all times, experimental and control group participants were given the opportunity to withdraw and receive standard hospital treatment.

CASE 12: COMPARING THE EFFICACY OF TWO INTERVENTION PROGRAMS FOR MOTHERS AND DRUG-EXPOSED INFANTS

Research Goals

This study was interested in investigating cognitive and affective developmental problems of infancy known to be associated with maternal drug addiction. All mothers selected to participate in the study had been drug-free for at least 2 months. Infants were between 6 and 12 months of age and had no known neurological problems. The investigation used a positive control design to compare the efficacy of a therapeutic infant day care program with the efficacy of a parent-education and job training program. Outcome measures included assessment of infant intelligence, mastery motivation, infant–mother attachment, and infant–mother interaction patterns.

The Semi-Randomized Clinical Trial

The researchers recognized that although some families might be willing to to submit to random assignment, others might only be willing to participate if they received the program they desired. This type of self-selection to treatment condition could result in the selection of biased samples. Because they had a large potential subject population, the researchers decided to use a semi-randomized clinical trial. Parents who refused random assignment were given the program they desired. The effect of the two treatments for families willing to be randomly assigned could then be compared to the effect of treatment for families who received a preferred treatment.

* * *

Identification and Recruitment of Subjects

Recruiting high-risk children or children with mental disorders, and their families for participation in research has the potential to violate participant privacy when prospective participants are identified through institutional or organizational records they believe are private. Once prospective participants have been identified, their vulnerable mental and social status also raises ethical concerns about potential coercion associated with subject recruitment procedures that offer payment to participants or ancilliary mental health services to organizations on which they are dependent for assistance. Prospective research subjects may also be harmed if recruitment procedures inadvertently reveal socially damaging information. Furthermore, the principle of justice, the fair and equitable distribution of research risks and benefits, poses special ethical challenges when research participants are recruited from poor or minority communities.

IDENTIFYING POTENTIAL PARTICIPANTS THROUGH INSTITUTIONAL RECORDS OR ORGANIZATIONAL MEMBERSHIP

In some types of research (e.g., some survey studies), prospective participants can only be identified through institutional records that may or may not be public (see Case 13). In these situations, children and their families may see direct contact by the investigator as an invasion of privacy. In other contexts, individuals may participate in public activities (e.g., Alcoholic Anonymous [AA] meetings) that they nevertheless view as ensuring some form of privacy (see Case 14). In such situations, during recruitment research staff can respect an individual's right to privacy by having the institution or organization make the initial contact. Optimally, in this first contact the institution or organization requests permission to release the individual's name or provides potential participants with a means of contacting the research investigator if he or she is interested in research participation (see Case 19). A less preferable method is to invite participation by letter and request that an individual send back a postcard only if he or she does not wish to be contacted (OPRR, 1993). The investigator then calls all persons who have not declined participation. In such cases, investigators must ensure that individuals are given ample opportunity to terminate telephone conversation at any point and that the call itself does not disclose personal information to other household members or colleagues that might prove damaging to the individual.

INCENTIVES FOR PARTICIPATION

Offering incentives for participation is often used as a means of recruiting subjects. The decision to offer inducements creates an ethical tension between fair compensation for the time and inconvenience of research participation and undue coercion to participate in procedures to which subjects might not otherwise consent (Fisher, 1993). Investigators must be particularly cautious when deciding on appropriate inducements for impoverished persons who may be willing to assume, or have their children assume, extraordinary burdens to receive payment (Levine, 1986). Subject payments should reflect the degree of risk, inconvenience, or discomfort associated with participation (OPRR, 1993). However, there is little consensus on what constitutes due and undue incentives for research participation (Macklin, 1981).

Levine (1986) suggested that investigators take a market approach to this problem, whereby research participation is viewed as a job requiring unskilled labor, and payment is determined at a level that will attract a sufficient number and diversity of participants. Investigators offering incentives must take special precautions when children and adolescents are recruited. This entails offering payments that do not unduly exceed the range of incentives the child normally experiences and, when feasible, ensuring that cash payments go directly to the minor (Fisher, 1993; SRCD, 1993; see also Case 15).

In some cases, recruitment may be facilitated when investigators provide community centers with services that might not otherwise be available. In these situations, the research team needs to ensure that both center staff and prospective participants do not see such services as contingent on participation in data collection efforts (see Case 16).

RECOGNIZING INDIVIDUAL VULNERABILITIES

In designing recruitment procedures, investigators need also consider the psychological implications of being targeted as a "subject" population (Fisher & Tryon, 1990). For example, siblings of autistic children may not see themselves as a vulnerable group prior to exposure to recruitment. Investigators can draw on empirical knowledge concerning self-concept, self-esteem, and other developmental strengths and vulnerabilities in the target population to create nonharmful recruitment procedures (see Case 17).

ENSURING FAIR REPRESENTATION
AND ACCESS TO RESEARCH BENEFITS

Investigators working with diverse populations have the responsibility to ensure that minority and lower socioeconomic populations have equal access to research benefits. They must also ensure that these populations, because of their vulnerability in the community, are not exposed to unfair distribution of research risks. This may present special challenges to investigators assessing mental health services for children and adolescents, because there may sometimes be serious questions raised as to the validity of existing measures to identify psychopathology across different populations. Such situations run the risk of under- or overdiagnosing children from minority and poor communities. Diagnostic errors can, in turn, result in minority and poor children being unfairly excluded from potentially advantageous treatment studies or unfairly overrepresented in research, such as drug studies, which may present greater than minimal risk. As illustrated in Case 18, recruitment strategies for diverse populations can be enhanced through the establishment of advisory committees made up of minority representatives from the community and the mental health professions. The accuracy of research inclusion and exclusion criteria can be additionally enhanced through the use of culture fair tests and assessments of environmental contexts.

CASE 13: PSYCHOLOGICAL AUTOPSY
BY RELATIVES OF ADOLESCENT SUICIDES

Research Goals

A national survey on adolescent suicide using follow-back procedures with surviving family members and friends was conducted. Psychological autopsy procedures require that families are contacted shortly after the suicide. Death notices are typically obtained through state health departments.

Protecting Family Privacy

To conduct a nationwide psychological autopsy study is often difficult because states differ in the accessibility of these records to the public. In considering how best to protect family privacy, the investigators recognized that their procedures might have to differ across states. Three approaches were used. Some states allowed a direct approach wherein parents of recently deceased children were sent a letter directly from the investigator with a self-addressed envelope and response form enclosed. Other states sent a letter informing the family that unless they notified the department that they did not wish to be contacted, a letter from the investigator would be sent within the next month. Other states took the responsibility of forwarding the investigator's request materials with a cover letter stating that "In order to ensure your privacy in this matter, we have asked the Department of Health to mail this letter for us. In the event that you should prefer not to participate in the interview, you will not be contacted again."

In all these procedures, only families who returned the postcard reflecting their interest were contacted. Follow-up interviews were conducted by telephone by a mental health professional who could make appropriate referrals for mental health services for those who wished them. In using this procedure, the investigators found that the majority of informants indicated that the interviews were helpful in giving them an opportunity to obtain perspective on the event. Others welcomed the opportunity to turn their tragedy into a positive contribution to suicide prevention efforts.

CASE 14: A CROSS-SECTIONAL COMPARISON OF PARENTING STYLES IN PARENTS WITH AND WITHOUT ALCOHOL USE DISORDERS

Research Goals

Developmental psychologists in a large urban city designed a cross-sectional descriptive study of parenting styles of alcoholic mothers and fathers. The purpose of the study had been greeted enthusiastically by several AA programs throughout the city and the program leaders had agreed to help with recruitment. Data to be obtained included extensive videotaped records of parent–child (2–5 years of age) interactions in a series of controlled (e.g., Strange Situation) and semi-controlled (e.g., eating lunch together, playing) situations. A matched sample of parents without identified alcohol abuse problems would also be tested.

Respecting Privacy Rights During Recruitment

The research team was aware that ethical issues regarding privacy and confidentiality (see Case 35) would be primary concerns in this study. To ensure that these issues were adequately identified and addressed they established an advisory committee of AA leaders, AA members, and practitioners specializing in substance abuse who met regularly with the researchers. The first issue discussed concerned recruitment.

Because AA meetings are devoted to preserving participant anonymity and helping alcoholics with their drinking problems, the committee members believed that in-person recruiting at an AA meeting would be intrusive and potentially counterproductive to the goals of AA. It was decided that a written brochure describing the study would be made available to all who attended. The committee members also pointed out that some members of AA would not want their spouses to know about the severity of their drinking problem. This raised discussion on how to ensure that contact with interested potential participants did not inadvertently inform others about their AA status. The committee decided that to further protect prospective participant privacy, the brochure would include a self-addressed "interest form" that gave the potential research participant several means of contacting or being contacted by the research team. For example, the interested AA member could contact the researchers by phone, attend several scheduled open meetings for potential participants at the lab, or have the research team contact him or her at home or at work by telephone or by mail. The brochure indicated that any written material or telephone calls to home or work would describe the study as one on general parenting practices.

CASE 15: ENDOCRINE SEQUELAE OF TRAUMA IN CHILD VICTIMS OF A NATURAL DISASTER

Research Goals

The purpose of this research was to study endocrine sequelae of trauma in child victims (6–12 years) of a natural disaster. Children whose families had lost their homes during a recent earthquake were the target of investigation. Families were staying in city shelters or with relatives. A short-term longitudinal design was used in which children were to be tested 2 weeks, 2 months, 6 months, and 12 months after the earthquake. At each test point, endocrine levels would be measured through blood sampling. Psychopathology and emotional status were measured through clinical interview and parent- and self-report questionnaires. The researchers planned to pay the families for each assessment period. Venipuncture was considered to be a minimal risk procedure for this population. (See Case 2 for further discussion of venipuncture.)

Offering Payments to Subjects

The investigators were concerned that a monetary inducement might be unduly coercive to families who had lost much of their personal property. On the other hand, because it is standard for participants to be paid for answering lengthy questionnaires over several testing periods, the investigators did not feel that participants should be deprived of monetary reward because of their economically vulnerable status. To guard against the potentially coercive nature of the inducement, a fair-market value for these tasks was determined. The investigators decided that the task was equivalent to activities for which one would be paid a minimum hourly wage. This meant that at each testing period children and parents would each be paid approximately $25 for the time they gave to the study. The research team also paid for transportation to and from the testing site. To further ensure that children's participation was not unduly coerced by family economic need, the children's payments were placed in individual accounts. (See also Case 24 concerning rational consent for disaster victims.)

CASE 16: DEVELOPMENT IN PUERTO RICAN AND DOMINICAN TODDLERS

Research Goals

Investigators designed a multiphase research program to study the socioemotional development of Puerto Rican and Dominican toddlers from lower income families living in a major metropolitan area. The first phase of the study would involve focus groups of Puerto Rican and Dominican mothers, fathers, and grandmothers discussing socialization goals and childrearing techniques. A content analysis of these discussions would form the basis of the second phase of research. This second phase included the construction and validation of culturally sensitive instruments to assess Puerto Rican and Dominican childrearing practices and the modification of existing Anglo-based measures of socioemotional development. These instruments would be used in the final phase of the project; a longitudinal study of the multiple determinants of psychological development in the toddler population. For this phase, the toddlers and their parents would be seen at 6-month intervals from the time they were 18 to 42 months of age.

Forming Investigator–Community Partnerships

A major concern to the research staff was how to overcome the fear and suspicion that many of the Puerto Rican and Dominican families felt toward participating in a project run by professionals from outside the community. They believed this problem could be overcome by the establishment of a long-term relationship with a community day-care center serving Hispanic families with preschool children. Trained graduate students affiliated with the research team could provide the center with psychological services (primarily developmental assessment and teacher consultation) and parents and staff would be invited to serve on a community advisory board to assist the research team in developing focus group questions to which participants would feel comfortable responding.

There was, however, the possibility that the provision of services might be unduly coercive to parents. For example, parents might feel that they and their children had to participate in data collection efforts in order for their children to benefit from the services. Furthermore, the center staff might feel obligated to urge the mothers' participation in the research to continue receiving the assistance provided by the university. The investigative staff resolved this issue by turning the assessment and teacher consultation service into a formal practicum experience for advanced graduate students. The practicum would be independent of the research project and be developed as a long-term relationship between the center and the university graduate program. Practicum students would not serve as research assistants for the project, thereby further underscoring the separation of receipt of services from participation in data collection. At each wave of testing, the voluntary nature of participation in the research project was repeatedly emphasized to the center staff and to mothers during informed consent procedures.

CASE 17: COMPARING THE EFFICACY OF FOSTER AND HOME-BASED PROGRAMS FOR CHILDREN WITH SED

Research Goals

This study compared the outcome of a therapeutic foster care program to that of an enhanced home-based intensive case management program for children with SED. The investigation used a positive controlled randomized design with multiple observations. Children with SED between 6 and 12 years of age were randomly assigned to one of the two treatment conditions. The domains of interest were provider behavior (e.g., services provided), family outcomes (e.g., family adaptability and cohesion), child outcomes (e.g., home, school and community functioning), and system outcomes (e.g., costs and service system changes). (See Case 20 for discussion of informed consent procedures. Also note special protections for wards of the state, described in 45 CFR 46.)

Recruitment for Out-of-Home Placement

From a purely research point of view, randomized assignment to conditions is desirable for maximum internal validity. However, in this project, random assignment meant that half the children would be assigned to a modality that placed them in out-of-home foster care while half would not be required to leave their home. From an ethical standpoint, the researchers wondered whether they had the right to remove children from their homes in the interests of science. The researchers decided to only recruit parents who already had referrals to existing foster placement programs. In this way, families already had the expectation that their children would be removed from home for some period of time. The research thus offered the possibility that through randomization their children might remain in the home.

CASE 18: COMPARATIVE EFFECTIVENESS OF ESTABLISHED TREATMENTS FOR CHILDREN WITH ADHD

Research Goals

The purpose of this study is to investigate the long-term comparative effectiveness of state-of-the-art medication versus state-of-the-art behavioral treatment versus the combination; and the long-term comparative effectiveness of these systematic, well-delivered treatments versus the routine care provided in the community for treatment of children with ADHD. This 2-year multimodal treatment study is being carried out at six sites throughout the United States with a common protocol in a cooperative agreement with NIMH. Children are randomly assigned to one of four arms: medication, an intense multicomponent behavioral treatment, the combination of the two modalities, or a community comparison (assessment and referral) group. The first three groups are treated for 14 months and all participants are periodically assessed for 2 years.

Ensuring Fair Representation and Access to Research Benefits for Minority Children

Previous studies had found that lower socioeconomic and minority populations tended to be underrepresented in long-term treatment studies. Because the goals of the study necessitated adequate recruitment of children from varying ethnicities, appropriate methods to do so equitably had to be developed. The steering committee that was developing the treatment protocol sought ways simultaneously to ensure a fair representation of minority children and to make the benefits of participation available to minority children. It established an Ethnicity, Culture, and Gender (ECG) Task Force that was chaired by a minority psychiatrist. This task force was charged with developing ways to communicate with minority leaders and to facilitate development of culture-fair assessment procedures. The task force arranged a number of consultations with experts on assessment of minority children and appropriate recruitment strategies. A half-day consultation was provided by a minority educator with extensive experience in dealing with minority communities and providing special services within these communities. The consultant discussed the fear among minority parents that diagnosis equals labeling, which in their experience leads to warehousing without services. She raised a number of questions about recruitment and diagnosis, which led to changes in the protocol, to prevent both over inclusion and unnecessary exclusion.

Concerns About Overdiagnosis and Overuse of Medications With Minority Children. The study includes provision of stimulants as one of the treatments, and this raised concerns among some professionals from the African-American community, who were troubled by the potential for overuse of medications with minority children. The consultant pointed out that some of the symptoms of ADHD could be mimicked by the normal reaction to a terrorizing environment. Therefore, a clinical semistructured interview was added to the protocol, in which a clinician assesses the environmental context of the child's symptoms; if the clinician thinks the child does not really have ADHD, he or she can override the diagnosis generated by the structured diagnostic interviews and rating scales.

Underrepresentation of Minorities When IQ Scores Are Used as a Cut-Off Criterion. The consultant also pointed out that the exclusion of children with an IQ below 80 might unfairly exclude some minority children whose actual learning potential is considerably better, but whose formal test scores are depressed by cultural disadvantage. This posed a problem because it was necessary to find a way to ensure that the children accepted in the study had sufficient verbal skill to participate meaningfully in the behavioral and cognitive-behavioral treatments. Several solutions were considered. One was to add a correction score to the IQ based on a normative study of cultural factors that spuriously affect test scores. However, field testing of this system disclosed inconsistent results and the suspicion that the norms were outdated. The solution eventually adopted was to give a culture-fair normed adaptive behavior interview to the parent of any child who did not score 80 or more on one of the WISC scales. If the child scored 80 or more on this supplementary test, he or she qualified. This allowed culture-fair inclusion while still ensuring ability to participate in treatment.

Participation of Parents Who Do Not Speak English. A related issue concerned the problem of parents who do not speak English well enough to participate in assessments and treatments. Initially, in the wish not to exclude this segment of the population, there was consideration of providing interpreters. The problems inherent in translation (e.g., potential invalidation of the norms for assessment instruments) precluded this option. In addition, the problems of conducting therapy in another language appeared insurmountable, especially because much of it would be in a group format for parent training. A further complication was how many additional languages should be considered: Although Spanish was the most obvious and common, one of the participating centers was in Quebec, where French is the norm. It was obvious that this issue had the potential of magnifying site differences in implementation. The ECG task force recommended the following solution. Because attempted translations would delay the initiation of the study and because of other problems previously noted, it did not seem feasible to include non-English speaking families in the main study. Instead, the sites with a significant non-English speaking population would join in submitting a supplementary grant application using the same protocol with appropriate translations and cultural adjustments so that the data would be comparable, but not confound or complicate the execution of this already complex study.

* * *

Casebook

Informed Consent Procedures

As noted previously, ethical codes for research with human subjects allow experimental risk under conditions in which the potential benefits to the participant or to members of society outweigh those risks. The acceptance of the balance of risks and benefits as a primary means of ethical justification implies that beneficence, the moral obligation to protect the welfare of research participants, does not take priority over other moral values in ethical decision making for human experimentation. According to Veatch (1987), current ethical codes have subordinated beneficence to the principle of autonomy: the right to self-determination. As a consequence, informed consent becomes the primary means of ensuring that participants are not victims of an imbalance tilting toward greater risks than benefits (Freedman, 1975).

ADDITIONAL PROTECTIONS FOR CHILDREN AND YOUTH INVOLVED AS SUBJECTS IN RESEARCH

Consent procedures for children and adolescents require special consideration for several reasons. Minors do not have the legal capacity to consent and, depending on the age of the child and the complexity of the research context, may lack the cognitive capacity to comprehend the purpose and nature of research (Fisher, 1993; Fisher & Tryon, 1990; Melton, Koocher, & Saks, 1983; Thompson, 1990). Children may also lack the power or skills to refuse participation (Fisher & Rosendahl, 1990; Keith-Spiegel, 1983; Koocher & Keith-Spiegel, 1990; Levine, 1986).

Guardian Consent. To ensure that the rights of minors are protected, federal regulations require that adequate provisions are made for soliciting consent of parents, legal guardians, or those who act *in loco parentis* before a child can participate in research. According to Federal Regulation 46.408[b], the permission of one parent is sufficient for minimal risk research or research involving greater than minimal risk but presenting the prospect of direct benefit to the individual subject. Permission of both parents, where feasible, must be sought for research involving greater than minimal risk with no prospect of direct benefit and for research not otherwise approvable. As illustrated in Case 19, determining guardianship can sometimes present ethical challenges for investigators.

Child Assent. The rights of minors are further protected through the requirement that provisions are made for soliciting the assent of the child, when he or she is capable (Federal Regulation 46.408[a]). Although the assent of a child is not a necessary condition for proceeding with the research, the objection of a child of any age is binding unless the research holds out the prospect of direct benefit that is important to the child and only achievable through the experimental procedures. In designing assent procedures investigators need to take into account the child's maturity, his or her unique strengths and vulnerabilities, and the context in which decision making will take place (see Case 20). Discussion of assent procedures in the absence of parental consent is provided in a later section in this casebook.

THE INFORMED, RATIONAL, AND VOLUNTARY REQUIREMENTS OF CONSENT

Informed consent procedures, as currently required by federal regulations and professional ethical codes, are designed to protect participant autonomy by ensuring that the decision to participate is informed, rational, and voluntary. This includes a clear and comprehensive statement about potential research risks and benefits (see Case 21).

The Informed Requirement of Consent. The informed aspect of consent refers to the investigator's obligation to fully disclose information about all procedures that might influence an individual's willingness to participate in a study. According to Federal Policy 46.116 such information must include:

- A statement that the study involves research, explanation of the purpose and duration of the research, and a description of the procedures.
- A description of any foreseeable risks or discomforts.
- A description of potential benefits to the participant or others.

- Disclosure of alternative procedures or treatments that may be advantageous to the subject.
- A description of the extent and limits of confidentiality.
- For research involving more than minimal risk, information regarding compensation and availability and nature of treatment if injury occurs.
- A statement describing the voluntary nature of the research, the right to refuse participation or withdraw participation at any time without penalty.

A further requirement of informed consent is that the information must be presented in a manner that is appropriate to the language usage and level of comprehension of the participant and/or his or her guardian (OPRR, 1993). In most cases, federal guidelines require that informed consent be documented. However, under certain circumstances this requirement may be waived (Federal Regulation 46.117[c][1]). Case 22, describing informed consent procedures in a war zone, illustrates such a circumstance. It should also be noted that the Office for Protection from Research Risks (OPRR) considers research in sensitive areas such as child abuse, illegal activities, or reportable communicable diseases as posing potential risks to subjects. Consequently, as illustrated in Case 23 where the need to report such information to authorities is legally mandated, subjects should be so informed before agreeing to participate in the study (OPRR, 1993).

The Rational Nature of Consent. The rational requirement of consent reflects recognition that the very condition of risk or mental disorder that identifies the child as a potential participant may compromise adequate comprehension of research risks and benefits (Fisher, 1993). For example, investigators conducting a study on the development of children of parents with chronic mental disorders need to take into account the impact of parental symptoms on the parent's capacity to understand the nature of the study and respond in the child's best interest. Alternatively, parents of a child with a mental disorder for which there has been no effective treatment may misinterpret a descriptive study as a means of attaining professional assistance or may mistake statements regarding potential benefits of participation for presumed benefits (Carroll et al., 1985; Fisher, 1991, 1993; Fisher & Rosendahl, 1990). Studying the impact of trauma on child victims and their families also requires special measures to ensure rational consent (see Cases 22 and 24).

The Voluntary Nature of Consent. Investigators studying children with mental disorders must be particularly sensitive to the potentially coercive nature of informed consent procedures. Vulnerable and/or disenfranchised families contacted while seeking services at a hospital, mental health center, or social service agency may be concerned that failure to consent will result in a loss of services for themselves or for their children (Fisher, 1991, 1993; Fisher & Rosendahl, 1990). Investigators also need to guard against potential conflicts of interest that may restrict the perceived voluntary nature of participation (see Case 25). As noted previously, investigators should take precautions that the opportunity to be randomly assigned to a treatment or no-treatment condition is not unduly coercive to a participant or guardian who is desperate to alleviate the adverse effects of a mental disorder. As discussed in the section on participant recruitment, the impact of subject payments on voluntary choice must also be considered.

THE ONGOING NATURE
OF INFORMED CONSENT

The OPRR (1993) conceptualizes informed consent as an ongoing educational process between investigator and prospective participant that should be monitored and discussed on more than one occasion. This is particularly relevant for the conduct of longitudinal studies, where the nature of the assessment instruments may change to fit the changing developmental status of the participants and where issues of confidentiality may shift as a child participant reaches adolescence. Viewing consent as an ongoing process is also of critical importance when videotaping is used. Given the potential threats to confidentiality posed by the use of videotaping, participant rights are best protected if individuals are given the opportunity to decline usage or select among possible uses of the tapes (e.g., data analysis, professional presentations) both before and after the taping sessions (see Case 26).

CASE 19: A LONGITUDINAL STUDY
OF THE PSYCHOSOCIAL DEVELOPMENT
OF MALTREATED TODDLERS OF DEPRESSED
MOTHERS

Research Goals

The purpose of this research program was to study the causes and consequences of child abuse and neglect from toddlerhood into early childhood. One of the long-range goals of the study was to identify vulnerability and protective factors contributing to the probability of maltreatment and its developmental sequelae. A second goal was to distinguish the developmental sequelae of child maltreatment from the effects of risks factors associated with lower socioeconomic status. Among variables measured were quality and nature of the home setting, a thorough demographic evaluation, parental ego strength and history of maltreatment, security of attachment, child aggressiveness, impulsivity, self-destructive behaviors, and other socioemotional and cognitive patterns of development. Families were contacted by service workers from local departments of social service. Only families who agreed to discuss participation with a member of the project staff were contacted.

Cases of Unclear Custody and Guardianship

When studying maltreated children, it is often difficult to decide the composition of the family and who is entitled to make decisions about the child. For example, some children are in foster placements, and it may be difficult to contact or meet with the biological parents because of their unstable living arrangements, incarceration, drug use, or other circumstances related to the removal of the child. In other cases, children are living with grandparents or other relatives because their parents are unable to care for them. Often, in these arrangements, grandparents have custody of the children, but may or may not have legal guardianship. Federal regulations (45 CFR 46) include special protections for wards, which would apply to children in foster care. However, unclear custody and guardianship situations raise the question of who is best able to make decisions about the child's participation in research. Is it reasonable to expect the biological parents to exercise informed consent about the child's participation if they were not able to care for the child appropriately? On the other hand, should the caregiver who has physical custody of the child be permitted to make decisions on the child's behalf if the biological parent is not aware of or has not consented to the child's participation?

Involving Both Custodial and Biological Parents in Decision Making

To address this problem, the researchers attempted to involve both the biological parent and the custodial parent in making decisions as much as possible. If both consented for the child to participate, child assent procedures were started. If either communicated they did not want the child to participate, the researcher went no further. In cases in which the biological parent was unavailable, the consent of the custodial parent was deemed sufficient if he or she had appropriate responsibility for the child.

Changing Guardianship

Because many of these families are disorganized and chaotic, guardianship may change over the course of a longitudinal investigation. For this reason, guardianship and custody arrangements were checked before each test point (e.g., every 6 months) and additional consent was obtained. Because a number of the interviews asked about maltreatment, the legal requirement to report child abuse was clearly communicated to biological and custodial parents, as well as children, at each testing point. The informed consent procedures also stated that if abuse was discovered the researchers would, if feasible, let the parents know that a report was to be made and assist them in making their own report if they wished. The researchers also recognized that threats to child welfare do not always clearly fall within the reporting requirements for child abuse; thus the consent form stated that if at any time the researchers had concerns about the immediate welfare of the children, they would discuss those concerns with parents in order to make sure that any needed help was made available.

CASE 20: COMPARING THE EFFICACY OF FOSTER AND HOME-BASED PROGRAMS FOR CHILDREN WITH SED

Research Goals

This study compared the outcome of a therapeutic foster care program to that of an enhanced home-based intensive case management program for children with SED. The investigation used a positive-controlled randomized design with multiple observations. Children with SED between 6 and 12 years of age were randomly assigned to one of the two treatment conditions. The domains of interest were provider behavior (e.g., services provided), family outcomes (e.g., family adaptability and cohesion), child outcomes (e.g., home, school, and community functioning), and system outcomes (e.g., costs and service system changes). Recruitment was limited to parents who already had referrals to existing foster placement programs (see Case 17). In this way, families already had the expectation that their child would be removed from home for some period of time. The research thus offered the possibility that through randomization their children might remain in the home.

Seeking Child Assent After Randomized
Assignment to Out-of-Home Placement

Only parents who had formerly agreed to foster placement were recruited for this study (see Case 17). Although parents were asked to sign consent forms prior to randomization and placement, the researchers were concerned that asking children to sign the assent forms prior to random assignment might make them feel that they were responsible for being placed outside the home. The investigators, therefore, described the study to the child prior to enrollment and determined his or her oral consent. It was only after randomization and placement that the child was asked to sign the assent form. If the child refused at that point, he or she was not included in the study, but would stay in the foster placement.

CASE 21: PHARMACOLOGICAL TREATMENT
OF HYPERACTIVE CHILDREN WITH MENTAL
RETARDATION

Research Goals

The purpose of this study was to assess the behavioral, cognitive, and side effects of fenfluramine (Pondimin) as an alternative to methylphenidate (Ritalin) in hyperactive children (5–13 years) with mental retardation. Five drug conditions were compared: Placebo, three doses of fenfluramine, and one dose of methylphenidate. Each drug condition was to be given for 2 weeks with order determined by a complex Latin square assignment. All parties having contact with the children, including their parents, teachers, and study personnel, were blind to the medication sequence. Prior to starting the protocol, each child was placed on a known placebo for 1 week.

Informing Parents About the Results of Research
Suggesting Neurotoxicity Effects in Animals

Fenfluramine is controversial in some circles, because of animal studies suggesting that doses given over a brief period can cause long-lasting depletion to serotonin content in certain midbrain structures. Some animal researchers argue that this suggests that the drug could have an irreversible effect on serotonin function in human beings. However, the results from animal studies are equivocal, no long-lasting serotonegic changes have been observed in humans, and the drug has been used in adults for over two decades without reports of adverse consequences related to CNS functioning (see also Case 4). This information was presented to the IRB, which determined that the benefits to individual subjects outweighed the potential risks. The IRB required the investigators to include a paragraph in the informed consent form indicating that animal research exists suggesting that fenfluramine may cause permanent changes to serotonergic structures and that there is some unknown risk that the drug could cause permanent neurological damage in the children taking part in this study.

Further Ensuring That Parents Have Adequate Comprehension of Potential Risks and Benefits

The investigators' previous experience indicated parents do not usually refuse to take part in the study solely because of the neurotoxicity issue. When asked how they feel about the risks involved, some parents have stated that they feel that they "have no choice." This does not mean that they feel coercion in the usual sense, but rather that they have tried a variety of treatments with little effect and are desperate for a "new" agent that might work for their children. The investigators have had some parents join the study solely because of the fenfluramine condition, as their children had unacceptable therapeutic responses to methylphenidate on prior occasions. Research staff were concerned that by warning the parents that fenfluramine may cause permanent neurological changes, they might be sending a message that this is a "powerful medicine" that may be effective where other drugs have failed. For example, some parents had asked whether a permanent change could be positive. The investigators were, therefore, careful to clarify to parents that there is no evidence that the fenfluramine is a more powerful agent than other treatments and that neuropharmacology is much too crude a science to be attempting to make permanent change in patients. (See Cases 40 and 56 for discussion of managing participant reactions to medication and debriefing parents on their child's reaction to the experimental conditions, respectively.)

CASE 22: THE PSYCHOLOGICAL IMPACT OF VIOLENCE ON CHILDREN LIVING IN A WAR ZONE

Research Goals

The purpose of this study was to assess the processes of adjustment required when life's conditions present chronic instances of danger. In particular, the investigators examined the developmental consequences of consistent exposure to political violence on Palestinian children and youth living on the West Bank during the Palestinian Uprising (*Intifada*). Children were interviewed and given questionnaires to determine the incidence of posttraumatic stress disorder (PTSD) in this population and to describe the children's socially adaptive and maladaptive methods of coping with danger.

Ethical Challenges for Research Conducted in War Zones

Conducting research on psychological sequelae of political violence with children and adolescents in war zones presents some special ethical challenges. Among these challenges are the stress to children of having to discuss their traumatic experiences, the closing of research sites, the stress of confronting children who have been physically injured or traumatized, and the appropriate suspicion participants may feel about giving information that may jeopardize themselves or their family.

Conducting research on the impact of the *Intifada* on children and youth in the West Bank presented numerous logistical and ethical issues, among them being "the problem" of informed consent. In the West Bank, secret police have posed as journalists and researchers to engage in political espionage and surveillance. As a result of information gathered in such a manner, individuals have been imprisoned or placed in administrative detention, or entire families have been subjected to house raids. Naturally, therefore, there are ample grounds for suspicion among the potential participants in legitimate research.

Oral Consent

Such suspicion has required contacting potential participants through local intermediaries known to and trusted by the participants. The intermediaries would explain the study to the parents and screen them to assure that they understood that their and their child's participation was voluntary. Moreover, oral, rather than written consent, was solicited. This oral consent procedure was necessary as parents were often reluctant to sign a form out of fear of retaliation from the army and because in a war zone area the researchers could not guarantee the security of any material with identifying information.

Informing Children About the Voluntary Nature of Participation

In some instances, children were suspicious of the researchers despite reassurances from their parents and teachers. Therefore, it was also very important to clarify to children their option not to participate in the study even after parents offered their consent. For example, on one visit to a kindergarten classroom in a refugee camp, one of the children whose parents had given consent came up to one of the researchers and began to hit her. Upon questioning by the child's teacher, it turned out that the child had spotted a tape recorder in the researcher's bag, which was associated in the child's mind with the arrest of her father. The child's father had been arrested after he had been "interviewed" by secret police who, posing as journalists, had used a tape recorder to interview him. The child was assured by her teacher that the investigators were not the enemy and that it was fine if she did not want to speak with them.

CASE 23: EVALUATION OF A MEDICATION–PLACEBO TREATMENT FOR ADOLESCENT ANXIETY DISORDERS

Research Goals

This study examined psychosocial correlates of an outpatient psychopharmacology treatment for adolescent anxiety disorders. Participants were given medication or a placebo over a period of 1 month. Participants came in each week for medical monitoring and for interviews. The psychosocial measures tapped a broad range of personal life experiences including cognitive processes, emotional stability, school and occupational activities, domestic, social, sexual, and illegal activities.

IRB Recommendations to Modify Parental Consent Forms

The investigators were faced with several questions concerning the content of the parental consent forms. The original version described the psychosocial interview in general terms (i.e., "Your child will be asked about his or her feelings and how he or she gets along with family and friends"). Several IRB members wanted the investigators to modify the consent procedures by including the following statements: "The interviews are sensitive in nature and include questions of illegal and sexual activity, and domestic violence" and "Your chid may find some of the questions painful or uncomfortable to answer." In addition, the IRB wanted the investigators to give each parent the right to review the questionnaires before their adolescents answered them.

The researchers were concerned that the content suggested for inclusion in the consent forms (i.e., illegal and sexual activity) was only a small part of the research and if highlighted would in fact mislead parents and participants as to the purpose of the study. They also believed that there were no data indicating that the questions they would be asking would be painful or uncomfortable to answer, and that including such a statement risked biasing the adolescents responses to these questions. They were also worried that showing parents the questionnaires would violate ethical guidelines on test security as well as potentially bias the adolescents' responses.

Responding to the IRB Recommendations

The investigators respected the parents' and adolescents' right to know the type of information asked during the interview. In order to respect these rights, but not distort the purpose of the study, they decided to provide a general list of all the different content areas that the child would be asked to talk about. They sought and received a Certificate of Confidentiality so that participant's illegal behaviors would be protected from subpoena, and informed parents and participants of this protection and the researcher's obligation to report child abuse.

The research team believed that given the absence of data on whether discussion of these events was "painful," framing the questions in such a context might bias responding. They also believed that given their decision to include all content areas touched by the questionnaires, parents and potential participants who did feel that discussion of sexual or illegal activities would be uncomfortable were fully informed that these questions would be asked. They did add the following sentence to the consent form: "During medical and psychiatric evaluations minor discomfort may occur when answering some questions. If you feel uncomfortable please tell the interviewer so that we may discuss it with you." The investigators recognized that patients (even in nonexperimental medical contexts) have the right to refrain from answering any question. They included a statement to this effect in the consent procedures, but also added that although the participant had the right to refrain from answering questions, medication-related physical questions were very important to the patient's well-being and should be answered whenever possible.

Finally, the researchers decided that having parents screen the assessment questions not only violated test security, but jeopardized the scientific validity of participant responses to these questions. They told the IRB that the research could not be conducted under those circumstances. The IRB concurred with this decision and with all the modifications mentioned here.

CASE 24: ENDOCRINE SEQUELAE OF TRAUMA
IN CHILD VICTIMS OF A NATURAL DISASTER

Research Goals

The purpose of this research was to study endocrine sequelae of trauma in child victims (6–12 years old) of a natural disaster. Children whose families had lost their homes during a recent earthquake were the target of investigation. Families were staying in city shelters or with relatives. A short-term longitudinal design was used in which children were to be tested 2 weeks, 2 months, 6 months, and 12 months after the earthquake. At each test point, endocrine levels would be measured through blood sampling. Psychopathology and emotional status were measured through clinical interview and parent- and self-report questionnaires. The researchers planned to pay the families for each assessment period. Venipuncture was considered to be a minimal risk procedure for this population. (See Case 2 for further discussion of venipuncture.)

Ensuring that Consent is Rational

The primary ethical issue faced by the researchers was, given their recent traumatic experiences, were the parents and children in a position to give rational consent? The research team was concerned that the trauma of the earthquake and stress associated with their subsequent displacement from their homes might impair both the parent and child's ability to rationally understand the nature of the research. To address this issue, the absence of immediate benefits and the voluntary nature of the study was stressed during the consent procedures. In addition, a simple comprehension test was piloted and developed to ensure that participants understood the basic elements of the consent forms. Parents or children who did not appear to fully comprehend the experimental procedures, risks and benefits, or the voluntary nature of participation were not included in the study. (See also Case 15 on ethical issues involving offering this population incentives for research participation.)

CASE 25: EVALUATING CHILDREN'S DECISION
TO CONSENT TO PREDICTIVE GENETIC TESTING

Research Goals

Predictive genetic testing is concerned with the probability that an individual will develop a genetically related disease. The purpose of this study was to examine psychosocial issues related to the decision of 9- through 16-year-olds with a family history of Huntington's disease to participate in predictive genetic testing. With advancing medical technology, questions remain as to how and when to tell children and families about the availability of tests and test results. This study was designed to learn how children and adolescents understand the process of genetic testing so that ethical guidelines could be put into place regarding the type and quality of information and explanation required to render true informed assent or consent.

Conflict of Interest

Participants in the study were simultaneously asked to consent to genetic testing and to an evaluation of their comprehension of the genetic testing consent form. The goal of the study was to develop guidelines for assent/consent procedures; thus there was no consent model for this study. These procedures had to be informed by developmental research on related matters. Ironically, the effectiveness of these consent procedures would be determined by the results of the study. Of principal ethical concern was the dual role and potential conflict of interest that might emerge if members of the research team conducted the informed consent procedures: The research team had obvious interest in participants consenting to the genetic testing so that follow-up research on the consequences of consent could be conducted. To ensure that families received the most unbiased explanation of the process, families were asked to nominate an "advocate" (such as a family physician), with no connection to the research, who could help the family evaluate the benefits and deterrents to participation. (See also Case 58 for decisions regarding debriefing.)

CASE 26: A LONGITUDINAL STUDY
OF PARENT–CHILD INTERACTIONS IN FAMILIES
WITH CHILDREN WITH CHRONIC MEDICAL
PROBLEMS AND HEALTHY PEERS

Research Goals

The investigators were conducting a longitudinal study comparing parent–child interactions in families with children with chronic medical problems and those with healthy children. At each age (infancy through 7 years), children and their parents came to the laboratory and videotaped observations of parent–child interactions were conducted.

Home observations conducted during the first year were also videotaped. Over the years, the researchers developed an extensive library of videotapes to which they often returned with new research questions. They also used these videotapes to train other professionals in their coding procedures, to describe their findings at professional meetings, and for inservice training for medical and allied staff within the health care system.

Ongoing Consent for the Use of Videotapes

Although videotape has enabled the researchers to study behavior in new and exciting ways, it also raises new ethical issues, particularly in the area of confidentiality. Although equipment now exists for visually "scrambling" faces on videotapes, in general visual identity is not disguised and in many cases the purpose of the research or teaching project is defeated by doing so (e.g., many times facial expressions are important data). Thus confidentiality must be protected primarily by restricting access to the tapes (see also Case 35).

The initial consent form gives parents several options: (a) to give permission for the taping only for research purposes; (b) to give permission for research plus in-hospital teaching; or (c) to give permission for any educational use. Parents check off the preferred alternative. At the end of testing, parents are offered the opportunity to view the videotape and, if they want, change their preferred alternative. Although they may not know how the researchers actually coded the tapes, it allows parents to see themselves as the researchers see them. This procedure has the advantage of making it clear to parents that saying "no" to requests for use of videotape is both permissible and expected.

Most parents chose to give consent for the broadest use, but a small number chose not to have their tapes used beyond the study per se. Only one parent asked that the videotape be destroyed when the research project was completed. Whenever the tapes have been used for teaching or demonstration, it is made clear to students and audiences that the material is confidential and that parents have given permission to use it for teaching purposes. Parents are also offered a copy of the tape if they provide a cassette for that purpose. Most families do want copies. The videotape, which serves as a record of the child's development over the first 7 years, is something the researchers can give back to families in exchange for their participation.

* * *

Casebook

Child Assent in the Absence
of Parental Consent

Federal regulations for solicitation of parental consent assume that the child comes from a reasonably secure and loving family (Gaylin & Macklin, 1982; Levine, 1986). However, significant numbers of high-risk or disordered children and adolescents have undetermined custody, nonrelative guardians, or state guardianship (Gibbs, 1990; Hendren, 1991). In addition, the adverse physical or social environments in which some of these children live may make obtaining parental consent difficult or dangerous for the child.

WAIVING THE REQUIREMENT
OF GUARDIAN CONSENT

Federal regulations provide guidelines for helping investigators and IRBs determine the conditions under which requiring parental consent does not reasonably protect the welfare of minor research participants (Federal Regulation 46.408[c]). Children from neglecting or abusing families may be included in this category. In other types of research (e.g., studies on adolescent sexual activity or substance abuse), the solicitation of parental consent may violate a teenager's privacy or even jeopardize his or her welfare (see Case 27). Current state laws granting adolescents the autonomy to make decisions concerning treatment for venereal disease, drug abuse, or emotional disorders have been used as a model to determine conditions under which guardian consent may be waived (Fisher, 1993; Holder, 1981).

In other situations, parental consent may be waived when the research cannot be practically carried out without the waiver. The study on juvenile detainees, described in Case 28, is an example of minimal risk research in which time limitations for conducting the research (prospective participants were often detained for only a few days) and inaccessibility of many parents during this period made conducting the research infeasible if parental consent was required. When research risks are minimal and informed consent infeasible, respect for the importance of family involvement in children's lives dictates that, in addition to child assent procedures, parental notification be offered as both a courtesy and a mechanism for providing additional information (45 CFR 46.115[d]; Nolan, 1992).

Passive Consent

Difficulties in acquiring guardian consent is not in itself sufficient to waive the requirement for guardian consent. Research that does not meet the requirement for waiver of parental consent should not utilize passive consent (when guardians are sent forms asking them to respond only if they do not wish their child to participate) as a means of overcoming low rates of parental response. Passive consent is not an ethical substitute for guardian consent because it does not meet the standards set by the principles of beneficence, respect for persons, and justice (Fisher, 1993). The use of passive consent procedures with vulnerable, poor, and disenfranchised populations can create an unjust situation in which such children are disproportionately deprived of the protections afforded by guardian consent when compared to their healthier and financially better off peers.

PARTICIPANT ADVOCATES

When parental consent is waived or when children or adolescents are wards of the state (see Case 29), federal regulations (45 CFR 46) require that an advocate for the minor be present to: (a) verify the minor's understanding of assent procedures, (b) support his or her preferences, (c) ensure that participation is voluntary, (d) check periodically whether the youth wants to terminate participation, (e) assess reactions to planned procedures, and (f) ensure that debriefing addresses all participant questions and concerns (Fisher, 1993; OPRR, 1993). The participant advocate should have no investment in the research project or role in subject recruitment (Fisher, 1993).

CASE 27: A STUDY OF PSYCHOLOGICAL STRESSORS AND DISORDERS IN GAY AND LESBIAN ADOLESCENTS

Research Goals

The purpose of this study was to examine psychosocial stressors and prevalence of anxiety and depressive disorders in 14- to 18-year-old gay and lesbian adolescents. Access to this population was obtained through a gay and lesbian community center. The adolescents who came to the center were from a broad section of schools in the community. This enabled the researchers to obtain a sample size that would not have been feasible if the general population of each school was sampled and students were asked to identify their sexual orientation on a written form. Most of the teens who attended the center had not told their parents of their sexual orientation and many were concerned that negative reprisals would result if their parents were told or if information was inadvertently released to their teachers or schoolmates. Center staff were very enthusiastic about the project and supportive of having students interviewed at the center.

Obtaining a Waiver of Parent/Guardian Consent

The researchers believed that parental consent would not be in the best interests of these adolescents because parental notification of the purpose of the study might place the child at psychosocial or physical risk. In addition, the developmental science knowledge base indicated that by 14 years of age adolescents had the cognitive capacity to understand the informed consent procedures (see, e.g., Melton et al., 1983; Weithorn, 1983). The researchers decided that this study would meet the DHHS 45 CFR 46.408[c] criteria for waiver of parent/guardian involvement when such involvement is not a reasonable requirement to protect the child, provided appropriate mechanisms for protecting the adolescents were substituted.

Selecting a Participant Advocate

As an appropriate mechanism for protecting participant's rights, the investigators looked for an adult to serve as a participant advocate to help ensure that the teen's consent was informed and voluntary. This was difficult because both the researchers and the staff at the community center might have a conflict of interest in having the teens participate. The center did have a relationship with a nearby community clinic where it referred teens who wanted medical or psychological assistance. A psychologist on staff at the clinic agreed to serve as an independent advocate for the participants, reviewing their comprehension and willingness to participate in the research. (See Case 37 for a discussion of child abuse reporting requirements for this population.)

CASE 28: ASSESSING MENTAL HEALTH SERVICE NEEDS AND SERVICE UTILIZATION AMONG JUVENILE DETAINEES

Research Goals

The purpose of this study was to assess the extent of impairment and alcohol, drug, or mental disorders (ADM) service needs of juvenile detainees. The first phase of the study included evaluation of ADM diagnosis, comorbidity, and functional impairment. The second phase was to determine the extent that juvenile detainees who needed ADM services received them while in custody of the criminal justice system or as part of their case disposition.

Waiving Parental Consent

The researchers believed that within the context of the importance of the data for future policy to benefit juvenile detainees, the research met the federal guidelines for waiving consent under (45 CFR 46.102[i], 46.116[d], and 46.408[b]). First, because the juveniles would undergo standard medical and psychological tests as part of detention, risks associated with the research clinical interview were not greater in and of themselves than those the youth would ordinarily encounter during the performance of routine physical and psychological tests. Second, there was a limited time frame (often only a few days) in which youths were detained before their case disposition. During this period, it was often difficult for justice system staff to contact parents. Accordingly, for a significant number of juveniles, the research could not be practically carried out if guardian consent was required. The investigators' IRB concurred with this decision and believed that the conditions outlined here served to adequately protect the participants.

Attempting to Obtain Guardian Consent When Feasible

The investigators decided that even though the requirement for guardian consent would be waived, they would pursue parental permission when possible. A human subjects liaison would be present during visiting hours and attempt to obtain consent from visiting parents for at least 24 hours. The 24-hour period was selected because it was important to interview juveniles before their detention hearings, after which 20% are usually released. Losing this group would bias the sample because such persons were probably arrested for less severe criminal offences or had less severe criminal histories. It was decided that the liaison would not attempt to call parents or guardians who had visited because there would be no way to confirm who the liaison was speaking to and such contact could lead to revealing information about the juvenile's arrest that might violate his or her privacy. If the parent or guardian refused participation, the youth would not be contacted. If the parent/guardian agreed to participation then the juvenile's informed assent was sought. If the juvenile refused assent they were not further contacted.

Consent Procedures and the Participant Advocate

If the liaison was unable to contact the guardian, a participant advocate was asked to intervene. The participant advocate was a psychologist who regularly met with the juvenile detainees, but who had no formal or informal connection with the research project. The participant advocate interviewed the youth, evaluated the juvenile's comprehension of procedures, determined if he or she wished to consent, and that consent was voluntary. If the participant advocate judged the youth as capable of informed, rational, and voluntary consent then the liaison approached the juvenile to obtain his or her assent. If the youth refused or the advocate determined that the detainee could not rationally or voluntarily respond to the consent procedure, he or she was not contacted further. In addition to describing the purpose and nature of the research, the juvenile consent procedures informed the participant of the research team's obligation to report information regarding child abuse, and that parents/guardians would be contacted concerning the adolescent's participation in the research (see later).

Parental Notification

After the youths had been tested, all parents or guardians were sent two forms from the address noted in the archival records. The first form was a project information sheet that explained the nature of the project, indicated that the information had already been collected, and that a participant advocate was involved to protect the child's rights. This form also ensured the parent of the confidentiality of the data, gave parents or guardians the right to withdraw the data, and encouraged them to contact the project director if they had any questions or concerns. The second form provided a list of social services available in their county. This list was not limited to ADM services because this might needlessly alarm the parents.

CASE 29: NEUROLOGICAL CORRELATES OF AIDS IN INFECTED INSTITUTIONALIZED CHILDREN

Research Goals

The purpose of this study was to examine the neurological correlates of AIDS in infected children whose mothers had transmitted the HIV virus during pregnancy. The children (8–12 years of age) were in a state hospital being treated for the last stages of AIDS. The mothers of most of the children were deceased and many of the youths were wards of the state. The research procedures included neuropsychological testing and MRI. The procedures presented no more than minimal risk and held out no direct benefits for the terminally ill child participants. The investigators believed that the research was likely to yield generalizable knowledge about the child participants' disorder that could be applied to the diagnosis and treatment of other children with AIDS contracted through maternal transmission.

Assessing Children's Ability to Comprehend the Risks and Benefits of Research

Once the decision had been reached that the benefits of the study outweighed the risks and that these risks were not unjustly distributed to this institutionalized population (see Case 6), the primary ethical issue became the children's own evaluation of risk–benefit and their desire to participate or not participate in the study. Because this research offered no direct benefit to the children, their dissent would override any legal guardian's consent. An important question, therefore, was whether these children were competent to assent.

Pediatric oncologists (Kamps et al., 1987) have suggested that experiencing the negative side effects of illness and medical procedures may make some children with cancer more likely than other children to evaluate the potential discomfort of the procedures. However, because AIDS is associated with cognitive deficits, the child's ability to comprehend information given during informed assent might be impaired. The researchers decided to conduct a preliminary study to assess the cognitive abilities of these children to understand (a) what the neuropsychological and MRI procedures would be like, (b) that the procedures would not be of any help to them, and (c) that they might help other children through their participation. This preliminary study indicated that a majority of the children could comprehend the assent information.

Participant Advocates

Several of the staff nurses who were not associated with the project, agreed to serve as participant advocates to evaluate each child's comprehension of the research procedures, their willingness to participate, and their understanding of the voluntary nature of the research. The assent procedures would include (a) a description of the risks involved in a language the child could understand, (b) a clear statement that these procedures would not help the patient's illness or make them feel better, and (c) a discussion of the voluntary nature of participation emphasizing that the child's care would not be affected by his or her declining to participate at any time. It was decided that those children whose impairments made it unlikely that they could understand these three points would be excluded from the study.

Discussing the Altruistic Aspects of Research Participation

A second concern was whether telling the child that the procedures held out no benefit for them would be psychologically harmful. Previous research with terminally ill children with cancer (see Kamps et al., 1987) suggested that the diagnosis of terminal illness cannot be concealed from patients in late childhood, that such children realize that death is a final event, and that they are able to face their own deaths. The researchers also drew on developmental research indicating that children of this age engage in prosocial (altruistic) behaviors. The researchers concluded that the opportunity to help other children might benefit the patients by giving them a sense of increased self-worth. It was, therefore, decided that the assent procedures would include discussion of how the child's participation could help doctors find medicines that might help other children in the future.

* * *

Casebook

Deceptive Research Practices

Debate regarding the ethical justification for or against deceptive research practices has focused on whether they should be conducted for the potential societal benefit or prohibited for their potential violations of participant autonomy, trust, and welfare (Baumrind, 1964, 1979, 1990; Bok, 1978; Fisher & Fryberg, 1994; Kelman, 1967). Arguments for deception emphasize the methodological advantage of keeping participants naive about the purpose of a study so that they can respond spontaneously to experimental manipulations, the potential scientific and social value of the research, and the efficacy of debriefing as a means of fulfilling the moral obligation of respect (Milgram, 1964; Resnick & Schwartz, 1973; Smith & Richardson, 1983). Arguments against deception emphasize the methodological problems associated with participant suspicion, the potentially harmful consequences of dehoaxing, and the researcher's fiduciary obligation to participants (e.g., Baumrind, 1990; Fisher & Rosendahl, 1990; Orne, 1962).

FACTORS IN THE CONSIDERATION
OF THE COST–BENEFIT BALANCE
OF DECEPTIVE RESEARCH

The use of deceptive techniques leads to the withholding of information about the real purpose of the research. It may also provide incomplete disclosure or false information regarding the experimental procedures. As a consequence, the use of deceptive techniques risks violating an individual's right to make autonomous decisions regarding his or her participation in research. According to the OPRR (1993), when considering the use of deception, investigators must first decide whether the information to be withheld would, if known, influence the individual's desire to participate in the research. Cases 30 and 31 illustrate situations in which investigators considered whether incomplete disclosure of the purpose and nature of the study would be a material factor in guardian consent decisions. Under some circumstances, the principle of nonmaleficence (to do no harm) may lead an investigator to withhold information from a participant regarding the full purpose and nature of the study. This is especially true if the reason why the child was selected for the research may rest on a risk factor of which he or she is unaware.

Because deceptive techniques always run the risk of reducing participant autonomy, appropriate protections for human subjects requires that such procedures only be considered when they are demonstrated to be scientifically valid and when nondeceptive alternatives do not meet methodological criteria to competently test the hypothesis under investigation. A deception study may be well designed and superior to methodological alternatives, but still may not meet ethical standards for implementation if the experimental hypothesis cannot be effectively translated into a body of scientific knowledge or into useful application (Fisher & Fryberg, 1994; Freedman, 1987; Seiber, 1990). Thus, evaluation of the scientific validity and value of an experiment plays a critical role in cost–benefit assessments of deceptive research.

Another factor to be considered when evaluating the costs and benefits of deceptive experimentation is the possibility of experimentally induced harm through psychological or physiological discomfort in response to certain planned procedures. For example, research designed to deceptively manipulate failure, disapproval, or to tempt participants to perform moral breaches can place children and youth at risk for anger, shame, and attributions of negative self-worth. Investigators in Cases 30 and 31 decided to use deceptive procedures after a careful consideration of the scientific and social value of the hypothesis, the limitations of alternative methodologies, and the minimal risk of harm involved in participation.

DEHOAXING

Investigators should reveal the true nature of the experimental deception at the end of the experiment when doing so contributes to the subject's welfare (i.e., "when it corrects painful or stressful misperceptions, or when it reduces pain, stress, or anxiety concerning the subject's performance," OPRR, 1993, p. 3). A more difficult decision is when debriefing could itself produce harm. When considering ethical justifications for dehoaxing or not dehoaxing a minor research participant, investigators need to weigh the child's autonomy rights against the obligation to protect the child's welfare. Such decision making needs to be conducted within the context of knowledge about the child's cognitive, moral, and social development. For example, investigators contemplating dehoaxing procedures must consider whether young children and even adolescents have the recursive thinking skills to understand the deception (Thompson, 1990). For example, Lepper, Ross, and Lau (1980) found that high school students who experienced induced failure in a deception study persisted in erroneously believing they had been responsible for the failure even after dehoaxing. Moreover, undergraduates asked to weigh the costs and benefits of deceptive research believed that college students would react to dehoaxing procedures with embarrassment or annoyance (Fisher & Fryberg, 1994). Investigators in Case 30 adjusted their dehoaxing procedures after they found that some young subjects playing what they believed was a competitive electronic game with another child were distressed to learn upon dehoaxing that their "opponent's" actions were computer generated.

Developmental research further suggests that children as old as 8 or 9 do not incorporate intentionality as a defining feature of the concept of deceit (Piaget, 1965; Wimmer, Gruber, & Perner, 1985). As a consequence, young children may not understand the experimental purpose of the deception and, if dehoaxed, simply conclude that researchers are adults who lie (Fisher & Rosendahl, 1990). Case 31 provides an innovative means of ensuring that children's experimentally induced misperceptions are corrected without exposing them to a sense of experimenter betrayal.

PARTICIPANT PARTNERS

The use of deceptive research techniques continues to be a source of controversy between those who believe that under minimal risk conditions deception is ethically justified when it is the only scientifically valid means of gathering information important to child welfare, and those who believe that, irrespective of the risk–benefit balance, it is always unethical to deprive individuals of information that might affect their autonomous choice to participate in research. The opinions of participants and their guardians regarding deceptive research procedures is as yet a relatively untapped resource to assist ethical decision making (Fisher & Fryberg, 1994; Fisher et al., in press). In the absence of knowledge concerning participant perspectives, investigators and their IRBs run the risk of underestimating the degree of potential distress associated with a particular experimental condition or of abandoning scientifically and socially worthwhile procedures on the erroneous assumption that prospective participants would experience them as harmful. Investigators in Cases 30 and 31 drew on the opinions and observations of parents and participants before and after they implemented their studies to help evaluate the costs and benefits of their research procedures.

CASE 30: INSTRUMENTAL AND HOSTILE AGGRESSION IN CHILDREN REFERRED FOR DISRUPTIVE BEHAVIOR DISORDERS

Research Goals

Investigators working with inpatient and outpatient 8- to 12-year-old boys, wanted to design an analog task that could distinguish between the children's use of instrumental and hostile aggression. A control group of males was recruited from the community. Participants were diagnosed with ADHD, conduct disorder, or oppositional defiant disorder. The investigators designed a computer game by which they could learn how these children respond to competitive situations. The boys wore headphones and believed they were playing the game in competition with an unknown peer who was presumably in an adjacent room. The boys were told that both they and their competitor could press one button to block their opponent's game (the measure of instrumental aggression) and a second button to send a noxious noise through the opponent's headphones (the measure of hostile aggression). In actuality the experimenter, sitting behind the boy, controlled the "opponent's" buttons, and used them to systematically provoke the participant with either tilts or noises. The boys could not see their scores and were told that the experimenter would tell them their score at the end of the game. When the game was over, all participants were informed that they were the winner.

Evaluating the Use of Deception in Light of Alternative Procedures

The investigators recognized that the use of deceptive research techniques poses a threat to participant autonomy. However, they believed that these deceptive conditions were safer for children than alternative methodologies that manipulated real-life competitive and potentially aggressive situations. Moreover, because of the paucity of research on children with disruptive behavior disorders, the relevance of the research to application, and the apparent intractability of aggression, the investigators believed this study had important potential benefits for treatment of disruptive behavior disorders. They found considerable support for their analog task from parents of children with these disorders and from professionals in psychiatric and educational settings.

Deciding Whether to Inform Parents About the Deceptive Nature of the Study

Having decided that the deceptive procedures were safe and scientifically valid, the investigators recognized the importance of ruling out the possibility that any child would have knowledge about the deception. For that reason, they considered the risks of informing or not informing parents about the deceptive procedures prior to their child's participation. They were particularly concerned that if even one parent revealed that the experimenters actually controlled the game, this knowledge would spread among the rest of the patients, thereby invalidating the study. At the same time, they considered it important to maintain the parent's trust and therefore did not want to provide any false information. In considering what the child would experience during participation in the research, the investigators reasoned that if they included a detailed description of the procedures, knowledge that the experimenters controlled the game would not significantly impact a parent's decision to allow her or his child to participate. As a result, the consent information did not say that the child would be playing against another child, but that he would be in a competitive computer game that at times would be easy and at times would be difficult. Parents were also informed that the child would leave the game feeling good about his performance.

Dehoaxing

In the first two studies, children and their parents were initially debriefed following data collection. However this raised several problems. First the debriefing contaminated the design for other patients. Second, children were at times distressed by the debriefing. Although dehoaxed parents did not raise objections to the deception itself, parents and teachers frequently asked that the investigators not debrief their child. As one parent stated, "We have worked so hard to build his trust in his therapist, I don't want him to think that people are lying to him." Similar sentiments were expressed by teachers and principals who were concerned that children would be confused or upset by the deception. The investigators went back to their IRB and received permission to only debrief parents about deception in later studies.

CASE 31: CHILDREN'S EYEWITNESS MEMORY
IN A FORENSICALLY RELEVANT CONTEXT

Research Goals

The goal of this study was to examine children's eyewitness memory in a forensically relevant context. The primary question of interest was whether children's reports about a babysitter's behavior would be affected by misleading suggestions. The study's purpose was to test children in a real-life context providing them with leading questions similar to those potentially used in investigations of child abuse. Four-year-old children visited a laboratory individually and played with a confederate posing as a babysitter. This play session was videotaped. Two weeks later the child returned to the laboratory to be questioned about the session. Prior to questioning, half of the children were introduced to a "police officer" who told them that the babysitter might have done some bad things and that he needed the child's help to find out what happened. All children were then questioned. The dependent variables concerned whether those children who had been exposed to a suggestive authority figure would be more likely to spontaneously report or confirm suggestions that the babysitter had acted badly.

Evaluating the Use of Deception in the Context
of Alternative Procedures

When designing the study, the investigators considered whether the research had social importance and whether they could accomplish their goals through a nondeceptive methodology. The investigators believed that empirically valid information about children's susceptibility to leading questions was seriously lacking and providing such information could have an important impact on investigative procedures for suspected child abuse cases. They also decided that alternative methodologies to deception (e.g., naturalistic observation, having a teacher actually do something wrong) were either impractical or unethical.

Deciding When to Inform Parents
About the Deceptive Nature of the Study

After concluding that the deceptive techniques were justified by the study's prospective value and that equally effective alternative procedures were not feasible, the investigators considered what information to include in the parental consent and child assent procedures. Knowledge that memory was a factor in the experiment might lead some parents to question their child in a manner that could influence the child's rehearsal strategies, thereby contaminating the research. The investigators also reasoned that for this first play session, knowledge that the study included a memory component would not significantly impact the parent or child's permission. Accordingly, on the first laboratory visit, participants and their parents were only told that the study concerned children's play behaviors. Parents, but not children, were informed about the videotaping. In addition, parents were asked not to discuss the study with their children until after the second session.

On the second day of testing, parental consent was again taken. This time the parents were told the true nature of the study and the specific questions the child would be asked. In this way, parents were aware of the deception before they signed the second consent form. The parent's right to decide not to have her or his child participate in this phase of the study was emphasized. Children were not told about the deception, but their assent procedures included information that they would be interviewed by an adult.

Dehoaxing

When the questioning was over, the children were debriefed. Developmental research on very young children's understanding of deception suggested the 4-year-old participants would not comprehend the true nature of the research. The researchers believed that the purpose of debriefing was to ensure that children did not leave thinking that the babysitter had actually done anything bad or that the police officer had lied. For this reason, children were shown a videotape of the first session where they could see that nothing bad had happened and that they had had an enjoyable play period. Just prior to the video, children in the negative deceptive condition were told that the police officer had been mistaken and that the babysitter had done nothing wrong. Children enjoyed watching the video. A week later, the researchers called parents to check to see whether their child had any negative reactions to the experiences. The parents reported that the children remembered the experiment as an enjoyable experience and did not appear to have negative impressions of the babysitter.

* * *

Casebook

Confidentiality

Research on children and adolescents with mental disorders often elicits sensitive information that an individual may not have previously revealed to others or that could produce risk or harm if known beyond the research setting. As discussed in previous sections of this casebook, ethical considerations regarding recruitment, informed consent, and deceptive research procedures can provide appropriate mechanisms for protecting participant privacy. Once a participant or his or her guardian has agreed to share personal information with a research team, investigators are obligated to ensure that information is not divulged to others in a manner that is inconsistent with the participant's understanding of the original agreement. Effective procedures for protecting confidentiality will ensure that a participant retains control over sharing her or himself physically, behaviorally or intellectually with others (OPRR, 1993).

PROCEDURES FOR PROTECTING
CONFIDENTIALITY

In many research contexts, investigators can use routine procedures for assuring the confidentiality of data. Subject codes rather than identifiers, secure storage and limited access to data, disposal of unnecessary identifying information, and appropriate supervision of research personnel are just some of the routine precautions that can be taken to protect participant confidentiality. Additional protections may be necessary when data are collected by professionals outside the research team or across geographically diverse sites (see Cases 32 and 33).

ADDITIONAL PROTECTIONS

Routine procedures for maintaining confidentiality may not be viewed as sufficient by researchers investigating especially sensitive or potentially stigmatizing information such as drug or alcohol abuse, HIV infection, or illegal behaviors. For example, there may be research contexts in which the maintenance of confidentiality cannot be guaranteed (i.e., the psychological impact of war, Case 22). In other research settings, one may not be able to provide services for children who, during the course of research, indicate they are in need of assistance (i.e., the absence of community resources for assisting children who report fear of gang violence, see Case 34). In these settings, failure to offer help to a child may undermine his or her trust in the implicit societal contract between adults and children: that adults will aid those who are vulnerable to their actions and choices (Fisher, 1994; Fisher, Higgins, Rau, Kuther, & Belanger, in press). In such situations it may be possible to collect data anonymously and explain to potential participants how knowledge produced by the research can lead to improvement or greater availability of services.

The Certificate of Confidentiality. When identifying information is required to conduct sensitive research (i.e., therapeutic or longitudinal research), there may be situations for which routine procedures for assuring confidentiality are not sufficient to protect the participant from harm. For example, data collected on violent behavior, substance abuse, or even parenting behaviors of individuals with mental disorders may be subject to subpoena stemming from criminal investigations or custody disputes (see Case 35). In these circumstances, an investigator conducting biomedical, behavioral, clinical, or other research can apply for a Certificate of Confidentiality under 301[d] of the Public Health Service Act. The Certificate provides the investigator immunity from any governmental or civil order to disclose identifying information contained in research records. The Certificate is granted when research is that which would be recorded in a patient's medical record or of such a "sensitive" nature that if released could result in stigmatization, discrimination, or legal action and that could damage an individual's financial standing, employability, or reputation (Hoagwood, 1994).

The Certificate may not, however, override state reporting laws on child abuse, although it can protect the confidentiality of information about past abuse divulged by research subjects (Hoagwood, 1994). Nor does the Certificate protect the researcher against disclosing child data to parents; such protection can only be assured through permission by the parent or guardian at the time of informed consent (Hoagwood, 1994). When an investigator is granted a Certificate, both the protections and limitations of protection should be explained to child and adolescent participants and their parents.

DISCLOSURES

Investigators studying mental disorders of childhood and youth may, during the course of research, become privy to information suggesting child abuse or threats of harm or violence to the participant or identified others.

Reporting Child Abuse.   Following the 1976 Child Abuse Prevention and Treatment Act, all 50 states have enacted statutes mandating the reporting of suspected child abuse or neglect. In all states, this law pertains to mental health professionals and in at least 13 states to researchers, as members of the general citizenry (Liss, 1994). Other states vary as to whether researchers are included in mandated reporting. Thus, until case law decisions can provide more guidance, investigators need to review their own state laws to determine if they or members of their research team are obligated to report child abuse and neglect (Fisher, 1991, 1993; Liss, 1994). At present, however, as Case 36 illustrates, it is not clear whether researchers are legally required to release to authorities research records pertinent to the abuse after it is reported. Once reporting obligations are determined, the principal investigator needs to ensure that research personnel are trained to recognize indicators of abuse and to follow appropriate procedures. Such obligations should be fully communicated to both parents and minor participants at the time of informed consent (Fisher, 1993). Investigators may also choose not to ask specific questions about child abuse in situations where the obligation to report such information might place the participant in greater social or physical risk (see Case 37).

Protecting the Participant From Self-Harm.   In the course of research, investigators interviewing or conducting standardized tests with high-risk children or youth with mental disorders may come on information suggesting they may be contemplating suicide. Investigators need to be prepared for such circumstances by determining specific criteria and procedures to be followed if research personnel suspect the possibility of self-inflicted harm. Participants and their guardians should be informed about these procedures prior to gaining permission to participate. As Case 38 poignantly indicates, when working with some impaired populations these criteria may need to be quite broad, and may require vetoing a child or adolescent's request that information not be released.

Protecting Third Parties From Harm.   An issue particularly relevant to developmental scientists who study family violence or delinquency is whether mental health researchers share with practitioner colleagues the responsibility to protect third parties about dangers posed by clients (Fisher, 1993). At present, it would be wise for investigators conducting such research to examine whether, given appropriate circumstances, their role in research might meet the duty to protect as outlined by *Tarasoff* v. *Regents of the University of California* (1976): (a) a "special relationship" with a participant, (b) the ability to predict that violence will occur, and (c) the ability to identify the potential victim (Appelbaum & Rosenbaum, 1989). As illustrated in Case 39, the presenting problems of some research participants (i.e., pedophiles) require advanced planning for protecting both the rights of the participants and the welfare of the community (Jenkins-Hall & Osborn, 1994; Monahan, Appelbaum, Mulvey, Robbins, & Lidz, 1993). In recent years, there has been considerable debate over the obligation to protect identifiable third parties from potential harm caused by the unsafe sex practices of an HIV positive research participant. Investigators should approach such a situation with exteme caution, taking into account the fact that some state laws prohibit certain licensed professionals from revealing a client's HIV status.

CASE 32: LEARNING AND NEUROLOGICAL CORRELATES OF HIV INFECTION IN CHILDREN WITH HEMOPHILIA

Research Goals

This was a multisite project designed to follow a cohort of children with hemophilia to trace the impact of the HIV virus on child and family coping. The study was initiated in the late 1980s, with children ranging in age from 6 to 11 years. These children had first received blood transfusions during the early period of AIDS awareness, and in most cases the blood donated during this period had not been tested for the HIV virus. As a consequence, 50% of the research participants were expected to develop AIDS during the course of the study. Once every 6 months, children and their parents would come in for measures of physical growth, neurological problems, neuropsychological testing, psychological assessments, and measures of family stress and parental coping. The study paid for the family's transportation (some families were at a great distance from the hospital). Parents were paid $100 and children $25 for each interview period. The aim of the study was to examine the relationship of hemophilia and HIV to learning problems, neurological functions, and the physiological profile of HIV infection.

Protecting Confidentiality When Medical
Data are Collected by Different Specialists
in a Multisite Collaborative Study

The study required MRIs, EEGs, blood tests, and psychological tests, all conducted by different specialists in different offices and sometimes in different buildings. One of the first ethical problems to arise was how to maintain confidentiality across the multiple settings at which the medical and psychological testing were conducted. Because the research grant provided funds for all testing, each child was given a research number and all information was billed to this number. Therefore, health information did not have to go to an insurer nor a private physician and the patient's name did not have to appear on clinical records transferred from different testing sites. To further ensure confidentiality, only numbers were used in any intersite transmittal of information. Results of all testing were discussed with parents and, if they providedwritten permission, results of testing could be sent to physicians or schools (e.g., when learning difficulties were discovered).

Informing Medical Personnel in Contact
With Blood Samples of the Child's HIV Status

An additional problem was whether the HIV status of the child should stay anonymous to various professionals on the project. For example, when parents gave permission, child autopsies were conducted. The ethical issue was that although all physicians take health precautions when working with patient blood, the AIDS status of the children did present an established risk to the pathologist conducting the autopsy. Was it fair not to make the pathologist aware of this risk? There was also some social risk for the family if the community learned that the child had died from AIDS. The investigators concluded that because the state laws forbade professionals from releasing information about HIV or other communicable diseases, revealing the child's AIDS status to the pathologist would not jeopardize the family's privacy in the community. The family was aware of this decision when they were asked to consent to autopsy. To further protect the family, no information was released to the hospital. Rather, the autopsy was billed directly to the research project's hemophilia billing number. (See Case 59 for discussion on ethical issues associated with informing children about their HIV status.)

Because the life course of each child was unknown at the time the study was funded, some children died before all the monies assigned for their research participation had been exhausted. With the parents permission, this money was donated to the state's Hemophilia Foundation in the name of the deceased child.

CASE 33: PHYSIOLOGICAL INDICATORS OF DEPRESSION AND ANXIETY IN DIABETIC CHILDREN

Research Design

The purpose of this study was to measure biological indicators of depression and anxiety in diabetic children (6–11 years of age). Children were admitted into the hospital for a 5-day program to teach patients and their families how to regulate their medication and diet. As part of the medical treatment program, blood tests to monitor sugar and insulin levels were routinely administered on an average of four times a day. The researchers needed to measure platelet serotonin and cortisol levels three times a day for 2 days at regular intervals to obtain information on physiological indicators of depression and anxiety, respectively. The investigative team developed a schedule for each child that would overlap as much as possible with his or her medical venipunctures (see Case 2).

Protecting Participant Confidentiality

The investigators wanted to guard against breaches of confidentiality concerning the child's physiological status (awareness of medical data by the research team) and the child's psychophysiological status (awareness of the psychological data by the medical team). The investigators decided that the best way to protect the rights of the participants was to collect the data anonymously. They spoke with the hospital medical team who agreed to administer the blood tests. In addition, following the medical team's analysis of the blood, the samples were given to the researchers with only a subject number. This number would allow hospital personnel to provide researchers with demographic and medical histories from patient charts without revealing personally identifying information. The researchers would not share with the medical team findings concerning individual patients. In addition, when recording their results, the researchers would use a separate coding system so that the patient's serotonin and cortisol levels could not be identified by hospital staff.

CASE 34: DEVELOPMENTAL CORRELATES OF EXPOSURE TO COMMUNITY VIOLENCE IN A SAMPLE OF MIDDLE AND HIGH SCHOOL STUDENTS

Research Goals

In this study, the investigators collaborated with several middle and high schools to develop a school-based intervention to help children minimize exposure to and distress associated with being victimized or witnessing community violence. The first year of the project was devoted to establishing baseline data from which several intervention strategies could be developed. Student responses to questionnaires provided data on the frequency of exposure to acts of violence observed or experienced personally as a victim or perpetrator; the psychosocial impact of these experiences; the relationship of individual coping styles to both involvement and reactions to violent acts; the degree to which parental and peer social support influences such involvement and/or distress; and student preferences for specific school-based programs. The investigators also conducted a survey of community services (e.g., police, legal services, social services) available to crime victims.

Confidentiality Versus Anonymity

The investigators believed that the greatest risk to participants at this baseline phase would be a violation of confidentiality resulting in a report to authorities about crimes in which students had been a victim, witness, or perpetrator. Confidentiality could be protected through subject codes, secure data storage, and obtaining a Certificate of Confidentiality. With a Certificate of Confidentiality, the investigators would not be required to respond to subpoenas regarding criminal activities.

However, school administrators and members of the investigative team felt a responsibility to help children if they knew of a specific serious incident that was troubling them. Because neither the survey on the availability and adequacy of community services for crime victims and witnesses nor the creation of a formal program for helping students would be completed until the following year, the investigators were concerned that any efforts to assist children would be premature and could have potentially negative consequences. Moreover, given the developmental status of the participants, having such identifying information could be counterproductive to the long-term goals of the school-based intervention program. Specifically, student knowledge that school personnel and members of the research team knew of, but did not report, specific crimes, might inadvertently serve as a model to students that such crimes should not be reported. Finally, given the community's concern about increasing neighborhood violence and the fact that there have been no court cases to test the scope of the Certificate of Confidentiality's protection, there was a slight risk that research records could be subject to subpoena. On this basis, the investigators decided that all information would be collected anonymously.

Collecting Data Anonymously Over Several Days

The battery of self-report instruments was time intensive, requiring approximately 2 hours to complete. Classroom schedules and student activities made collecting the data in one period impossible. The investigators, therefore, developed the following procedure for collecting the data anonymously over several days. On the first day of testing, each student was given three stickers with the same number written on each sticker. This became the student's subject number, known only to the student. The numbers were distributed randomly across classes to prevent any chance of inferring a student's identity from his or her subject number. On the first day of testing, participants were asked to place one of the stickers on their answer sheet and to keep the remaining stickers for the following test days. On subsequent test days, students placed these stickers on the last page of the test booklet. Each day, the participants were reminded to keep their numbers confidential. The investigators were aware that some students might lose their numbers. For added protection students were asked to select a "code name" for themselves (e.g., "Batman," "Catwoman," "Bingo") and to print the code name on the back of each test booklet. Students enjoyed this task.

CASE 35: A CROSS-SECTIONAL COMPARISON OF PARENTING STYLES IN PARENTS WITH AND WITHOUT ALCOHOL USE DISORDERS

Research Goals

Developmental psychologists in a large urban city designed a cross-sectional descriptive study of parenting styles of alcoholic mothers and fathers. The purpose of the study had been greeted enthusiastically by several Alcoholic Anonymous (AA) programs throughout the city and the program leaders had agreed to help with recruitment. Data to be obtained included extensive videotaped records of parent–child (2–5 years of age) interactions in a series of controlled (e.g., Strange Situation) and semicontrolled (e.g., eating lunch together, playing) situations. A matched sample of parents without identified alcohol abuse problems would also be tested.

Procedures for Protecting Confidentiality

The research team was aware that ethical issues regarding privacy (see Case 14 for how these issues were addressed during subject recruitment) and confidentiality would be primary concerns in this study. To ensure that these issues were adequately identified and addressed, they established an advisory committee of AA leaders, AA members, and practitioners specializing in substance abuse who met regularly with researchers to brainstorm on ethical issues.

The Certificate of Confidentiality and Information Regarding Child Abuse. Alcoholism is sometimes associated with other forms of substance abuse; thus the investigators felt it was important to obtain information regarding current usage of both alcohol and drugs. To protect participants the research team applied for and received a Certificate of Confidentiality to provide immunity from subpoena of research records that might contain information about illegal drug-related behavior. They designed informed consent procedures to communicate this information to prospective participants. The consents also indicated that the Certificate had not yet been tested in court and that the researchers were under legal obligation to report information that suggested child abuse.

The research team and advisory committee thought it a strong possibility that some of the research participants may have abused their children on alcoholic binges prior to their participation in the study. Although any such abuse would be tragic, the researchers and committee members believed that abuse-related questions concerning previous behaviors would place the researchers in the role of "investigator" and subject parents to revealing information that the researcher knew might provide incriminating evidence that would have to be reported to authorities. It was decided that no such questions would be asked.

The Use of Videotape. A third concern involved the use of videotape in the parent–child interactions. The researchers believed that the data could not be adequately coded in the detail needed to provide scientifically valid and valuable information unless raters had access to multiple viewings of the behaviors. The investigators decided that to ensure the scientific integrity of the research, videotapes would be used (with the permission of the parent). Informed consents would indicate that the tapes would only be viewed by research personnel and kept in a secure area, that the parent would be given an opportunity to with-draw the videotapes from data collection after the session had been filmed, and that the parent would have the opportunity to request to have the video destroyed at the completion of the data analysis phase of the study. In addition, all written materials regarding data collection would contain only a subject number with the code for that subject number restricted to the primary investigator. (See Case 26 for further discussion on informed consent for videotaping.)

Responding to a Spouse's Request to View Videotapes. D u r i n g the study, the husband of a participant parent approached a research staff member and asked if he could view the video data of his wife and child. The staff member told him that all data were confidential and were used only for research purposes. He persisted by saying that the videotape was about his own family and therefore should be available to him. The staff person referred him to the psychiatrist on the project. In contacting the psychiatrist, the husband indicated that he was initi-ating divorce proceedings and was asking for child custody rights on grounds that the mother was incapable of giving adequate care to the child. The psychiatrist explained the confidentiality of the data and refused the request. At this point, the psychiatrist also informed the husband of the availability of the institution's legal office. The husband took the posture that he should have gone immediately to the legal office and would do so. However, he did not make any further attempts to obtain the "evidence on his wife."

CASE 36: AN EPIDEMIOLOGICAL STUDY OF PATTERNS OF MENTAL HEALTH SERVICE USE BY RURAL ADOLESCENTS

Research Goals

The purpose of this study was to look at the development of psychopa-thology and patterns of service use from prepuberty to late adolescence in rural families representing a broad range of socioeconomic levels. Over the course of 3 years, service usage was evaluated every 3 months. Children and their families were seen yearly for full psychiatric evalu-ations. (See also Case 47 for a discussion of participant referrals.)

Reporting Child Abuse

During a psychiatric interview, a prepubertal child revealed that a man in the neighborhood had repeatedly inspected the boy's genitals for disease and had the boy do the same. The interviewer reminded the boy about the consent form that had stated that child abuse would be reported and told him that his parents would be informed. The parents were called and reminded of the researcher's obligation to report child abuse to local authorities. The parents agreed to file a joint report with the PI. The parents were also told that there was no evidence in the psychiatric interview that the boy was clinically impaired by this experience.

Releasing Research Data as Evidence of Abuse Allegations

Although the man involved in the abuse admitted his guilt, the local grand jury decided there was not enough information for prosecution. The investigating police officer approached research team members to ask if they would release reports and interview tapes as evidence. This request brought up issues regarding the research team's responsibility to the child, the child's parents, other research subjects, and potential participants.

Team members reviewed their informed consent procedures. The consent form stated that child abuse would be reported to the authorities, but did not say that information gained during the research interview would be released. In addition, the researchers had obtained a Certificate of Confidentiality and had promised both parents and children that all other information would be confidential.

The researchers realized that to release the interview tapes they would need the consent of both the parents and the child. Their notes on follow-up interviews with the child indicated that he did not show signs of psychopathology related to the abuse and that he had expressed a desire to be finished with the legal process related to it. The researchers were concerned that if they, as mental health professionals, requested permission for the release of information, the child or his family might feel pressured or obligated to consent.

An additional consideration was the welfare of other participants in the study. Given that the research was being conducted in a small town, other participants would be aware that information was released and might be concerned that their data were not secure. The credibility of the entire research enterprise and fiduciary responsibility of the scientists would then be in question. Taking all these matters into account, the researchers decided not to ask the parents for permission to release the information and to tell the police investigator that they would not provide any additional information.

CASE 37: A STUDY OF PSYCHOLOGICAL STRESSORS AND DISORDERS IN GAY AND LESBIAN ADOLESCENTS

Research Goals

The purpose of this study was to examine psychosocial stressors and prevalence of anxiety and depressive disorders in 14- to 18-year-old gay and lesbian adolescents. Access to this population was obtained through a gay and lesbian community center. The adolescents who came to the center were from a broad section of schools in the community. This enabled the researchers to obtain a sample size that would not have been feasible if the general population of each school was sampled and students were asked to identify their sexual orientation on a written form. Most of the teens who attended the center had not told their parents of their sexual orientation and many were concerned that negative reprisals would result if their parents were told or information was inadvertently released to their teachers or schoolmates. Center staff were very enthusiastic about the project and supportive of having students interviewed at the center. (See Case 27 for a description of assent procedures when the requirement for parental consent is waived.)

Excluding Questions About Child Maltreatment and Informing Participants of the Requirement to Report Child Abuse

The investigators considered the confidentiality of the data a critical ethical responsibility in this study. They recognized that one threat to confidentiality was their obligation to report information they might learn about suspected child abuse. Although the issue of maltreatment in the families of gay and lesbian youth is important, asking such questions would place the participants at risk of exposing their sexual orientation (associated with their participation in the study) to protective services and ultimately to their parents and community. This had the potential to stigmatize the youth, limit employment and/or health insurance opportunities, and in some cases could put the youths at risk for violent reactions from family members. The investigators therefore decided that no questions directly related to child abuse would be asked. The consent forms did however inform the teens that the researchers were required to report child abuse if they learned of it.

CASE 38: THE DEVELOPMENT
OF A SCREENING PROGRAM TO IDENTIFY
ADOLESCENTS AT RISK FOR SUICIDE

Research Goals

This project involved a two-stage screening program to identify adolescents at risk for suicide. The project targeted adolescents in Grades 10 through 12. One of the ethical provisions of the informed consent was to give the adolescent a veto over investigators informing either a parent or a treatment agency about problems identified during the investigation unless the youth gave an indication of suicidality or indicated she or he had experienced child abuse.

Respecting Versus Overriding an Adolescent's
Request Not to Report Impaired Functioning

During the course of research, a youth screened positive and, on interview, was found to meet criteria for major depressive disorder and alcohol abuse. The youth gave no indication that he was or had been suicidal (i.e., he responded negatively in at least five places to questions about whether he had ever had suicidal ideation or had ever made a suicide attempt). After the assessment was completed, the adolescent was told that he appeared to be suffering from significant psychiatric problems and that his mother should be informed of this and that treatment should be sought. He stated that he would not give his approval for this, that he did not believe that he needed treatment, and that his mother should not be told. Abiding by the protocol, no further action was taken. Seven months after the survey was completed, the youth committed suicide.

The research team reviewed the protocol and applied to their IRB for an amendment to the effect that information about significant impairing diagnosis (i.e., any condition that would lead to personal psychiatric distress and/or impaired social or educational functioning) should be passed on to the child's caretaker regardless of the adolescent's consent. The only exception would be if there was evidence that imparting this information to the caretaker would lead to abuse, in which case information would be passed to the appropriate child welfare agency.

CASE 39: EVALUATION OF A COMMUNITY-BASED TREATMENT PROGRAM FOR CHILD MOLESTERS

Research Goals

This project compared the effectiveness of two methods of community-based treatment for child molesters. The first approach treated deviant sexual cognitions with rational emotive therapy (RET). The second approach provided RET plus behavior therapy, with a focus on identifying and treating recidivist tendencies with relapse prevention. Participants had engaged in illegal sexual offenses and were predominantly referred to the program by probation officers, mental health professionals, lawyers, and judges.

Stated Limitations on Confidentiality

Investigators received a Certificate of Confidentiality providing them protection against the obligation to release current criminal activity. The informed consent procedures indicated that the research staff would report known instances of the commission of a specific sexual offense against a specific person. The investigators sought to balance the responsibility to provide effective treatments and evaluations of such treatments against the obligation to protect the community from identifiable danger. They took the position that they were required to report only those instances when there was an identifiable victim. They went to great lengths to develop interview and treatment procedures that would preclude their coming into possession of specific information about victims, parents, or guardians. Participant-clients were given repeated instructions to discuss their behaviors in a general manner without revealing names or specific locations of events.

The Duty to Protect

The major potential threat to community members occurred when an acute client crisis signaled impending relapse or an actual reoffense. Participant-clients who experienced an acute crisis were encouraged to stay at the community center under supervision until it was determined that the crisis had been resolved. In cases of impending relapse, the participant's mental status, frequency and duration of deviant thoughts or fantasies, offense-related behaviors (i.e., cruising), accessibility of a victim, and the means to cause harm were assessed. Clients were assisted in developing a course of action and their behavior in and out of the center was monitored. As indicated during informed consent procedures (administered throughout several phases of the project), if a client did not follow the terms of the plan, the appropriate authorities were notified.

Terminating Participation and Reporting the Termination to Authorities

A 27-year-old client who had numerous sexual contacts with children communicated to his therapist difficulties in controlling his urges to act out with underage males. He was judged to be in need of intensive therapy and it was recommended that he make regular contact with the center on a daily basis until his sexual urges were under control, that he begin behavior therapy (aversive conditioning) immediately, and that he begin daily self-reporting of urges and fantasies. After several individual sessions, the client began group work using a cognitive behavioral model. In addition, he was receiving individual behavior therapy three times a week, and his sexual urges seemingly were becoming more controllable. He had not acted out up until this point.

At about 6 months into treatment the client began having physical symptoms of fatigue and depression. He reported to a hospital where he was tested and diagnosed as HIV positive. The client was instructed that he would need to have a more regimented treatment plan to ensure no sexual acting out. The client felt discriminated against and began to be noncompliant with treatment. The client began high-risk behaviors (cruising, peeping, exposing himself). The client was given further individual sessions, behavioral contracts, and warnings regarding his compliance with treatment. After several rule infractions, the client was terminated from the treatment program. His probation officer was informed of the termination and the need to closely supervise this client. The client was eventually arrested for masturbating in a public restroom in the presence of a child.

*   *   *

Casebook

Modifying Procedures During the Course of Clinical Trials

Although the risks and benefits of clinical trials research are carefully thought out during the design stage and approved by an IRB, often during the course of therapeutic research, therapists or parents may raise questions about a child or adolescent's reaction to an experimental condition. Federal regulations require that the progress of clinical trials research is adequately monitored to ensure the continued protection of research participations (Federal Policy 46.111 [a][6]). The OPRR (1993) further recommends that placebos be stopped or protocols modified when there is sufficient evidence that the treatment is producing significant benefits or unacceptable side effects. Thus, at all phases of clinical trials research, an investigator must continue to assess the balance of participant risks and benefits within the context of maintaining a formal relationship between data and conclusions that can yield scientific facts about the value of the therapeutic approach. Case 40 illustrates how procedures for managing side effects in a drug study can be incorporated into the statistical analysis of treatment efficacy. In Case 41, investigators consider altering the timing of a placebo washout condition to protect participants from negative social consequences tied to termination of an effective experimental treatment.

BREAKING THE BLIND IN A SINGLE OR DOUBLE MASKED STUDY

Studies evaluating the efficacy of a therapeutic strategy will often compare the outcome of individuals randomly assigned to this therapy condition to that of individuals randomly assigned to a conventional treatment or a placebo. To rule out the influence of experimenter or participant expectation in randomized clinical trials (RCT), individual treatment assignments are not known by research staff and/or participants (double blind and single blind studies respectively). In such studies, investigators are required to develop procedures that will allow the blind to be broken in case of emergency, that is, when a participant has a negative reaction to his or her experimental assignment (OPRR, 1993).

Ethical challenges arise in determining the criteria under which the blind should be broken. For example, sometimes during a crossover design (in which each participant experiences the experimental and control treatment at randomly assigned times) teachers, parents, or clinical staff may become concerned that a child's behavior is deteriorating. This deterioration may be the result of a negative reaction to an experimental medication. In such instances, the child should be taken off the medication and possibly withdrawn from the study. Alternatively, the change in behavior may be a return to baseline levels, following a particularly successful treatment phase of the study. In such instances, breaking the blind precipitously would unnecessarily compromise the scientific integrity of the study.

One way to assure that neither scientific rigor nor participant safety is sacrificed when questions regarding the child's reaction to an arm of the study are raised is to compare the child's current behavior to his or her baseline behavior assessed prior to the onset of the clinical trials (often during a nonblind placebo washout phase). If the child's behavior is commensurate with baseline measures, then the blind need not be broken immediately. The situation should be discussed with the parents and, with their agreement, the child's behavior should be carefully monitored to ensure that it does not go below baseline levels (see Case 42).

In therapeutic research conducted in successive waves with child or adolescent participants, maintaining the blind even after a patient has completed his or her participation in the study may be a necessary means of avoiding investigator bias. Although this ensures the scientific integrity of the research, it may deprive the participant of necessary information concerning follow-up treatment. In these situations, investigators may arrange for treatment disclosures to former participants conducted by an independent person who provides safeguards against former participants sharing this information with investigators (see Case 43).

RESPONDING TO REQUESTS FROM CLINICAL STAFF TO MODIFY RESEARCH PROCEDURES

One way in which clinical trials studies differ from standard clinical treatment is in the primacy of the research staff over the therapist in decisions regarding patient care (see Imber et al., 1986). For example, although the therapist can make recommendations, ultimate responsibility for assessing treatment qualifications of potential patients, the mode of treatment a patient will receive (i.e., decided through random assignment), when a patient should be withdrawn from a particular clinical arm, and whether referral for additional care is appropriate rests with the research team rather than the treating clinician. It is important that when a clinician suggests a child is having a negative reaction to planned procedures, investigators guard against conflicts of interest that may bias decision making against the best interests of the clinical trials participant. One way to accomplish this is to weigh the concerns of therapists in equal balance with scientific requirements when making decisions about withdrawal or modifications in research procedures for individual participants.

Manualized Therapy. To ensure the scientific validity of most clinical trials studying psychosocial or behavioral interventions, treatments must be administered in a uniform manner by therapists who have been carefully trained to meet certain behavioral criteria. At the same time, to assure the clinical applicability of the experimental treatment, treatment manuals must allow for an acceptable balance between adherence to treatment procedures and opportunities for clinical judgment.

On some occasions, a therapist may express concern that the manualized treatment is inadequate for the needs of a particular patient (see Case 44). If the research staff agree with the therapist's concerns, then the patient should be withdrawn from the study and offered an available alternative treatment. If the research staff does not agree that the manualized treatment is inadequate for this patient, they should explore with the therapist potential ways in which treatment guidelines can be applied to promote the patient's welfare. When these concerns cannot be reconciled, an independent senior clinician, with no clinical or administrative responsibilities in the study, should be authorized to make the final decision regarding the patient's continued involvement in the research (Imber et al., 1986).

Random Assignment. One particular distinction between clinical trials research and standard treatment is the restrictions such research imposes on the subjectivity and flexibility of clinical decision making (Imber et al., 1986). This may raise problems for clinical staff involved in the recruitment or treatment of participants in therapeutic research who may believe that a specific arm of the research may provide greater benefits for a particular patient (see Case 45). In this situation, the investigator should review with the staff member the scientific and ethical bases for the study. In most circumstances, this involves discussing how, for the population under investigation, the experimental treatment has not been empirically established to be superior to either the control treatment or any available treatment. At the same time, the investigator should reconsider whether the patient's particular mental health profile would place the child or adolescent at special risk if he or she participated in the study in lieu of receiving available standard treatment. The purpose of randomization is to rule out bias in selection of subjects for experimental and control groups; thus under no circumstances can a therapist's recommendation provide a basis for assignment to one arm of an RCT.

CLINICAL CARE DURING A TREATMENT FOLLOW-UP PERIOD

The ability to document the extent to which the effects of an experimental treatment will persist over time should be a critical component of clinical trials research. Clearly, an important means of assessing the direct and societal benefits of a treatment is to determine its long-term impact on patient mental health. This has led some investigators to view any response to requests for additional or supplementary treatments following the clinical trials as contaminants of the research process. At the end of the treatment phase, these investigators may encourage participants who have responded positively to the experimental treatment to delay as long as possible seeking additional medical or psychological support.

Increasingly, however, this position is seen as inadequate from both a scientific and ethical perspective. From a scientific perspective, refraining from supplementary care following a successful treatment may not be an indication of a positive reaction to treatment. It is just as likely that a positive reaction would lead patients to continue to utilize mental health professionals as resources for life adaptation when needed (see Cases 45 and 46). In addition, because it is ethically unacceptable to request that protocol failures refrain from seeking additional treatment, a comparison of the use of adjunctive therapies by participants in different arms of the clinical trials can be an excellent empirical source for determining the continued efficacy of a treatment after it has been terminated. Finally, given the vulnerability of children and adolescents with mental disorders, a request not to seek further treatment may be unduly coercive to participants and their families, especially if they see honoring this request as a condition for their participation in the research.

CASE 40: PHARMACOLOGICAL
TREATMENT OF HYPERACTIVE
CHILDREN WITH MENTAL RETARDATION

Research Goals

The purpose of this study was to assess the behavioral, cognitive, and physiological side effects of fenfluramine (Pondimin) as an alternative to methylphenidate (Ritalin) in hyperactive children (5–13 years) with mental retardation. Five drug conditions were to be compared: a placebo, three doses of fenfluramine, and one dose of methylphenidate. Each drug condition was to be given for 2 weeks with order determined by a complex Latin square assignment. All parties having contact with the children, including their parents, teachers, and study personnel, were blind to the medication sequence. Prior to starting the protocol, each child would also take a known placebo for 1 week. (See Case 4 for a discussion of risk–benefit assessment.)

Managing Physiological Side Effects

With a dose study such as this, the appearance of side effects is a fairly common problem. Parents are given a verbal and written description of the most common side effects at the beginning of the study. Parents are also provided office and home phone numbers of the PI and the inpatient pharmacy in the event of an emergency. Both the PI and the inpatient pharmacy have sealed envelopes with a medication code for each child should untoward effects or an emergency occur. (See Cases 21 and 56 for discussions of parental consent and debriefing procedures, respectively.)

Perhaps the most common phone calls received concern routine colds and infections that the children get, with inquiries about whether any prescribed medication is likely to interact with study medications. In these cases, the investigators check to ensure that adverse interactions cannot occur between the study medication and the newly prescribed drug (usually amoxicillin). If the child is badly affected by the illness and his or her behavior appears to be atypical, the study medication is often suspended altogether until he or she is feeling better. If illness has occupied a significant portion of a treatment phase, a week or more of the study medication may be added to extend that phase so that a sufficient sample of "uncontaminated" behavior is available.

Another problem is the appearance of side effects with the medium or high dose of fenfluramine. A few of the subjects have become very drowsy, dizzy, or tearful with the higher doses. If these appear unacceptable to the parents, the investigators try to get the child in for testing the next morning and then suspend the remainder of medication for that treatment phase. If the side effects are intolerable in the parents' view, the medication is simply terminated immediately. In the latter case, it is possible to obtain rating scale data, but the investigators have to forego collecting cardiovascular measures or performance tests. If a child has an unacceptable reaction to medication early on in the trial, the PI checks to see what condition caused the reaction. If this occurred with low or medium doses of fenfluramine, then any higher doses are eliminated from the trial for that child.

Managing Behavior Regression

Another problem occasionally encountered is significant regression of behavior when the child begins the placebo phase. The schools are often more likely to complain about such deterioration than parents. Most complaints are likely to occur during a placebo phase immediately after a particularly successful treatment phase. The schools sometimes place considerable pressure on parents to terminate the medication condition or involvement with the study with implied or emphatic threats to suspend the child if his or her behavior does not improve. In such circumstances, the investigators usually try to collect at least 1 week of data, while reassuring the parties concerned. However, the child is brought in earlier, if necessary, to protect him or her from adverse disciplinary consequences (see Case 41).

Minimizing Risk and Threats to Internal Validity

All of these problems pose threats to the internal validity of the study. Any change in the length of treatment intervals can have implications for changes on certain dependent variables, such as body weight. Weight gain or loss, for example, will be affected by the duration of the treatment interval. Also, the dropping out of subjects having side effects with fenfluramine necessarily is somewhat selective, and this could create the false impression that higher doses are better than, in fact, is the case. That is, only subjects able to tolerate all three doses would be represented in the final analysis of dosage effects. One way to counter this false impression is to present the number of subjects showing their *optimal* response at each dose or, alternatively, the numbers able to *tolerate* each treatment. In this case, dropouts presumptively will appear to do better at lower doses.

CASE 41: ASSESSING PSYCHOSOCIAL TREATMENT AS AN EFFECTIVE AUGMENTATION TO MEDICATION FOR CHILDREN WITH ADHD

Research Goals

These investigators were interested in learning whether psychosocial treatment could improve the efficacy of medication for children with ADHD. Children were randomly assigned to a medication only, a medication with psychosocial treatment condition, or a placebo with psychosocial treatment condition. The treatments started in September so that teacher as well as parental reports could be used as outcome measures. To see if the child was benefiting from the medication, or if he or she could do well without medication, at the end of the treatment period, children in the medication conditions were given a placebo challenge. Parents and teachers were not informed when this challenge would take place.

Altering the Timing of a Placebo Challenge

At the end of the first year of the study, a mother of a child on a placebo challenge called to say her child was doing poorly, and that his functioning had so deteriorated that he had performed terribly on a statewide exam during that week. His performance on the exam would affect his school placement during the following year. The teacher reports corroborated that the child had deteriorated on placebo.

The mother was informed that the child had been on placebo and he was placed back on medication. At the mother's request, the investigators informed the principal about the placebo trial and asked if the school would be willing to retest the child on an alternative form of the statewide test. The principal agreed.

Because this was likely to happen to other participants, with approval from their IRB, the research team modified their protocol. At the beginning of the school year they received each child's end of the year achievement test schedule and pushed the date of the placebo challenge up if it interfered with school testing. The investigators believed that the minimal effect this change could have on the "purity" of the data collection procedures was worth not putting the child in a precarious position.

CASE 42: EVALUATING THE EFFECT OF A NEW ANTIDEPRESSANT FOR ADOLESCENTS WITH CHRONIC DEPRESSION

Research Goals

The purpose of this study was to test the effect of a new antidepressant against a placebo for adolescents with chronic depression. The patients had not responded to any treatment over the course of at least four admissions to a state hospital. Patients were randomly assigned by a computer program to a 12-week medication or placebo group. Both groups received supportive psychotherapy. All participants were given a placebo for the first 2 weeks of the study to wash out effects of other medications. Those who continued to have depression after the 2 weeks were entered into the study.

Responding to a Physician's Request to Break the Medication Blind

During the sixth week of the study, one of the attending physicians voiced concern about a patient's behavior. The physician believed the child was having a negative reaction to the treatment and wanted to break the medication/placebo code to change the patient's medication. The researchers deliberated on the wisdom of taking the child out of the study. They decided to compare the child's behavior to the placebo washout condition. They found that the child's current behavioral and psychosocial indicators were not lower than they had been at baseline condition. The researchers, therefore, decided to keep the child in the clinical trial for another 2 weeks, closely monitored by staff. The child's behavior improved, and at the end of the study it was found that he had been in the medication group.

CASE 43: LONGITUDINAL RESEARCH ON THE EFFICACY OF A PSYCHOPHARMACOLOGICAL TREATMENT FOR ADOLESCENT SCHOOL REFUSAL

Research Goals

This was a double-blind placebo-controlled study evaluating the efficacy of imipramine compared to placebo, each in combination with cognitive-behavioral therapy. Participating adolescents (12–18 years) met criteria for anxiety disorder and major depression and had missed at least 20% to 30% of school days in the previous month. Adolescents and their parents participated in eight scheduled treatment appointments that included cognitive-behavioral therapy and medication management (e.g., vital signs, monitoring side effects). Of the 25 adolescents who entered the protocol, 21 completed the study over the 5 years it was conducted.

Reasons for Not Breaking the Blind at the End of Each Participant's Treatment

When the study was designed and approved by the IRB it had been decided that breaking the blind for each adolescent after he or she completed the study would compromise the research because members of the research team would be biased by knowing how individual adolescents responded to the different treatment combinations. For example, if one adolescent responded to imipramine in combination with therapy in a certain way, another adolescent who responded similarly might be expected to be in the imipramine condition as well. This could influence how an adolescent was treated by the research staff and how his or her symptoms were viewed. Consequently, during the informed consent process for participation in the first year of the study, each family was told that they would only be able to find out to which treatment condition (imipramine or placebo) their adolescent had been randomly assigned after the entire study had been completed.

Toward the end of their participation in the study, all participants were tapered off the study medications, which usually took about 10 to 16 days (depending on the medication dosage). At this time, adolescents and/or their families were offered referral options for ongoing treatment. Because the blind was not broken for subjects at the end of their participation in the study, families and future treatment providers did not know if imipramine had proven helpful to the adolescent or if they had done well on psychosocial intervention with placebo.

Reasons for Breaking the Blind at the End of Each Participant's Treatment

After the first year of the study, some team members continued to feel strongly that the research should not be potentially compromised by breaking the blind for individual subjects. Other team members thought families should have access to treatment information upon completion of the study based on several reasons. First, by not providing medication information the family and next treatment provider would not have all the information necessary to design an optimal treatment plan. Second, adolescents who were doing well on the study medication should have the opportunity to continue with current treatment. If they were taking imipramine with a remission of symptoms, discontinuation of the medication could lead to a relapse of symptoms. If they were responding well to placebo, imipramine might be prescribed unnecessarily. Conversely, if a subject was doing poorly under either condition another medication could be considered. The members of the research team believed treatment decisions are important and should be made with as much information as possible.

Upon reevaluation, the research team felt that the method of preserving the blind was hindering families' treatment decisions because a vital piece of information was missing. Once this was decided, the research team worked out the following plan for how to best execute the option of breaking the blind for individual subjects while maintaining the integrity of the research. All final ratings regarding each adolescent's treatment response would be required to be returned to the research team prior to the blind being broken. This assured that adolescents and parents were not influenced in how they completed their final ratings by knowing the treatment condition.

Once the rating scales were completed, families would have the option of contacting a psychiatrist who had knowledge of the child's experimental condition assignment. This team member, who did not have contact with participants during the study, was responsible for monitoring laboratory results (e.g., imipramine serum levels) of all participants. Families could contact the psychiatrist directly or have their physician contact the psychiatrist to obtain information about whether their adolescent had been randomized to imipramine or placebo. Families were given specific instructions to not let any of the team members know to which medication condition their adolescent had been assigned. Once this policy was initiated, many families decided to break the blind and they honored their promise not to share information with the research team members.

CASE 44: BEHAVIORAL OUTCOMES
OF A PSYCHOSOCIAL INTERVENTION
FOR PATIENTS WITH CHILDHOOD AUTISM

Research Goals

In a study on the efficacy of a psychosocial intervention for patients with childhood autism, hospital therapists were given a treatment manual to ensure that treatment would be conducted in a standardized manner across therapists. Clinical staff were trained on the manual and expected not to deviate from its techniques during the course of the study.

Responding to Staff Concerns
About Manualized Therapy

At several points in the study, some of the clinical staff raised concerns about "manualized" therapy when they felt that there was a clinical issue that needed to be addressed outside the manual guidelines. The investigators handled these concerns as follows. First, no deviations from the manual would be considered unless they involved what the therapist believed was a clinical crisis. If that situation arose, the therapist would discuss the nature of the crisis with the research team and efforts were made to address the therapist's concern within the context of the manual.

If, after attempting to implement the research team's recommendations, the therapist felt that the crisis was still not being adequately handled, a second independent therapist, not affiliated with the research team, would be asked to evaluate the issue. If the second therapist decided that the patient was in crisis and not able to respond to the research protocol, the patient would be pulled from the study and receive the treatment recommended by the therapist and expert. The number of such patients were reported in the summary of results. This situation arose for only a very small percentage of the experimental population, so it was not included as a factor in the analysis.

CASE 45: ASSESSING THE EFFICACY
OF A PROBLEM-SOLVING INTERVENTION
TARGETING SUICIDAL ADOLESCENTS
AND YOUNG ADULTS

Research Goals

This study evaluated the effectiveness of a time-limited, outpatient problem-solving intervention targeting suicidal adolescents and young adults. Participants were randomly assigned to either the experimental treatment or the treatment-as-usual control condition. Patients engaged in the experimental treatment attended 14 days of intensive group meetings at the treatment facility. The treatment was structured on a problem-solving and social competence paradigm. A comprehensive intake assessment and biannual follow-up was conducted over a 2-year period. It was predicted that both groups would improve over time, but that those in the experimental group would gain significantly better problem-solving skills immediately after the intervention and during the follow-up period, whereas controls would evidence degradation of any initial problem-solving gains. (See Case 8 for discussion on selecting an appropriate control condition.)

Responding to Staff Requests to Assign
Patients to Specific Arms of the Research

The few problems that did arise revolved primarily around potential staff overinvolvement. In certain cases, treatment staff wanted to have their patients enter the experimental treatment in order to get what they believed to be the best possible care. Despite infrequent requests, no exceptions to randomization were allowed and in each case the scientific/research commitment and related agenda of the project were reviewed. As an additional step to ensure that those randomized to the control group were not lost in the system, and also to alleviate staff anxieties and ensure appropriate clinical care, at the end of the first phase of the study, the initial follow-up appointment with an identified staff member was confirmed for the patient. In addition, provisions were made so that this clinical staff member could remain constant across the 3-year research period.

Access to Treatment During Long-Term Follow-Up

Following referral and confirmation that inclusion criteria had been met, all subjects willing to participate reviewed and signed a statement of informed consent detailing the purpose, procedures, and goals of the study. Random assignment to a group was noted and discussed in detail with all participants at this time. An additional area of emphasis during this initial interview was the long-term nature of follow-up that would integrate periodic telephone and mail-out procedures as needed. Given the severity of the problems that precipitated treatment and the issues addressed in the course of treatment, the investigators did not restrict access to treatment augmentation during the follow-up period. Rather, they logged ongoing treatment of any kind as a follow-up variable along with recurrence or reemergence of suicidal or self-destructive behavior.

Because one of the primary goals of the intervention program was to prevent a recurrence or reemergence of suicidal behavior, they viewed effective treatment as enabling the individual to access available resources when and if needed. Accordingly, all individuals completing treatment (as well as control subjects), were apprised of available resources both in terms of emergency services and available longer term individual or group treatment. To the investigators' surprise, relatively few individuals actually accessed longer term treatment. However, a number of participants did from time to time access emergency services as needed. The investigators viewed this as evidence of successful intervention and treatment and, as noted, integrated it into the follow-up assessment batteries as a variable.

CASE 46: A PREVENTIVE EDUCATION PROGRAM
FOR PARENTS OF AUTISTIC CHILDREN

Research Goals

The purpose of this study was to assess the comparative efficacy of two 24-session behavior management programs for parents of autistic children ages 5 to 15. One program focused on teaching parents behavior modification techniques. The other taught parents how to teach their children self-management skills. Pretest and outcome measures included laboratory-based assessment of child behaviors and cognitive status as well as parental self-reports on stress and family environment. Posttesting was conducted at 6 months and 1 year following the end of the intervention.

Responding to Requests for Assistance
During a Follow-Up Period

The researchers struggled with what to do if, during the follow-up period, parents called in for consultation regarding their child's behavior problems. The researchers felt a dual obligation to avoid contaminating the follow-up assessment and to continue to be a resource for participating parents. They looked to previous research for guidance. In earlier work they had discovered that helping parents with specific problems did not appear to generalize to other parenting behaviors. They, therefore, reasoned that when a parent called in a crisis situation, recommending highly specific actions to ease the crisis would not contaminate an intervention aimed at enhancing the ability to use a broad range of behavioral principles. To further protect the scientific integrity of the study, they informed participants from both experimental groups that following the 24 treatment sessions the research team would be available for emergency phone contact, but not for treatment. The number of times parents called for postintervention assistance was then included as an outcome variable.

* * *

Casebook

Offering Services Beyond Those Required by the Research Protocol

During the course of research with high-risk or disordered children and adolescents, experimental methods may tap previously undetected emotional, cognitive, or social problems for which formal assessment or treatment lies outside the research protocol. When encountered during the implementation of nontreatment explanatory or descriptive studies, the detection of these vulnerabilities may raise ethical issues concerning the validity of risk estimates, participant autonomy, and scientific responsibility (Fisher, 1993, 1994). When such evidence arises during the conduct of therapeutic research, the possibility of offering adjunctive referrals or treatment raises ethical concerns about the balance between participant protections and establishing the validity of the therapeutic approach under appropriately controlled experimental conditions. Both situations place the investigator in what Veatch (1987) coined the *scientist-citizen dilemma*: the need to reconcile the researcher's professional commitment to the production of scientific knowledge with his or her humanitarian commitment to participant welfare. Case 47 poignantly illustrates this dilemma when a research team struggles with their humanitarian responsibility to an impoverished family.

The mental health scientific tradition, like other human subjects' research traditions, has typically drawn on an act utilitarian metaethical position when responding to reporting or referring decisions that may threaten the internal validity of an experiment (Beauchamp, Faden, Wallace, & Walters, 1992; Mill, 1861/1957). As a result, when a conflict has arisen between scientific rigor and the discovery that a participant may need assistance outside the research protocol, the investigator's responsibility to produce data that can benefit members of society has often been seen to supersede his or her obligation to the individual participant (Fisher, 1994). However, as the cases in this section illustrate, in recent years researchers have struggled with developing procedures that can allow them to meet the dual obligations of scientific responsibility and participant care (Fisher, 1993, 1994; Fisher, Higgins, Rau, Kuther, & Belanger, in press).

ESTABLISHING CRITERIA FOR EVALUATING RISK

The Validity of Risk Estimates. When considering the implications of providing referrals or treatments to research participants outside the research protocol, investigators must consider whether the research-derived information provides a valid means of identifying specific developmental disorders or risks. Investigators must be wary of the potential to overestimate or underestimate the predictive power and diagnostic validity of assessment instruments, especially those that may have the psychometric properties to adequately identify group differences but not meaningfully diagnose individual psychopathology (Fisher, 1993, 1994). Case 48 provides a candid discussion of problems that can arise when adjunctive treatments are offered to low-risk parents on the basis of information derived from experimental procedures designed to broadly categorize the quality of infant–parent relationships.

Adjunctive Treatment as an Experimental Variable. In research utilizing assessment instruments with diagnostic validity, research staff may discover that participants or their family members meet diagnostic criteria for mental disorders for which the research does not directly provide treatment. Uncovering such information raises concerns about the impact of recommending collateral treatment on the scientific validity of the research design. The investigators in Cases 49 and 50 approached such challenges through innovative use of a referral procedure that was incorporated as a variable in the statistical analysis of treatment results.

REFERRALS AS STANDARD PRACTICE

Studies on the developmental patterns of substance abuse, poverty, depressive symptomotology, and other developmental risk factors will yield information suggesting a child or adolescent's welfare may be in jeopardy. Investigators conducting such studies should, at the design stages of the research, decide what information will or will not be shared with participants and their families, and how that information will be assessed with respect to referral decisions (Fisher, 1993). Recent work suggests that many middle and high school students believe that it is ethically permissible to break confidentiality and for parents or other concerned adults to be contacted, if during the course of research, a teenage participant reveals suicidal ideation, and to a lesser extent information about physical abuse, sexual abuse, or sexually transmitted diseases (Fisher et al., 1994).

Clarifying the Scope and Limitations of Referral Procedures.
When working with children and adolescents, it is particularly important to clarify during the informed consent stages how risks will be identified, and if and to whom referrals will be made (Fisher, 1993, 1994). For example, researchers should not promise children or adolescents absolute confidentiality if they anticipate that some of the participant's responses may need to be shared with parents or guardians (see Case 51). On the other hand, investigators may plan to offer adolescents, or even younger children, the opportunity to self-refer (see Asher, 1993; Fisher et al., in press). Parents should be informed at the outset of this possibility (see Case 48). As illustrated by both Cases 52 and 53, self-referral procedures raise ethical dilemmas regarding the investigator's responsibility to follow-up the adolescent's response to referral recommendations. Investigators working with high-risk families need to also be prepared for requests by parents for research-derived clinical assessments that may help participants involved in domestic violence situations and the legal system (see Cases 54 and 55).

Providing Routine Referral Information.   Providing referral information need not be dependent on an assessment of imminent risk. Investigators working with children and adolescents will often uncover risk factors (i.e., low self-esteem, peer rejection, moderate alcohol use, sexual activity) that do not fit into any established diagnostic criteria, but that have been identified as potential marker variables for a cluster of developmental problems. In such research contexts, research staff can provide each participant and their guardians with a list of community agencies offering psychosocial evaluations and treatment of developmental problems (Fisher & Rosendahl, 1990). Some investigators conducting longitudinal studies, have developed innovative newsletters or brochures to keep participants and their families aware of mental health resources in the community (e.g., *Newsletter of the Adolescent and Family Development Project* published by Arizona State University in Tempe and the *Yellow Pages for Young Adults* published by the Simmons College Research Project, Boston, MA).

CASE 47: AN EPIDEMIOLOGICAL STUDY OF PATTERNS OF MENTAL HEALTH SERVICE USE BY RURAL ADOLESCENTS

Research Goals

The purpose of this study was to look at the development of psychopathology and patterns of service use from prepuberty to late adolescence in rural families representing a broad range of socioeconomic levels. Over the course of 3 years service usage was evaluated every 3 months. Children and their families were seen yearly for full psychiatric evaluations (see also Case 36).

Providing Assistance to an Impoverished Family

On one visit to an isolated family, the interviewers became aware that the family had little food and that all electricity had been cut off because a $30 bill had not been paid. The investigators felt a humane obligation to help this family who had little food and no heat during the winter.

Integrity of the Research. Their concern for the integrity of the research made this choice difficult. Would assisting the family affect variables such as socioeconomic level or service usage that were critical to the study? The researchers determined that some minimal economic assistance would not substantially change the economic status of the family and that they would still remain on the lowest rung of the economic ladder of the study sample. They also recognized that by alerting some members of the community to the family's problems, the adolescents might utilize services about which the family might not have ordinarily been aware. The researchers reasoned, however, that because their research was on service usage, increasing knowledge about the availability of services for this family would not substantially alter the study.

Protecting the Privacy Rights of Participants. The final issue concerned the privacy and autonomy of the family itself. The family was proud and parents did not consider themselves a family that took charity. Fortunately the individuals hired to conduct the interviews were from the local community. They were therefore able to assess ways in which the family could be assisted without invading their privacy or making their plight known to the community. The local interviewers succeeded in having the electricity bill paid anonymously and a truck load of wood delivered to the house. They also put the family in contact with a social service provider who could help them assess their needs.

CASE 48: A LONGITUDINAL STUDY ON THE TRANSITION TO PARENTHOOD FOR PARENTS AND INFANTS IN A LOW-RISK POPULATION

Research Goals

The purpose of this longitudinal study was to track the psychosocial correlates of the transition to parenthood for mothers, fathers, and infants from pregnancy through early childhood. During the first year of the child's birth, researchers obtained data on stresses and strains in the marital relationship. At the end of the first year of life, infant–parent attachment security was measured.

Offering an Intervention to Parents of Infants Classified as Insecurely Attached

During the course of research the investigators found that many of the mothers of infants rated "insecurely" attached were in troubled or isolated marriages. Although they recognized that such an attachment classification did not provide diagnostic information on individual infants, they decided to share information with the parents about the infant's attachment status (see Case 61 for the rationale for this decision).

Having decided to tell parents that their child might be at risk for poor socioemotional development, the investigators debated whether they were obligated to provide a service referral. They were concerned that it might be cruel to provide such information without some form of support. However, because this study was conducted in a small rural town, there were no preventive education services available to the parents. The investigative team, therefore, decided to offer an intervention program.

Designing an Intervention for Low-Risk Parents

Having decided to offer a program for parents of infants classified as insecurely attached, the investigators faced the problem that no such intervention model existed. What type of program should be offered parents? Previous research on depressed mothers suggested that insecure attachment is a function of the parent's "personality organization" rather than parenting knowledge. On this basis it was decided that personal coping styles rather than parenting styles should be the focus of intervention. However, another problem soon arose. Although all parents were free to participate, the fathers were more hesitant. This created an intervention targeted to mothers which could lead to negative stereotyping of a mother who already was in a vulnerable relationship with her spouse.

A related problem was the fact that with a focus on personality, the intervention ran the risk of intruding on the privacy of the mother in a way that she had not intended when she signed up for the initial study on parenting. A final concern was whether intervention for "normal parents" with no known clinical disorders should be based on work with disturbed mothers and infants. Given the obligation they felt to inform parents of their research findings, and the potential anxiety that this information might raise, the research team decided that their concerns about the risks of offering a short-term counseling program were offset by the potential alleviation of anxiety and enhancement of parenting practices that the intervention might provide.

Evaluating the Efficacy of the Intervention

Because they were designing a new type of prevention program, the investigators believed they were obligated to evaluate its impact on parenting practices and infant attachment. Mothers who wished to participate were asked to sign an additional informed consent for the evaluation phase. The intervention was conducted and the researchers found no significant change in parent–child relationships. In addition, during the time that they undertook the intervention, new research in the area suggested that evidence for the linkage between insecure attachment and serious behavior problems had become weaker rather than convincingly stronger. Moreover, it was apparent after speaking to mothers and fathers about the researchers' concerns and the service they were making available, that few really wanted to hear about them; many reacted defensively. The researchers concluded that in the future they would not initiate an intervention based on parental correlates of child attachment categorization. Instead, they would tell parents during informed consent procedures that such information would not be shared because of the lack of diagnostic validity of the measures for individual children and families.

CASE 49: COMPARING THE EFFICACY OF THREE PSYCHOSOCIAL INTERVENTIONS FOR INPATIENT DEPRESSED ADOLESCENTS

Research Goals

This research team used an RCT approach to compare the efficacy of three psychosocial interventions for inpatient adolescents diagnosed with depression. The outcomes of 12-week cognitive-behavioral, interpersonal, and family therapy treatments were compared. The protocol called for psychological evaluations of both adolescents and their parents across all three treatments.

Offering Treatment to Parents

The psychological evaluations indicated that a small proportion of parents were clinically depressed. The ethical question was whether offering treatment to the parents would invalidate the results of the study. One consideration was that the family therapy condition required parental participation that could be jeopardized if parents were incapacitated by their depression. A second consideration centered on the external validity of the research. That is, if parent treatment was not offered, the experimental conditions might be very different from actual clinical practice. In this regard, the researchers concluded that a therapist who ascertained that a parent was clinically depressed would probably refer that parent for treatment.

On this basis, the research team decided that parents with clinical depression would be referred for medical treatment. Medical treatment, rather than psychosocial treatment, was selected so as not to confound the comparison of the family therapy and two individual therapy interventions. However, if the family intervention was found to be effective, it would be available to control group participants and their families. In most cases, the medical treatment for parents consisted of administration by a nurse of noratriptaline. This service would not be paid for by the research, but through regular third-party reimbursement. The parental treatment was then entered as a variable in the statistical analysis making it a 2 (parental medication) × 3 (psychosocial treatment) design.

CASE 50: EVALUATION OF A SCHOOL-BASED SOCIAL SKILLS PROGRAM FOR PREVENTION OF BEHAVIORAL AND ACADEMIC PROBLEMS

Research Goals

In a longitudinal study, children (6–10 years of age) were screened for participation in an intensive school-based intervention aimed at the prevention of conduct disorder, substance abuse, and academic failure. Screening was based on the presence of cross-setting disruptive behavior. A diagnostic survey of this cohort revealed that approximately 67% of the children satisfied diagnostic criteria for ADHD. In addition, children met criteria for other disruptive behavioral disorders as well as mood and anxiety disorders. The experimental intervention being tested in the study was a generic psychosocial skills program. The program included training parents and teachers in behavior management and problem-solving skills facilitation methods and training children in problem-solving skills.

Referring Children Diagnosed With Psychiatric
Disorders for Medical Treatment

The diagnostic information made available to the investigators posed an ethical dilemma. ADHD, mood, and anxiety disorders are medical diagnoses that often require treatment with psychotropic medications. The investigators were concerned that withholding assessment information pertaining to the possible existence of a psychiatric disorder would deprive a child of an accepted medical treatment that could provide amelioration of the child's symptoms. The investigators questioned whether the psychosocial intervention provided by the study was adequate to the task of "treating" the more seriously disordered experimental subjects. Was it ethical to retain a representative sample of high-risk children as controls, many of whom may possess diagnosable mental disorders?

The investigators considered informing parents about those children who met diagnostic criteria for a clinical disorder, referring them for treatment, and excluding them from the study. However, this would result in the exclusion of children who might be in most need of the school-based experimental intervention. On the other hand, not identifying children with clinical disorders might also result in differential exclusion or attrition. For example, parents of high-risk subjects in the control condition might be more likely to compensate for their child's problems by seeking specialized clinical service. If so, children who remained untreated in the control group would become an unrepresentative sample.

Adjunctive Clinical Treatment
as an Experimental Variable

The solution arrived at by the investigators was to make referrals when appropriate and include the adjunctive clinical treatment as a variable. This strategy not only provided an acceptable ethical response to the question of disclosing results of probable clinical disorders, but could also increase the precision and clinical significance of the experimental intervention. To the extent that medication, for example, exerts a powerful effect on outcome variables in the study, inclusion of medication as an explanatory variable in the analysis permits determination of the differential effect of medication on outcome.

At the beginning of the study, parents of both experimental and control subjects whose test results suggested a psychiatric disorder were informed that behaviors identified in their children were consistent with certain clinical diagnoses. Parents in both conditions were next invited to an educational inservice program in which information on diagnostic and treatment issues were reviewed. They were informed, for example, that the use of stimulant medication was a safe and effective treatment of ADHD. They were given the opportunity to ask questions and informed that on request they could have access to the project's child psychiatrist who, after an independent clinical evaluation, would discuss the need for ancillary service and/or assist them in identifying appropriate services.

Records of subsequent treatment, including type, quantity (dosage), and duration were carefully charted. Analytically, adjunctive medication therapy was treated as a time-varying covariate reflecting the type, quantity, and duration of treatment within the assessment interval. This provided the opportunity to assess the effects of the treatment intervention over and above those of medication effects.

CASE 51: PSYCHIATRIC DISORDERS OF PHYSICALLY ABUSED ADOLESCENTS

Research Goals

This study sought to compare the psychiatric disorders of physically abused adolescents recruited from a state central register of abuse to a matched community control sample recruited utilizing random selection procedures. Ninety-nine physically abused adolescents and 99 control adolescents, ages 12 to 18, and their families were interviewed utilizing standardized semistructured and structured measures administered by clinically trained interviewers blind as to group status. Psychiatric risk factors for adolescent psychopathology, other than abuse, including parental psychiatric disorders were entered into a multiple logistic regression model which was used to test the additional risk of psychopathology due to abuse.

Need for Services and Duty to Inform

During the course of study interviews, research interviewers became alarmed due to disclosure by an 18-year-old male adolescent of current suicidal ideation and a past suicide attempt involving aspirin ingestion, undisclosed to parents or professionals. Interviewers communicated their concern, heightened by the adolescent's report of alcohol abuse and risk-taking behavior, to the grant social worker.

A meeting held by grant staff to evaluate the risk for the adolescent resulted in a treatment plan that included reaching out to the adolescent and his parents in order to define the risk of suicide and to implement treatment referrals. The grant social worker contacted the adolescent and his parents, indicating a general concern and requesting a meeting with them.

Subsequent meetings with the mother and the adolescent, held both individually and conjointly, resulted in referral for treatment to a treatment program. After reevaluation by the treatment program, he was hospitalized for alcohol abuse and suicide risk. Contact by the mother to the grant social worker 1 year later revealed that the adolescent had graduated from high school, was living on his own, and employed full time. (See Cases 54 and 55 regarding utilization of research protocols for forensic purposes and parental requests for services.)

CASE 52: THE INCIDENCE AND PREVALENCE OF DEPRESSIVE SYMPTOMATOLOGY IN NONREFERRED HIGH SCHOOL STUDENTS

Research Goals

The purpose of this school-based study was to examine the incidence and prevalence of depressive symptomotology in a sample of nonreferred adolescents. Data were collected through standardized self-report instruments administered in the schools.

Establishing Criteria for Suicide Risk

The investigators were aware that the study of depression would yield data on suicidal ideation. They decided that before they initiated the research they would set criteria for determining when a student should be considered a suicide risk. Because they were using standardized assessment instruments rather than clinical interviews, they recognized that some students could be "faking" their responses. They decided that their criteria should only be viewed as a "screening device" and that students who met the criteria should be further evaluated by the school psychologist. They also believed that because they were studying adolescents, immediate referral to the school psychologist, rather than immediate contact with the parent was the best way to protect the adolescents' privacy rights. The researchers indicated this policy on the parental consent and adolescent assent forms.

Investigator Responsibility Following Referral

The research team then debated whether they had a responsibility to the student after the referral to the school psychologist had been made.

For example, what if the school psychologist could not see the child? What if the child refused to see the school psychologist? Given the tentative nature of a suicide risk assessment made on the basis of responses to a few items on a self-report questionnaire, they decided that their best course of action was to follow-up with both the school psychologist and the child. If the school psychologist reported that he or she had seen the student the researcher team would stop there. If the adolescent had not been seen, the researchers would contact the adolescent and discuss with him or her the importance of seeing the psychologist and also provide a referral to a clinic outside the school. Ongoing monitoring by the research team continued if the adolescent did not make contact with a mental health professional to encourage the student to talk with someone.

CASE 53: A LONGITUDINAL COMMUNITY-BASED STUDY ON ADOLESCENT DRUG AND ALCOHOL USE

Research Goals

A sample of 454 families was interviewed three times at 1-year intervals to identify risk and protective factors associated with adolescent substance use and abuse. Adolescents and their parents were interviewed individually. The 3-year longitudinal study did not include a treatment component.

Providing Routine Referrals

The research team recognized that adolescents using drugs and alcohol might have mental health needs requiring clinical services. Because the study was a longitudinal investigation of the natural course of substance use and abuse, the researchers believed that offering interventions to adolescents suffering from a myriad of psychological problems would threaten the internal validity of the study. At the same time, they recognized that some adolescents and/or their families might have joined the study in the hopes of learning more about their problems.

The investigators decided that before every interview they would routinely provide parents and adolescents with a referral list of community agencies specializing in adolescent substance abuse and family therapy. These lists were provided before the interview started to avoid the risk of labeling any participant as a *problem*. Interviewers were also trained to end the interview by asking participants if they would like to receive a call from a member of the project staff. Participants who indicated they would, were called during the next week to discuss their concerns. If they wished an appointment was set up to follow up on these concerns, and these appointments were used to make referrals to community agencies if appropriate. The investigators believed these routine procedures did not impair the scientific validity of their longitudinal descriptive study because the research team was not telling participants that they should seek such treatment, nor were they providing either assessments or treatment.

Determining What Levels of Drug or Alcohol Use Constitute a Clear and Immediate Danger to Participant Welfare

The investigators wanted to develop procedures to determine under what circumstances they would intervene and give feedback to subjects (or their parents) about risk associated with the adolescent's level of alcohol or drug use. They did not want to contaminate their longitudinal study by interfering in the natural course of drug and alcohol use, nor violate the adolescents' right to privacy. At they same time, they felt an ethical responsibility to intervene when usage levels constituted a clear threat of imminent harm.

The parental consent and adolescent assent forms explicitly told parents that with the exception of information involving child abuse, all other information would be held confidential. Participants and their parents were further informed that if the researchers believed the adolescent was in imminent danger, they would directly approach the adolescent to assist him or her in getting help. The researchers then needed to decide under what circumstances such a recommendation should be made.

Alcohol Abuse. Adolescent drinking was a difficult issue because, in the absence of extreme behaviors or side effects, there are few guidelines on when excessive drinking in adolescence presents an immediate danger. For example, the biological impact of alcohol is dependent on individual physiological and psychological characteristics. The researchers decided to handle the problem of excessive drinking through stories in a quarterly newsletter sent to participating adolescents and their families. For example, one story was titled "When Does Drinking Become a Problem" and listed several standard behaviors associated with problem drinking. In this way, the researchers felt they could inform subjects about the risks of problem drinking without jeopardizing the integrity of the research through labeling any individual participant as having a problem.

Drug Abuse.   In contrast to the uncertainty associated with diagnosing problem drinking behavior, some drugs have known toxic effects. For example, during a standard interview a female participant reported the use of a dangerous inhalant to get high almost every day. A call to the local poison control center revealed that this drug was potentially fatal. Interview responses from both the young woman and her mother revealed a high level of current conflict between the two and gave no indication that the mother was aware of her daughter's inhalant use. A member of the project staff had several telephone calls with the adolescent over a period of several weeks. The adolescent reported that she had discontinued her inhalant use after a friend told her about the recent death of a peer engaging in this activity. The staff member discussed with her the potential consequences of this behavior and the family problems that the adolescent perceived were causing the use. The staff member also expressed concern about future use. The adolescent promised to continue abstaining from inhalant use and this was confirmed in a second phone call several days later.

Follow-Up.   During the second phone call, the researcher raised the possibility of setting up a meeting with the project psychologist, the adolescent, and her mother to discuss the adolescent's unhappiness. The adolescent agreed to this plan and confirmed that she did not believe there would be any danger to her if her mother were contacted to make such an appointment. A psychologist from the project staff then contacted the mother, who agreed to a meeting. However, despite multiple telephone calls over a 3-month period, the mother never scheduled an appointment. Attempts at reminders and follow-ups were unsuccessful. The last contact with the adolescent occurred 2 years after this incident during routine tracking of subjects for maintaining the longitudinal sample. At that time she indicated she was not taking any dangerous drugs and was willing to continue participation in the study.

CASE 54: PSYCHIATRIC DISORDERS
OF PHYSICALLY ABUSED ADOLESCENTS

Research Goals

This study sought to compare the psychiatric disorders of physically abused adolescents recruited from a state central register of abuse to a matched community control sample recruited utilizing random selection procedures. Ninety-nine physically abused adolescents and 99 control adolescents, ages 12 to 18, and their families were interviewed utilizing standardized semistructured measures administered by clinically trained interviewers blind as to group status. Psychiatric risk factors for adolescent psychopathology, other than abuse, including parental psychiatric disorders were entered into a multiple logistic regression model that was used to test the additional risk of psychopathology due to abuse.

Guidelines for Provision of Appropriate Clinical Back-Up

General guidelines established prior to study implementation outlined the roles and responsibilities of research staff in identifying, assessing and intervening if adolescents participating in the study were judged to be at risk. Although investigators had procured a federal Certificate of Confidentiality, the investigators took the stance that current physical abuse, if disclosed, would be reported to the appropriate child protective services agency (the state Department of Social Services), and adolescents and families were instructed during the informed consent portion of the interview regarding reporting mandates relevant to current abuse and safety issues.

Interviewers, clinically trained psychology doctoral candidates blind as to group status, were trained to sensitively assess subject reaction to participation in this in-depth, multiple-interview protocol, and (a) alert research staff if the child was at risk either for ongoing physical abuse or due to a mental health crisis, and (b) provide to the family and/or individual interviewee the name of the grant social worker for feedback and/or referrals. Similarly, PIs, blinded as to abuse status, in the course of providing a "best estimate" of adolescent and parental psychopathology, were responsible for ascertaining if an adolescent or a parent were at current risk and then alerting the grant social worker, who was not blinded as to group status, either to follow through by getting additional information or to intervene with the family to implement referrals for treatment. In such cases, coordinator, social worker, and interviewers met to discuss the case and to decide on an appropriate intervention. The grant social worker then undertook responsibility for contacting those families to provide the necessary services (without fee), including case management, referrals, and feedback/evaluation within the confines of confidentiality. (See Cases 51 and 55 for discussion of the duty to inform about the utilization of research-based assessments for forensic purposes.)

Parental Partner Violence and Maternal Request for Services

During the course of the last interview, a mother became very tearful, sobbing when she was asked to respond to questions from the "Family Disagreements Interview Assessment." Assessment of the family by the grant social worker, initiated on request from the mother and the interviewers, revealed issues of spousal and child abuse throughout the course of the 24 years of the parental marriage. A report by the then 14-year-old daughter to Child Protective Services 2 years prior to research interviews had resulted in a cessation of the physical violence toward both the adolescent and the mother by the father. Orders of protection had been obtained at the time of adolescent physical abuse investigation which prohibited both spousal and child abuse violence. However, verbal and emotional abuse by the father to the mother had continued unabated, according to the mother's report.

Although the mother had reached out in the past to various agencies, she had been unwilling to follow through in an effective manner to utilize their services. Building on the rapport she had developed with the grant interviewers, the mother developed a relationship with the grant social worker, meeting with her three times for feedback and assessment purposes. She subsequently demonstrated an ability to obtain, request, and telephone this individual, and to accept treatment referrals over the course of the next 3 years. She also recontacted the social worker to discuss her ambivalence regarding staying within the abusive situation or moving on. Psychosocial evaluations based on grant research data were written at her request for submission to treatment personnel, always respecting the limits of confidentiality, including having obtained written informed consent from her to release information about her. She subsequently called the study social worker to state that she had developed the confidence to divorce her abusive husband. She also appropriately sought treatment for her daughter when she later became symptomatic at the time of her mother's initiation of divorce proceedings.

CASE 55: PSYCHIATRIC DISORDERS OF PHYSICALLY ABUSED ADOLESCENTS

Research Goals

This study sought to compare the psychiatric disorders of physically abused adolescents recruited from a state central register of abuse to a matched community control sample recruited utilizing random selection procedures. Ninety-nine physically abused adolescents and 99 control adolescents, ages 12 to 18, and their families were interviewed utilizing standardized semistructured and structured measures administered by clinically trained interviewers blind as to group status. Psychiatric risk factors for adolescent psychopathology, other than abuse, including parental psychiatric disorders, were entered into a multiple logistic regression model that was used to test the additional risk of psychopathology due to abuse. (See Cases 51 and 54 for discussion of the duty to inform parents and provide parent-requested clinical back-up services.)

Defining Treatment Needs for Utilization by Legal Systems

During the course of interviews, a 17-year-old male and his parents revealed to research staff that he had been arrested at the end of an airport runway when, while intoxicated with a hallucinogenic drug, he attempted to place dynamite on a grassy area. Subsequent to the second interview with mother and son, the mother called grant staff requesting termination of the interviews because of her son's need to have a mental health assessment for use in his legal defense.

Meeting as a treatment team, the study interviewers, coordinator, and one of the PIs formulated a treatment plan recognizing that the research staff were the first mental health professionals ever involved with the son and his family, despite previous attempts by his school to refer him for mental health services due to truancy and drug abuse. Based on this plan, the parents were contacted by the project coordinator offering the services of the PI, a general psychiatrist, and child and adolescent psychiatrists.

The adolescent, his parents, and his criminal defense attorney made appropriate follow-through on this suggestion, subsequently involving the PI who, after interviewing them and reviewing all study data, prepared a forensic psychiatric report that was submitted and utilized by the court for rehabilitative disposition planning for the adolescent. Both the adolescent and his parents complied with the treatment recommendations.

*   *   *

Casebook

Debriefing and Dissemination

Research on mental disorders of childhood and adolescence has the potential to uncover information that can directly benefit participants and their families. For example, a child's response to a new medication tested during a clinical trial can provide valuable information for future treatment decisions. Sharing such information with parents and (following parental permission) with practitioners responsible for treating the child promotes participant welfare and their right to learn about the nature, results, and conclusions of the research (see Case 56). On the other hand, as illustrated in Case 57, investigators must consider the extent to which postexperimental information will enhance or interfere with the child's ongoing treatment program. The potential benefits and harms of debriefing should be evaluated during the design stages of the research and the breadth and limitations of information sharing communicated to parents during the informed consent stage.

THE RIGHT "NOT TO KNOW"

In some situations, disclosure of a person's medical or psychiatric status may have the potential to cause psychosocial harm. For example, in the area of human genetic research, participants may find out things about themselves or family members (e.g., that they carry a recessive gene for a debilitating disorder) that they might not wish to know or that may compromise their insurability. In such situations, the potential consequences of disclosure should be discussed with children, adolescents, and their families prior to the initiation of research procedures. Except in cases in which early treatment is available that can improve prognosis, participants and their families can be given the right "not to know" the results of the genetic testing (OPRR, 1993; Case 58). However, when HIV testing is conducted, individuals whose test results are associated with personal identifiers must (under most circumstances) be informed of their HIV status and provided the opportunity to receive appropriate counseling (OPRR, 1993; Case 59). The requirement to inform individuals of their serostatus rests on the position that opportunities for early intervention outweigh the risks of disclosure.

Federal guidelines are unclear concerning the role of parents and guardians in determining the child or adolescent participant's right to know or not know the results of genetic or HIV testing. In both Cases 58 and 59, investigators chose to prioritize the autonomy rights of the children in such situations, while carefully explaining their decision to parents during the informed consent stage.

ESTIMATING THE GENERALIZABILITY OF RESEARCH RESULTS TO PRACTICAL APPLICATIONS

Descriptive or explanatory studies utilizing large numbers of subjects to generate group means can provide information about cognitive, socioeomotional, behavioral, or physiological patterns characterizing children and adolescents with low or high risk for mental disorders. Parents, practitioners, and policymakers are increasingly relying on this knowledge base to make decisions about preventive and remediative strategies for promoting the mental health of children and youth. As a consequence, investigators need to limit possible misapplications of findings derived from group data to clinical or policy decisions that affect the lives of individual children and youth (Fisher, 1993). For example, developmental research based on group means has demonstrated relationships between parental practices and certain cognitive and social competencies (e.g., parental teaching styles and school performance; maternal sensitivity and infant–mother attachment). However, because the predictive validity of these relationships for identifying later cognitive and socioemotional adjustment in individual infants and children has yet to be empirically verified, investigators must proceed with caution when deciding whether or not to share with parents such research-derived information regarding their child's developmental status (see Case 60).

Consideration for the Cultural Dimensions of Children's Lives. Given the diversity of the populations encountered in research on child and adolescent mental disorders, a measure of a psychological construct may or may not have the same or even similar psychometric properties or patterns of relationships with other variables in different populations

(Laosa, 1990). Investigators must, therefore, be sensitive to the extent to which the norming sample used to standardize test scores reflects a participant's cultural group or age cohort and be aware of the limitations of conclusions drawn from instruments using nonrepresentative norms (Fisher & Lerner, 1994). For example, current measures to assess child psychopathology may be biased toward over identifying children of certain subgroups as deviant (Edelbrock, 1994) and some normative expectations about adult–child relationships and social adaptation may vary across different subcultural groups (Fisher, Jackson, & Villaruel, in press; Laosa, 1990). As illustrated in Case 61, investigators have a responsibility to ensure that a scientific inference valid for one population does not lead to incorrect judgments regarding another population. This caution must be reflected in the design of research as well as the dissemination of research findings.

CASE 56: PHARMACOLOGICAL
TREATMENT OF HYPERACTIVE CHILDREN
WITH MENTAL RETARDATION

Research Goals

The purpose of this study was to assess the behavioral, cognitive, and physiological side effects of fenfluramine (Pondimin) as an alternative to methylphenidate (Ritalin) in hyperactive children (5–13 years) with mental retardation. Five drug conditions were to be compared: a placebo, three doses of fenfluramine, and one dose of methylphenidate. Each drug condition was to be given for 2 weeks with order determined by a complex Latin square assignment. All parties having contact with the children, including their parents, teachers, and study personnel, were blind to the medication sequence. Prior to starting the protocol, each child would also take a known placebo for 1 week. (See Cases 4, 21, and 40 for discussion of risks, parental consent procedures, and risk management, respectively.)

Summary Letters to Subjects' Physicians

On entry into the study, parents were told that the PI would prepare a summary letter to the parent and with permission to the child's physician on the child's completion of the study. The content of these letters always included: (a) the reason for admitting the child to the study; (b) duration of treatment, medication doses, and the time of day medication was given; (c) measures of drug change; (d) medication-related changes observed in the study; and (e) any recommendations for treatment based on the child's reactions to the experimental conditions.

Some children responded to neither of the active medications during the study, and in these cases the PI was at least able to recommend that the child's doctor avoid treatments that appeared to be unhelpful. Under these conditions, the PI sometimes developed a hunch about an alternative treatment that might be useful. As an example, a trial of antidepressant medication might be recommended in a case where a child with ADHD had a parent with major depression. In such cases, the PI clarifies that the recommendation is not grounded in empirical tests of this drug for this particular child. Also, some parents appear to have inadequate parenting skills. In those cases, the PI may explore the possibilities of counseling for the parents. In such instances, an addendum may be appended to the parent's copy of the letter to the doctor with specific clinics suggested.

CASE 57: LONG-TERM MEMORY IN DOWN SYNDROME INFANTS AND INFANTS WITH AVERAGE INTELLIGENCE

Research Goals

The purpose of this study was to compare learning and memory in infants with Down syndrome to infants with average intelligence. Participants were recruited through contacts made with parents by an early intervention for Down syndrome infants. Previous research suggested that for infants with average intelligence contingency experiences are important boosters for development. This study was designed to determine whether very young Down syndrome infants have the capacity for contingency learning and whether they can retain that learning for an extended period. Over the course of 2 days, infants were trained in an operant conditioning task to kick a mobile above their crib. One week later they were tested again to ascertain retention of the mobile conjugate reinforcement. The Bayley Mental Scales of Infant Development Indices were administered to examine relationships among mental and psychomotor skills, learning, and retention.

Sharing Test Results With Parents

As part of the agreement to recruit subjects, administrators at the intervention program from which the Down syndrome infants had been recruited requested that investigators not use the name "Bayley Scales of Infant Development" or provide parents with any feedback on their infants' scores on this test. The organization was concerned that such feedback would interfere with the organization's normal assessment process for each client that included a Bayley and subsequent parent conference.

The investigators felt that this request was in the best interests of the parents because feedback from the organization concerning the Bayley tests could be coordinated with other services, whereas a report from the researchers would not. The investigators did not, however, want to mislead parents into thinking that participation in the research would provide them with additional information about their infants. Therefore, during the consent procedures the parents were informed they would receive no feedback regarding their child's performance relative to other infants with Down syndrome or nondisabled infants, but would received a "final report" of the study providing information on group performance.

CASE 58: CHILDREN'S DECISION TO CONSENT TO PREDICTIVE GENETIC TESTING

Research Goals

Predictive genetic testing is concerned with the probability that an individual will develop a genetically related disease. The purpose of this study was to examine psychosocial issues related to the decision of 9- to 16-year-olds with a family history of Huntington's disease to participate in predictive genetic testing. With advancing medical technology, questions remain as to how and when to tell children and families about the availability of tests and test results. This study was designed to learn how children and adolescents understand the process of genetic testing so that ethical guidelines could be put into place regarding the type and quality of information/explanation required to render true informed assent or consent. (See Case 25 for discussion of issues involving consent to participate in this study.)

Informing Children About the Results of Genetic Testing

A difficult dilemma for the research team was whether children should be routinely told the results of their genetic testing or whether that decision should be left to the parents. The decision rested heavily on the fact that the child and adolescent needed to be knowledgeable about their status to facilitate their seeking the medical attention and guidance on reproductive risks they might need in the future. In addition, the children in this study were at least 9 years old and were knowledgeable about the purpose of the study through the assent procedures. The investigators believed that if the child agreed to participate, she or he had the right to know the test results.

After a great deal of debate, and a recognition that they might lose volunteer participants if disclosure of test results to children was required, the investigators decided they were willing to sacrifice potential selection bias in data collection caused by parental refusal for the right of the minor participants to be informed of their test results. The decision rested heavily on the fact that, as a research study, the team would not be providing routine medical care. They believed that by collecting data on participant refusers, they might also be able to understand and interpret the selection bias.

The Subjects' "Right Not to Know"

According to federal guidelines, individuals participating in human genetic research generally retain the right not to receive information about their genetic status except in rare instances where early treatment could improve their prognosis. In the case of Huntington's disease, no such treatment is available. Therefore, children were also given the option of not knowing the results of the genetic testing.

The research team gave the child the following options: (a) refuse to learn of the results of the genetic testing, (b) learn the results of the genetic testing through his or her parent, or (c) learn it through the research team. If the child did choose to learn about the test results through his or her parents, after a week, the research team checked in with the family. If the parents had not discussed the results, the team offered to talk with the whole family about the tests. If parents chose to tell their children, a follow-up session with a research staff member was held to ensure that the children/adolescents understood and properly assimilated the explanation.

Sharing Information When Participants
Withdraw From a Study

The investigators also considered what they should do if the parents withdrew the child before the results could be relayed. The team had valuable information that was potentially being withheld from the minor participant, yet they did not want to infringe on parental prerogative and the right to withdraw from the study. The research team decided that under such conditions the registry that maintained test results of all individuals being tested for the disorder would notify the minor of the availability of information on the positivity of the gene test when the minor became 18 years of age. A description of this procedure was included in the consent and assent procedures.

CASE 59: LEARNING AND NEUROLOGIC CORRELATES OF HIV INFECTION IN CHILDREN WITH HEMOPHILIA

Research Goals

The goal of this multisite study was to follow a cohort of children with hemophilia to trace the impact of the HIV virus on child and family coping. The study was initiated in the late 1980s with children ranging in age from 6 to 11 years. These children had first received blood transfusions during the early period of AIDS awareness, and in most cases the blood donated during this period had not been tested for the HIV virus. As a consequence, 50% of the research participants were expected to develop AIDS during the course of the study. Once every 6 months children and their parents would come in for measures of physical growth, neurological problems, neuropsychological testing, psychological assessments, and measures of family stress and parental coping. The study paid for the family's transportation (some families were at a great distance from the hospital). Parents were paid $100 and children $25 for each interview period. The aim of the study was to examine the relationship of hemophilia and HIV to learning problems, neurologic functions, and the physiological profile of HIV infection. (See Case 32 for discussion of confidentiality issues.)

Telling Children About Their HIV and AIDS Status as it Emerged During the Study

The most difficult issue was whether and how one should tell children about their HIV and AIDS status as it might emerge over time. The research team believed that it would not be ethical to keep this information confidential from the child if the parents were provided the information. Therefore, the informed consent procedures indicated that children would be told their HIV status over the course of the research. Parents indicated support for this position. How the child was to be told varied depending on the child's cognitive and developmental status and parental preferences. Some parents wanted to tell the child first themselves; others wanted to have a family meeting with the researchers.

The type of information communicated to the child varied depending on their developmental level. For the younger children, the name AIDS was not necessarily mentioned. They were told they had an illness that sometimes makes people very sick. As some of the children became adolescents and interest in sexual relations emerged, with permission of the parents, psychologists on the research team would speak with patients about the risks of HIV infection to potential partners. The parents were enthusiastic about this and the researchers held several retreats on this topic with the adolescent patients.

CASE 60: A LONGITUDINAL STUDY ON THE TRANSITION TO PARENTHOOD IN A LOW-RISK POPULATION

Research Goals

The purpose of this longitudinal study was to track the psychosocial correlates of the transition to parenthood for mothers, fathers, and infants from pregnancy through early childhood. During the first year of the child's birth, researchers obtained data on stresses and strains in the marital relationship. At the end of the first year of life, infant–parent attachment security was measured.

Informing Parents About Their Infant's Attachment Status

During the course of research the investigators found that many of the mothers of infants rated "insecurely" attached were in troubled or isolated marriages. Although insecure attachment had been empirically associated with developmental problems, this association was only probabilistic, not deterministic. That is, it provided information that a group of insecurely attached infants may be more likely than secure infants to develop behavior problems, but did not provide information about the probability that an individual infant will develop problems.

An ethical issue that arose was whether the research team should alert parents to the fact that their child was at risk when nothing about the individual child could be predicted. Would the at-risk label create problems itself? In addition, there was no known intervention for changing an infant's attachment security classification. As a research group, they debated this dilemma for some time. The critical issue that eventually led the researchers to inform the parents about the child's status was that parents had been told when they enrolled in the study (during pregnancy) that developmental concerns about the children would be shared with parents. The researchers felt that although only a very few families may have signed up for this reason, it was the parents right to know the information that the researchers had as long as the limited predictive value of this information was also communicated. (See also Case 48 concerning whether to develop an intervention for these parents.)

CASE 61: DEVELOPMENTAL CORRELATES OF OPPOSITIONAL BEHAVIOR

Research Goals

Investigators were conducting a descriptive study of classroom behavior and peer competence as correlates of oppositional behavior in nonreferred children from lower socioeconomic backgrounds. The study was conducted in a school system serving approximately equal numbers of children from African-American and Anglo/Euro-American backgrounds. Oppositional behavior and conduct disorder were identified through teacher responses to standardized measures. The manuals for these measures reported that African-American children had been included in the standardization groups.

Differential Patterns of Teacher Reports for Children From Different Cultural Backgrounds

During the first phase of the experiment, the investigators found that teachers were five times more likely to rate the African-American children above the cut-off point for oppositional behavior than they were the Anglo/Euro-American children. The researchers were concerned that either there was a high percentage of African American students with unidentified oppositional disorder or the measure was not diagnostically valid for this population. The test they had selected was the most widely used assessment instrument for oppositional disorders and in selecting the test the researchers had identified other empirical investigations that had included African American samples. However, although the teacher-report questionnaire was standardized on a sample including African American children, no specific norms were cited for this population. To their knowledge, no other test for oppositional behavior had been developed specifically for this population.

Converging Measures

The investigators decided to add two additional measures of child behaviors: a parental report measure and an experimenter behavioral observation. They developed the coding system for the observations from traditional theory and from interviews with both African-American and Anglo/Euro-American parents about behaviors in the child's home environment. The observations were videotaped and the behaviors of all children coded by both an African-American and Anglo/Euro-American trained observer.

Dissemination

The observational and parental reports, although reflecting a somewhat higher level of oppositional-related behaviors in African-American students, did not parallel the high proportions yielded from the teacher observations. When they reported their results, the researchers included data from all three measures, described the differences in patterns and correlations of the three measures with other outcome variables, and discussed limitations for conclusions drawn from this study when applied to the diagnosis of oppositional disorder in African-American youth.

*   *   *

Casebook

References and Suggested Readings[1]

Abramovitch, R., Freedman, J. L., Thoden, K., & Nikolich, C. (1991). Children's capacity to consent to participation in psychological research: Empirical findings. *Child Development, 62*(5), 1100–1109.*

Ackerman, T. F. (1990). Protectionism and the new research imperative in pediatric AIDS. *IRB: A Review of Human Subject Research, 12*(5), 1–5.

Alexander, J. R., Lerer, B., & Baron, M. (1992). Ethical issues in genetic linkage studies of psychiatric disorders. *British Journal of Psychiatry, 160,* 98–102.

Aman, M. G., & Kern, R. A. (1989). Review of fenfluramine in the treatment of the developmental disabilities. *Journal of the American Academy of Child and Adolescent Psychiatry, 28,* 549–565.*

American Association of Child and Adolescent Psychiatry. (1992). Use of passive consent in child/adolescent mental health research—effect of letter from Dr. Charles R. McCarthy, Director of the Office for Protection from Research Risks, NIH. *Research Notes in Child Adolescent Psychiatry, 10.*

American Psychological Association. (1992). Ethical principles of psychologists and code of conduct. *American Psychologist, 47,* 1597–1611.

Appelbaum, P. D., & Rosenbaum, A. (1989). *Tarasoff* and the researcher: Does the duty to protect apply in the research setting? *American Psychologist, 44,* 885–894.

Asher, S. R. (1993, March). *Inviting children to self-refer.* Paper presented as part of the invited symposium on "Ethical issues in the reporting and referring of research participants" at the biennial meeting of the Society for Research in Child Development, New Orleans.*

Atkins, M. S., Stoff, D. M., Osborne, M. L., & Brown, K. (1993). Distinguishing instrumental and hostile aggression: Does it make a difference? *Journal of Abnormal Psychology, 21,* 1993.*

Bach, M. L., Oberg, C. N., Bryant, N. A., & Boleman, J. L. (1992). Ethics and medicaid: A new look at an old problem. *Journal of Health Care for the Poor and Underserved, 2,* 427–447.

Balk, D. E. (1993). Ethics, bereavement and researchers. *The Forum Newsletter, IXX*(4), 20–23.*

Barkley, R. A. (1991). Introduction to the special issue: Child psychopharmacology. *Journal of Clinical Child Psychology, 20*(3), 226–231.

Barkley, R. A. (1991). Diagnosis and assessment of attention deficit-hyperactivity disorder. *Comprehensive Mental Health Care, 1,* 27–43.

Baer, M. D. (1993). Quasi-random assignment can be as convincing as random assignment. *American Journal on Mental Retardation, 97,* 373–375.

---

[1]Empirical articles providing detailed description of ethical practices or empirically derived information relevant to ethical decision making are marked with an asterisk.

Baumrind, D. (1964). Some thoughts on ethics of research: After reading Milgram's "Behavioral study of obedience." *American Psychologist, 26,* 887–896.

Baumrind, D. (1979). IRBs and social science research: The costs of deception. *IRB: A Review of Human Subjects Research, 1,* 1–4.

Baumrind, D. (1990). Doing good well. In C. B. Fisher & W. W. Tryon (Eds.), *Ethics in applied developmental psychology: Emerging issues in an emerging field* (pp. 17 - 28). Norwood, NJ: Ablex.

Bayer, R., Feldman, S., & Reich, W. (1981). *Ethical issues in mental health policy and administration.* Rockville, MD: U.S. Department of Health and Human Services.

Beauchamp, T. L., Faden, R. R., Wallace, R. J., Jr., & Walters, L. (1992). *Ethical issues in social science research.* Baltimore, MD: Johns Hopkins University Press.

Bell-Dolan, D. J., Foster, S. L., & Sikora, D. M. (1989). A reliable sociometric measure for preschool children. *Developmental Psychology, 25,* 306–311.*

Belter, R. W., & Grisso, T. (1984). Children's recognition of rights violations in counseling. *Professional Psychology: Research and Practice, 15,* 899–910.*

Bocker, J. V. (1990). Treating adolescent sexual offenders. *Professional Psychology: Research and Practice, 21*(5), 362–365.

Bok, S. (1974). The ethics of giving placebos. *Scientific American, 231,* 17–23.

Bok, S. (1978). *Secrets: On the ethics of concealment and revelation.* New York: Pantheon.

Bok, S. (1992). Informed consent in tests of patient reliability. *JAMA, 267*(8), 1118–1119.

Bradley, E. J., & Lindsay, R. C. L. (1987). Methodological and ethical issues in child abuse research. *Journal of Family Violence, 2*(3), 239–255.*

Bromley, M. A., & Riolo, J. A. (1988). Complying with mandated child protective reporting: A challenge for treatment professionals. *Alcoholism Treatment Quarterly, 5*(3–4), 83–96.

Boroch, R. F., & Cecil, J. S. (1979). *Assuring the confidentiality of social science research data.* Philadelphia: Univerity of Pennsylvania Press.

Burbach, D. J., Farha, J. G., & Thorpe, J. S. (1986). Assessing depression in community samples of children using self-report inventories: Ethical considerations. *Journal of Abnormal Child Pyschology, 14*(4), 579–589.

Campbell, M. (1987). Consent issues with disturbed and/or retarded children. *Psychopharmacology Bulletin, 23*(3), 379–381.

Capaldi, D., & Patterson, G.R. (1987). An approach to the problem of recruitment and retention rates for longitudinal research. *Behavioral Assessment, 9*(2), 169–177.

Carroll, M. A., Schneider, H. G., & Wesley, G. R. (1985). *Ethics in the Practice of Psychology.* Englewood, NJ: Prentice-Hall.

Castellanos, F. X., Elia, J., Kruesi, M. J. P., Gulotta, C. S., Mefford, I. N., Potter, W. Z., Ritchie, G. F., & Rapoport, J. L. (in press). Cerebrospinal fluid monoamine metabolites in ADHD boys. *Psychiatry Research.*

Ceci, S. J., & Peters, D. (1984). How blind is blind review? *American Psychologist, 46,* 1491–1494.*

Ceci, S. J., Peters, D., & Plotkin, J. (1985). Human subjects review, personal values, and the regulation of social science research. *American Psychologist, 40*(9), 994–1002.

Chandler, M., Fritz, A. S., & Hala, S. (1989). Small-scale deceit: Deception as a marker of two-, three-, and four-year-olds' early theories of mind. *Child Development, 60,* 1263–1277.*

Chase-Lansdale, P. L., Brooks-Gunn, J., & Paikoff, R. L. (1991). Research and programs for adolescent mothers: Missing links and future promises. *Family Relations, 40,* 396–403.

Chassin, L., Barrera, M., Bech, K., & Kossak-Fuller, J. (1992). Recruiting a community sample of adolescent children of alcoholics: A comparison of three subject sources. *Journal of Studies on Alcohol, 53*(4), 316–319.*

Christakis, N. A. (1992). Ethics are local: Engaging cross cultural variation in the ethics for clinical research. *Social Science Medicine, 35*(9), 1079–1091.

Cicchetti, D., & Manly, J. T. (1990). A personal perspective on conducting research with maltreating families: Problems and solutions. In G. Brody & I. Sigel (Eds.), *Methods of family research* (Vol. 2, pp. 87–133). Hillsdale, NJ: Lawrence Erlbaum Associates.*

Conte, J. R. (1987). Ethical issues in evaluation of prevention programs. *Child Abuse and Neglect, 11*(2), 171–172.

Curry, J. F. (1992). Implementation issues in adolescent inpatient research. *Comprehensive Mental Health Care, 2*(1), 27–43.

DeKraai, M. B., & Sales, B. D. (1991). Liability in child therapy and research. *Journal of Consulting and Clinical Psychology, 59*(6), 853–860.

Department of Health and Human Services (DHHS). (1983, March 8). Additional protections for children involved as subjects in research. *Federal Register, 48*(46), 9814–9820.

Department of Health and Human Services (DHHS). (1991, August). Title 45 Public Welfare, Part 46, *Code of Federal Regualtions, Protection of Human Subjects.*

Department of Health, Education, and Welfare (DHEW). (1978). *The Belmont Report: Ethical principles and guidelines for the protection of human subjects of research* (DHEW Publication No.[OS] 78–0012, Appendix I, DHEW Publication No.[OS] 78–0013, Appendix II, DHEW Publication [OS] 78–0014). Washington, DC: U.S. Government Printing Office.

Des Jarlais, D. C., & Friedman, S. R. (1987). AIDS prevention among IV drug users: Potential conflicts between research design and ethics. *IRB: Review of Human Subjects Research, 9*, 6–8.

Edelbrock, C. (1994). Assessment of child psychopathology. In C. B. Fisher & R. M. Lerner (Eds.), *Applied developmental psychology* (pp. 294–315). New York: McGraw-Hill.

Egeland, B. (1991). A longitudinal study of high-risk families: Issues and findings. In R. H. Starr & D. A. Wolfe (Eds.), *The effects of child abuse and neglect: Issues and research* (pp. 33–56). New York: Guilford.

Eichelman, B., Wikler, D., & Hartwig, A. (1984). Ethics and psychiatric research: Problems and justification. *American Journal of Psychiatry, 141*(3), 400–405.

English, A. (1989). AIDS testing and epidemiology for youths: Recommendations of the work group conference: "AIDS in adolescents: Exploring the challenge." *Journal of Adolescent Health Care, 10*(3, Suppl), 52–57.

English, A. (1991). Runaway and street youth at risk for HIV infections: Legal and ethical issues in access to care. Special issue: Homeless youth. *Journal of Adolescent Health, 12*(7), 504–510.

Eth, S. (1992). Ethical challenges in the treatment of traumatized refugees. *Journal of Traumatic Stress, 5*(1), 103–110.

Fassler, D. (1992). Ethical issues in child and adolescent psychiatry. *Journal of the American Academy of Child and Adolescent Psychiatry, 31*(3), 392.

Fisher, C. B. (1991). Ethical considerations for research on psychosocial interventions for high-risk infants and children. In *Psychological Practice: Marketing, Legal, Ethical and Current Professional Issues* (pp. 92–94). Washington, DC: The National Register.

Fisher, C. B. (1993). Integrating science and ethics in research with high-risk children and youth. *Social Policy Report: Society for Research in Child Development, 7*(4), 1–27.

Fisher, C. B. (1994). Reporting and referring research participants: Ethical challenges for investigators studying children and youth. *Ethics & Behavior, 4*, 87–95.

Fisher, C. B., & Brennan, M. (1992). Application and ethics in developmental psychology. In D. L. Featherman, R. M. Lerner, & M. Perlmutter (Eds.), *Life-span development and behavior* (pp. 189–219). Hillsdale, NJ: Lawrence Erlbaum Associates.*

Fisher, C. B., & Fryberg, D. (1994). Participant partners: College students weigh the costs and benefits of deceptive research. *American Psychologist, 49*, 417–427.

Fisher, C. B., Higgins, A., Rau, M. B., Kuther, T., & Belanger, S. (in press). Referring and reporting research participants at-risk: Views from urban adolescents. *Child Development, 67.*

Fisher, C. B., Jackson, J. F., & Villarruel, F. (in press). The study of ethnic minority children and youth in the United States. In W. Damon (Series Ed.) & R. M. Lerner (Vol. Ed.), *Handbook of child psychology: Vol. 1. Theoretical models of human development* (5th ed.). New York: Wiley.

Fisher, C. B., & Lerner, R. M. (1994). Foundations of applied developmental psychology. In C. B. Fisher & R. M. Lerner (Eds.), *Applied developmental psychology* (pp. 3–20). New York: McGraw-Hill.

Fisher, C. B., & Rosendahl, S. W. (1990). Risks and remedies of research participation. In C. B. Fisher & W. W. Tryon (Eds.), *Ethics in Applied Developmental Psychology: Emerging Issues in an Emerging Field* (pp. 43–60). Norwood, NJ: Ablex.

Fisher, C. B., & Tryon, W. W. (1990). Emerging ethical issues in an emerging field. In C. B. Fisher & W. W. Tryon (Eds.), *Ethics in Applied Developmental Psychology: Emerging Issues in an Emergig Field* (pp. 1–14). Norwood, NJ: Ablex.

Freedman, B. (1975). A moral theory of informed consent. *Hastings Center Report, 5,* 32–39.

Freedman, B. (1987). Scientific value and validity as ethical requirements for research: A proposed explication. *IRB-A Review of Human Subjects Research, 9*(6), 7–10.

Freedman, B., Fuks, A., & Weijer, C. (1993). In loco parentis: Minimal risk as an ethical threshold for research upon children. *Hastings Center Report, 23*(2), 13–19.

Gaylin, W., & Macklin, R. (1982). *Who speaks for the child: The problems of proxy consent.* New York: Plenum.

Gensheimer, L. K., Rossa, M. W., & Ayers, T. S. (1990). Children's self-selection into prevention programs: Evaluation of an innovative recruitment strategy for children of alcoholics. *American Journal of Community Psychology, 18*(5), 707–723.

Geraty, R. D., Hendron, R. L., & Flaa, C. J. (1992). Ethical perspectives on managed care as it relates to child and adolescent psychiatry. *Journal of the American Academy of Child and Adolescent Psychiatry, 31*(3), 398–402.

Gibbs, J. T. (1990). Mental health issues of black adolescents: Implications for policy and practice. In A. R. Stiffman & L. E. Davis (Eds.), *Ethnic issues in adolescent mental health* (pp. 21–52). Newbury Park, CA: Sage.

Goldberg, S. (1993). Some costs and benefits of psychological research in pediatric settings. In G. Koren (Ed.), *Textbook of ethics in pediatric research* (pp. 63–73). Malabar, FL: Krieger.

Goodman, G. S., & Tobey, A. E. (1994). Ethical issues in child witness research. *Child Abuse and Neglect, 18*(3), 290–293.

Gottesman, I. I. (in press). Schizophrenia epigenesis: Past, present, and future. *Acta Psychiatrical Scandinavia.*

Grisso, T. (1992a). Minors assent to behavioral research without parental consent. In B. Stanley & J. E. Sieber (Eds.), *Social Research on Children and Adolescents* (pp. 109–127). Newbury Park, CA: Sage.

Grisso, T. (1992b). Science and advocacy. American Psychological Association: When worlds collide: Law and ethics in conflict. *Forensic Reports, 5*(2), 179–188.

Grisso, T., & Appelbaum, P. S. (1991). Mentally ill and non-mentally ill patients' abilities to understand informed consent disclosure for medication: Preliminary data. *Law and Human Behavior, 15,* 377–388.

Grisso, T., & Appelbaum, P. S. (1992). Is it ethical to offer predictions of future violence? *Law and Human Behavior, 16*(6), 621–633.

Grisso, T., Appelbaum, P. S., Mulvey, E. P., & Fletcher, K. (1995). The MacArthur treatment competence study. II: Measures of abilities related to competence to consent to treatment. *Law and Human Behavior, 19,* 127–148.

Grisso, T., & Vierling, L. (1978). Minors' consent to treatment: A developmental perspective. *Professional Psychology, 9,* 412–427.

Gustafson, K. E., McNamara, J. R., & Jensen, J. A. (1992). Informed consent: Risk and benefit disclosure practices of child clinicians. *Psychotherapy in Practice, 10*(4), 91–102.*

Gustafson, K. E., McNamara, J. R., & Jensen, J. A. (1994). Parents' informed consent decisions regarding psychotherapy for their children: Consideration of the therapeutic risks and benefits. *Professional Psychology: Research and Practice, 25*(1), 16–22.*

Gwadz, M., & Rotheram-Borus, M. J. (1992). Tracking high-risk adolescents longitudinally. *AIDS Education and Prevention, Fall*(suppl), 69–82.

Hall, D. (1988). Reviewing research involving children: The practice of British research ethics committees. *IRB: A Review of Human Subjects Research, 10*(2), 1–5.

Hall, D. (1991). The research imperative and bureaucratic control: The case of clinical research. *Social Science and Medicine, 32*(3), 333–342.

Hayvren, M., & Hymel, S. (1984). Ethical issues in sociometric testing: The impact of sociometric measures on interactive behavior. *Developmental Psychology, 20,* 844–849.*

Hendren, R. L. (1991). Determining the need for inpatient treatment. In R. L. Hendren & I. N. Berlin (Eds.), *Psychiatric inpatient care of children and adolescents: A multi-cultural approach* (pp. 37–64). New York: Wiley.

Hendrix, D. H. (1991). Ethics and intrafamily confidentiality in counseling with children. *Journal of Mental Health Counseling, 13*(3), 323–333.

Herceg-Baron, R. (1981). Case study: Parental consent and family planning research involving minors. *IRB: A Review of Human Subjects Research,* 5–7.

Hoagwood, K. (1994). The Certificate of Confidentiality at NIMH: Applications and implications for service research with children. *Ethics & Behavior, 4,* 123–131.

Hoagwood, K., Jensen, P. S., & Leshner, A. (1991). Ethical issues in research on child and adolescent mental disorders: Implications for a science of scientific ethics. In S. Henggeler & A. Santos (Eds.), *Innovative services for difficult to treat populations* (pp. 541–561). Washington, DC: American Psychiatric Press.

Holder, A. R. (1981). Can teenagers participate in research without parental consent? *IRB: A Review of Human Subjects Research, 3*(2), 5–7.

Hughes, T., & Helling, M. K. (1991). A case for obtaining informed consent from young children. *Early Childhood Quarterly, 6*(2), 225–232.

Imber, S. D., Glanz, L. M., Elkin, I., Sotsky, S. M., Boyer, J. L., & Leber, W. R. (1986). Ethical issues in psychotherapy research: Problems in a collaborative clinical trials study. *American Psychologist, 41,* 137–146.*

Jackson, J. F. (1993). Multiple caregiving among African Americans: The need for an emic approach. *Human Development, 36,* 87–102.

Jenkins-Hall, K., & Osborn, C. A. (1994). The conduct of socially sensitive research: Sex offenders as participants. *Criminal Justice & Behavior, 21,* 325–340.*

Jensen, J. A., McNamara, J. R., & Gustafson, K. E. (1991). Parents' and clinicians' attitudes toward the risks and benefits of child psychotherapy: A study of informed consent content *Professional Psychology: Research and Practice, 22*(2), 161–170.*

Kamps, W. A., Akkerboom, J. C., Nitschke, R., Kingma, A., Holmes, H. B., Caldwell, S., & Humphrey, G. B. (1987). Altruism and informed consent in chemotherapy trails of childhood cancer. Special issue: Psychosocial aspects of chemotherapy in cancer care: The parent, family, and staff. *Loss, Grief and Care, 1*(3–4), 93–110.*

Kaser-Boyd, N., Adelman, H. S., & Taylor, L. (1985). Minors' ability to identify risks and benefits of therapy. *Professional Psychology: Research and Practice, 16*(3), 411–417.

Keith-Spiegel, P. (1983). Children and consent to participate in research. In G. B. Melton, G. P. Koocher, & M. J. Saks (Eds.), *Children's competence to consent* (pp. 179–211). New York: Plenum.

Kelman, H. C. (1967). Human use of human subjects: The problem in conducting research on maltreated children: Illustrations form a longitudinal study. *Child Abuse and Neglect.*

Kinard, E. M. (1985). Ethical issues in research with abused children. *Child Abuse and Neglect, 9,* 301–311.

Kinard, E. M. (in press). Methodological issues and practical problem in conducting research on maltreated children: Illustrations from a longitudinal study. *Child Abuse and Neglect.*

Koocher, G. P., & Keith-Spiegel, P. C. (1990). *Children, ethics, & the law: Professional issues and cases.* Lincoln: University of Nebraska Press.

Kopelman, L. (1981). Estimating risk in human research. *Clinical Research, 29,* 1–8.

Korn, J. H. (1987). Judgments of acceptability of deception in psychological research. *Journal of General Psychology, 114*(3), 205–216.

Korn, J. H., & Hogan, K. (1992). Effect of incentives and aversiveness of treatment on willingness to participate in research. *Teaching of Psychology, 19,* 21–24.

Kruesi, M. J. P., Swedo S. E., Coffey, M. L., Hamburger, S. D., Leonard, H., & Rapoport, J. L. (1988). Objective and subjective side effects of research lumbar punctures in children and adolescents. *Psychiatry Research, 25,* 59–63.

Langer, D. H. (1991). Legal rights for adolescents as research subjects. In R. M. Lerner, A. Peterson, & J. Brooks-Gunn (Eds.), *Encyclopedia of adolescence* (pp. 591–593). New York: Garland.

Laosa, L. (1990). Population generalizability, cultural sensitivity, and ethical dilemmas. In C. B. Fisher & W. W. Tryon (Eds.), *Ethics in applied developmental psychology: Emerging issues in an emerging field* (pp. 227–252). Norwood, NJ: Ablex.

Larossa, R., Bennett, L. A., & Gelles, R. J. (1981). Ethical dilemmas in qualitative family research. *Journal of Marriage and the Family,* 303–313.

LeBaron, S., Zeltzer, L. K., & Fanurick, D. (1989). An investigation of cold pressor pain in children: *I. Pain, 37*(2), 161–171.

Leikin, S. L. (1989) Immunodeficiency virus infection, adolescents, and the institutional review board. *Journal of Adolescent Health Care, 10*(6), 500–505.

Lepper, M. R., Ross, L., & Lau, R. R. (1986). Persistence of inaccurate beliefs about the self: Perseverance effects in the classroom. *Journal of Personality & Social Psychology, 50,* 482–491.

Lerner, R. M., & Tubman, J. G. (1990). Plasticity in development: Ethical implications for developmental interventions. In C. B. Fisher & W. W. Tryon (Eds.), *Ethics in applied developmental psychology: Emerging issues in an emerging field* (pp. 113–132). Norwood, NJ: Ablex.

Levine, R., (1986). *Ethics and regulation of clinical research* (2nd ed.). Baltimore, Munich: Urban & Schwarzenberg.

Lewis, C. E., Lewis, M. A., & Ifekwunigue, M. (1978). Informed consent by children and participation in an influenza vaccine trial. *American Journal of Pediatric Health, 68,* 1079–1082.

Lewis, M. (1990). Assessing social intervention: Scientific and Implications. In C. B. Fisher & W. W. Tryon (Eds.) *Ethics in applied developmental psychology: Emerging issues in an emerging field* (pp. 113–132). Norwood, NJ: Ablex.

Linehan, M., Armstron, H., Suarez, A., Allmon, D., & Heard, H. (1991). Cognitive-behavioral treatment of chronically parasuicidal borderline patients. *Archives of General Psychiatry, 48,* 1060–1064.

Linn, L. S., Yager, J., & Leake, B. (1988). Psychiatrists' attitudes toward preventive intervention in routine clinical practice. *Hospital and Community Psychiatry, 39*(6), 637–642.

Liss, M. (1994). State and federal laws governing reporting for researchers. *Ethics & Behavior, 4,* 133–146.

Litt, I. F. (1992). Ethics and research on adolescents. *Journal of Adolescent Health, 13,* 640.

Macklin, R. (1981). "Due" and "undue" inducements: On paying money to research subjects. *IRB: Review of Human Subjects Research, 3,* 1–6.

Mann, T. (1994). *Informed consent for psychological research: Do subjects comprehend consent forms and understand their legal rights?* Unpublished manuscript, Stanford University, Stanford, CA.

Margolin, G. (1982). Ethical and legal considerations in marital and family therapy. *American Psychologist, 37*(7), 788–801.

McGrath, P. A. (1993). Inducing pain in children: A controversial issue. *Pain, 52*(3), 255–257.

Melton, G. B. (1981). Effects of state law permitting minors to consent to psychotherapy. *Professional Psychology, 12*(5), 647–654.

Melton, G. B. (1989). Ethical and legal issues in research and intervention. Conferences: "AIDS in adolescents: Exploring the challenge." *Journal of Adolescent Health Care, 10*(3 suppl), 36–44.

Melton, G. B. (1990). Certificates of confidentiality under the public health service act: Strong protection but not enough. *Violence & Victims, 5,* 67–71.

Melton, G. B., Koocher, G. P., & Saks, M. J. (1983). *Children's competence to consent.* New York: Plenum.

Mezworski, T., Tolan, W. J., & Belsky, J. (1988). Intervention in insecure infant attachment. In J. Belsky & T. Nezworski (Eds.), *Clinical implications of attachment* (pp. 352–386). Hillsdale, NJ: Lawrence Erlbaum Associates.

Michaels, M. L., Roosa, M. W., & Gensheimer, L. K. (1992). Family characteristics of children who self-select into a prevention program for children of alcoholics. *American Journal of Community Psychology, 20*(5), 663–672.

Milgram, S. (1964). Issues in the study of obedience: A reply to Baumrind. *American Psychologist, 19,* 848–852.

Miller, R. D., & Weinstock, R. (1987). Conflict of interest between therapist-patient confidentiality and the duty to report sexual abuse of children. *Behavioral Sciences and the Law, 5*(2), 161–174.

Mill, J. S. (1957). *Utilitarianism.* New York: Bobbs-Merrill. (Original work published 1861)

Mishkin, B. (1982). The report and recommendations of the national commission for the protection of human subjects: Research involving children. *Advances in Law and Child Development, 1,* 63–96.

Mishner, J. M. (1992). Ethical assessment and moral reasoning in child therapy. *Child and Adolescent Social Work Journal, 9*(1), 3–19.

Monahan, J., Appelbaum. P. S., Mulvey, E. P., Robbins, P. C., & Lidz, C. W. (1993). Ethical and legal duties in conducting research on violence: Lessons from the MacArthur Risk Assessment study. *Violence & Victims, 8,* 387–396.

Morton, K. L., & Green, U. (1991). Comprehension of terminology related to treatment and patients' rights by inpatient children and adolescents. *Journal of Clinical Child Psychology, 20,* 392–399.

Munir, K., & Earls, F. (1992). Ethical principles governing research in child and adolescent psychiatry. Special section: Ethicical issues in child and adolescent psychiatry. *Journal of the American Academy of Child and Adolescent Psychiatry, 31*(3), 408–414.

Nannis, E. D. (1991). Children's understanding of their participation in psychological research: Implications for issues of assent and consent. *Canadian Journal of Behavioral Science, 23*(2), 133–141.

National Research Council. (1993). *Understanding child abuse and neglect.* Washington DC: National Academy of Sciences.

Nolan, K. (1992, Summer). Assent, consent, and behavioral research with adolescents. *AACAP Child and Adolescent Research Notes,* 7–10.

Nuremberg Code. (1946). *Journal of the American Medical Association, 132,* 1090.

Office for Protection from Research Risks (OPRR), Department of Health and Human Services, National Institutes of Health. (1993). *Protecting human research subjects: Institutional review board guidebook.* Washington, DC: U.S. Government Printing Office.

Olson, R. A., Huszti, H. C., & Mason, P. J. (1989). Pediatric AIDS/HIV infection: An emerging challenge to pediatric psychology. *Journal of Pediatric Psychology, 14*(1), 1–21.

O'Leary, K. D., & Borkovec, T. D. (1978). Conceptual, methodological, and ethical problems of placebo groups in psychotherapy research. *American Psychologist, 33,* 821–830.

O'Neill, P., & Hern, R. (1991). A systems approach to ethical problems. *Ethics and Behavior, 1*(2), 129–143.

Orne, M. T. (1962). On the social psychology of the psychological experiment: With a particular reference to demand characteristics and their implications. *American Psychologist, 17,* 776–783.

O'Rourke, K., Snider, B. W., Thomas, J. M., & Berland, D. (1992). Knowing and practicing ethics. *Journal of the American Academy of Child and Adolescent Psychiatry, 31*(3), 393–397.

Parker, L. S., & Lidz, C. W. (1994). Familial coercion to participate in genetic family studies: Is there cause for IRB intervention? *IRB: Review of Human Subjects Research, 16*(1, 2), 6–12.

Pentz, M. A. (1994). Primary prevention of adolescent drug abuse. In C. B. Fisher & R. M. Lerner (Eds.), *Applied developmental psychology* (pp. 435–474). New York: McGraw-Hill.

Pettifor, J. L. (1980). Private wise: Privacy of information. *Canadian Psychology, 21*(4), 187–190.

Piaget, J. (1965). *The moral judgement of the child* (M. Gabian, Trans.). New York: The Free Press. (Original work published 1932)

Porter, J. P. (1987). How unaffiliated/nonscientist members of institutional review boards see their roles. *IRB: A Review of Human Subjects Research, 9*(6), 1–6.

Prentice, E. D., & Antonson, D. L. (1987). A protocol review guide to reduce IRB inconsistency. *IRB: A Review of Human Subjects Research, 9*(1), 9–11.

Putnam, F. W. (1984). The study of multiple personality disorder: General strategies and practical consideration. *Psychiatry Annals, 14,* 58–61.

Rae, W. A., & Worchel, F. F. (1991). Ethical beliefs and behaviors of pediatric psychologists: A Survey. *Journal of Pediatric Psychology, 16*(6), 727–745.

Resnick, J. H., & Schwartz, T. (1973). Ethical standards as an independent variable in psychological research. *American Psychologist, 28,* 134–139.

Rogers, J. L., Howard, K. I., & Vessey, J. T. (1993). Using significance tests to evaluate equivalence between two experimental groups. *Psychological Bulletin, 113,* 553–565.

Ross, L., Lepper, M. R., & Hubbard, M. (1975). Perseverance in self-perception and social perception: Biased attributional processes in the debriefing paradigm. *Journal of Personality and Social Psychology, 32,* 880–892.

Rotheram-Borus, M. J., & Koopman, C. (1992). Protecting children's rights in AIDS research. In B. Stanley & J. E. Sieber (Eds.), *Social research on children and adolescents* (pp. 143–161). Newbury Park, CA: Sage.

Rudd, M., Rajab, M., Orman, D., Stulman, D., Juiner, T., & Dixon, W. (in press). Effectiveness of an outpatient intervention targeting suicidal young adults: Preliminary results. *Journal of Consulting & Clinical Psychology, 65.*

Sarason, S. (1984). If it can be studied or developed, should it? *American Psychologist, 39,* 739–754.

Scarr, S. (1990). Ethical dilemmas in recent research: A personal saga. In C. B. Fisher & W. W. Tryon (Eds.), *Ethics in applied developmental psychology: Emerging issues in an emerging field* (pp. 29–42). Norwood, NJ: Ablex.

Schetky, D. H. (1992). Ethical issues in forensic child and adolescent psychiatry. *Journal of the American Academy of Child and Adolescent Psychiatry, 31*(3), 403–407.

Schoeman, F. (1982). Protecting intimate relationships: Children's competence and children's rights. *IRB: A Review of Human Subjects Research, 4*(6), 1–5.

Sieber, J. E. (1990). How to be ethical in applied developmental psychology: Examples from research on adolescent drinking behavior. In C. B. Fisher & W. W. Tryon (Eds.), *Ethics in applied developmental psychology: Emerging issues in an emerging field* (pp. 61–78). Norwood, NJ: Ablex.

Silva, M. C., & Sorrell, J. M. (1988). Enhancing comprehension of information for informed consent: A review of empirical research. *IRB: A Review of Human Subjects Research, 10*(1), 1–5.

Small, A. M., Campbell, M., Shay, J., & Goodman, I. S. (1994). Ethical guidelines for psychopharmacological research in children. In J. Hattab (Ed.), *Ethics and child mental health* (pp. 244–253). Jerusalem, Israel: Gefen.

Smith, S. S., & Richardson, D. (1983). Amelioration of deception and harm in psychological research. *Journal of Personality & Social Psychology, 44*, 1075–1082.

Society for Research in Child Development. (1993). Ethical standards for research with children. In *Directory of Members* (pp. 337–339). Ann Arbor, MI: Author.

Spiker, D., Kraemer, H. C., Scott, D. J., & Gross, R. T. (1991). Design issues in a randomized clinical trial of a behavioral intervention: Insights from the Infant Health and Development Program. Special issue. *Journal of Developmental and Behavioral Pediatrics, 12*(6), 386–393.

Stiffman, A. R., & Davis, L. E. (Eds.). (1990). *Ethical issues in adolescent mental health.* Newbury Park, CA: Sage.

Sullivan, T., Martin, W. L., & Handelsman, M. M. (1993). Practical benefits of an informed consent procedure: An empirical investigation. *Professional Psychology: Research and Practice, 24*(2), 160–163.

Tarasoff v. Regents of the University of California, 131 Cal. Rptr., 14, 551 P 2d 334, 1976.

Thompson, R. A. (1990). Behavioral research involving children: A Developmental perspective on risk. *IRB: A Review of Human Subjects Research, 12*(2), 1–6.

Urquiza, A. J. (1991). Retrospective methodology in family violence research: Our duty to report past abuse. *Journal of Interpersonal Violence, 6*(1), 119–126.

Veatch, R. M. (1987). *The patient as partner.* Bloomington: Indiana University Press.

Veatch, R. M. (1991). Commentary: Beyond consent to treatment. *IRB: A Review of Human Subjects Research, 3*(5) 7–8.

Weissbrod, C. S., & Mangan, T. (1987). Children's attitudes about experimental participation: The effect of deception and debriefing. *Journal of Social Psychology, 106*, 69–72.

Weissberg, R. P., Caplan, M., & Ratiner, C. (1994). *The reactions of young adolescents to a sociometric rating-scale assessment.* Unpublished manuscript.

Weithorn, L. A. (1983). Children's capacities to decide about participation in research. *IRB: A Review of Human Subjects Research, 5*(2), 1–5.

Weithorn, L. A., & Campbell, S. B. (1982). The competency of children and adolescents to make informed treatment decisions. *Child Development, 53*, 1589–1598.

Wells, K., & Sametz, L. (1985). Involvement of institutionalized children in social science research: Some issues and proposed guidelines. Special issue: Mental health services to children. *Journal of Clinical Child Psychology, 14*(30), 245–251.

Westcott, H. L. (1994). On sensitivity and ethical issues in child witness research. *Child Abuse and Neglect, 18*(3), 287–290.

Wilson, J. R., & Crowe, L. (1991). Genetics of alcoholism: Can and should youth at risk be identified? Special Focus: Alcohol and youth. *Alcohol Health and Research World, 15*(1), 11–17.

Wimmer, H., Gruber, S., & Perner, J. (1985). Young children's conception of lying: Moral intuition and denotation and connotation of "to lie." *Developmental Psychology, 21*, 993–995.

Part IV

Bridging Science and Ethics

10

A Bioethicist's Perspective

Evan G. DeRenzo
National Institute of Health

The moral complexities integral to the performance of human subjects research are intensified when research involves children and adolescents. These complexities are multiplied yet further when the subjects are not only healthy minors but are, also, children and adolescents with psychiatric and/or behavioral problems. One is humbled in the face of these complexities. Nonetheless, research into the psychiatric and behavioral disorders of childhood and adolescence must move forward if we are going to progress in our ability to prevent, treat, and cure these life-sapping conditions. In fact, this volume is a direct result of the social mandate (Institute of Medicine, 1989) to act expeditiously to increase our research knowledge about mental disorders in children and adolescents. Widespread recognition of this need is manifest through society's financial and political support of this highly specialized human subjects research.

Such support demonstrates our acknowledgment that some risks are worth taking. Future patients will benefit from increased understanding of these vexing clinical problems. Parents want to involve their severely troubled children in studies that hold out the potential for direct benefit. To achieve these ends, we strike a compromise in the inherent ethical tensions between the duty-based and virtue-grounded goals of clinical care and the utilitarian aims of research. We do so in the hope that we will gain important knowledge with little harm or burden to the children, adolescents, and families who participate in our studies and to the research enterprise itself.

The difficult moral decisions involving individual protocols and subjects, however, are not made easier by our willingness to compromise on the larger, more abstract, questions. Working through the ethical concerns posed by specific protocols and the clinical management of particular, participating minors remains a process of exquisite moral, clinical, and scientific intricacy. Over the last 30 years, as we have appreciated more acutely these inherently competing claims, we have accepted that these decisions require broad social input and have opened the human subjects research process to public scrutiny through the creation and empowerment of the institutional review board (IRB) system (MacKay, in press).

Also, at least in partial response to this heightened appreciation for the thorny moral problems posed by modern medical care and research, we have seen the introduction into the medical setting of a new health care role, that of the clinical bioethicist (Fletcher, Quist, & Jonsen, 1989; Hoffmaster, Freedman, & Fraser, 1989; La Puma & Schiedermayer, 1994). One of the primary responsibilities of a clinical research bioethicist is to develop and implement strategies to untangle and resolve the morally complex questions and situations that arise, daily, in the performance of human subjects research. Like the philosopher, the clinical bioethicist poses questions relevant to the moral conduct of research and to the moral life of the setting in which it occurs. But unlike the philosopher who is "concerned with clarification and with understanding rather than with offering solutions, because at the end of the day that philosopher does not have to carry professional responsibility for the consequences of any solution that might be suggested" (Evans, 1994, pp. 555–556), such is not the case for the applied research ethicist. The distinction between theoretical and applied ethics is that the clinical bioethicist is additionally obliged to be pragmatic and oriented toward solutions.

Like the scientist, however, who dares not fall in love with her or his own hypotheses, the clinical research ethicist dares not fall in love with her or his own moral pronouncements. The clinical research ethicist must vigilantly guard against complacency in accepting one's own or other's moral answers. Instead, the clinical research ethicist works collaboratively with others to identify an ethically permissible range of options, facilitates decision making by assuring that there is input from a wide array of moral perspectives and that thoughtful and interactive deliberations take place. Such a process increases the likelihood that sound clinical judgments on the part of a well-integrated multidisciplinary research and health care team will result (Bulger, Heitman, & Reiser, 1993). Mere application of philosophic abstractions is unsatisfactory. Clinical conditions change rapidly, ethical norms evolve, and what is believed to be scientifically appropriate or efficacious one day can be demonstrated to be inaccurate, ineffective, or even harmful the next.

Thus, in a chapter such as this, it is impossible to review exhaustively all the issues requiring consideration when evaluating a particular protocol or considering entry or continued study participation of a particular subject. Instead, the discussion here raises but a few issues that merit general consideration. The chapter concludes with recommendations on ensuring that such considerations can be openly and fully engaged, if never fully and definitively concluded.

Also, there is insufficient space to recount the full discussion that grounds our assumptions about the ethical permissibility of involving children and adolescents in biomedical research. (For a thorough philosophic discussion of this debate, the reader is referred to Ackerman, 1979; Bartholomew, 1976; Freedman, 1975; Gaylin, 1982; McCormick, 1974, 1976; National Commission, 1977; Pence, 1980; Ramsay, 1970, 1976, 1977, 1980.) Instead, this chapter takes as its starting point the relevant codes and regulations which set the ethical framework for the performance of such studies.

SELECTED ETHICAL ISSUES TO CONSIDER

Risk Analysis

In the performance of human subjects research into mental disorders of children and adolescents, we have rejected the stringency of the Nuremberg Code. The Nuremberg Code requires the voluntary consent of each research subject, thereby precluding research with minors (Annas & Grodin, 1992). Instead, the biomedical community in the United States and throughout most of the world has adopted a more permissive attitude about balancing our duties and obligations to individual child-subjects against our need to have present children to serve the good of future others.

To apply this consequentialist analysis without producing unacceptable harms, researchers in the United States have restricted the full force of the utilitarian imperative by placing tighter boundaries on permissible exposure to research risks and setting more explicit goals for benefit in research with minors than with adults (Brock, 1994; Levine, 1986, 1989; Munir & Earls, 1992; OPRR, 1993; Protection of Human Subjects, 1991). That is, the federal regulations, 45 CFR 46 (Protection of Human Subjects, 1991) that set the framework for judging the ethical permissibility of any study set rigorous limits on placing minors at risk as a result of their research participation. In general, such risks must be overtly balanced in favor of potential direct benefits to the minor subjects. This framework forces researchers, IRBs, and clinical bioethicists, among others, to focus sharply on risk assessment and minimization.

But risk can only be assessed and minimized in relation to how it is defined. How risk is defined for children and adolescents, however, is a matter of interpretation. Add in the unknowns of the influences of mental disorder and our task of making precise and accurate judgments about what is appropriately defined as minimal risk, or only a minor increment above, becomes highly complex.

The regulatory definition of minimal risk (45 CFR 46, 46.102) requires that research participation should not pose risks of harm or discomfort greater than what might be expected in ordinary life experiences. But whose life? In a strict interpretation, this refers to the daily life of a healthy child or adult. A broader, more intuitively reasonable interpretation, and one, perhaps closer to the initial intent of the definition's authors (R. Levine, 1995), is that the definition should take into account a particular subject's circumstances. That is, where subjects are healthy children, the more stringent definition adheres. Where the subjects are ill or disabled, risks commensurate with these children's ordinary experiences may be allowable. Certainly at higher risk levels, it seems clear that where children are ill or disabled, we permit research to take into account their particular experiences. Therefore, it seems illogical to set a higher standard for minimal risk research, including minimal risk research that holds out the prospect for direct benefit, than for research above this threshold with no expected direct benefit.

In the regulatory language concerning children in research studies that hold out no prospect of direct benefit (45 CFR 46, 46.406), as the risk tolerance is allowed to rise to a minor increment above minimal risk, the procedural guidance directs that the "intervention or procedure presents experiences to subjects that are reasonably commensurate with those inherent in their actual or expected medical, dental, psychological, social or educational situations" (p. 15). Thus, for example, in a study of cystic fibrosis in children, it is arguably not unreasonable to expect a child who regularly experiences bronchoscopes for clinical care to submit to this procedure for research purposes.

Further muddling attempts to strictly delineate minimal risk, it can even be argued (Thompson, 1990) that the seemingly more liberal interpretation, depending on how one views the scope of ordinary daily life, is already built into the definition of minimal risk. This interpretation may hold up even when literally and narrowly read in relation to healthy, normal minors. Thompson (1990) suggested that this tolerance results from our standard understanding of minimal risk for minors that applies a traditional, linear, Piagetian model of vulnerability. That is, the underlying assumption of the standard model for determining minimal risk in children is that there is an inverse relationship between vulnerability and cognitive maturity. As the child's ability to comprehend the reasons for his or her own participation in the study increase and the child's life experiences become more varied as a result of increasing age, potential for harm decreases.

Perhaps, however, this assumption is flawed. Perhaps, instead, we should consider potential harms within a nonlinear or curvilinear developmental model (Thompson, 1990). Focusing on psychological risk, for example, by applying a nonlinear developmental model within a more flexible regulatory interpretation of minimal risk, we may need to consider more carefully that:

> these regulations suggest that as a child's normative life experiences change with age—in accord with the child's growing competencies and experiential background—norms defining research risk must comparably be revised to encompass these changing experiences. . . . For example, extended periods apart from parents with unfamiliar adults might be questionable in research with infants, but certainly not for older children and adolescents. Conversely, procedures that would be allowed with young children because they are part of that child's ordinary life experiences might not be permitted at later ages, when these experiences are not as typical. . . . For example, infants and toddlers commonly experience brief or prolonged separations from their caregivers (e.g., with a babysitter, in day-care, etc.), and they are often distressed by these experiences. . . . By the "minimal risk" regulation, research involving infants' involuntary separations from their caregivers is permissible. . . . Young children regularly experience invasions of their bodily and personal privacy by parents, teachers, and other adults. It is unclear, however, whether this justifies privacy violations in the research context. (p. 7)

What may be at stake is analogous to what Katz (1993) referred to as dignity rights or what Ramsay (1970) referred to as the distinction between being harmed and being wronged. For if we accept a nonlinear, developmental model of human growth, even a narrow and literal definition of risks of daily life for healthy, normal children may pose risks we have not yet sufficiently contemplated to the psychological well-being of minors in the research setting. That is, cognitive integration of such normal unpleasantries as invasions of privacy may be quite differently processed in the research setting than at home. For example, if we accept that optimal development of trust in healthy, normal minors requires that they can trust that those responsible for their care will do what is best for them as particular individuals, Evans (1994) may be correct that threats to this trust pose risk of serious and potentially long-lasting harms well beyond what we would consider minimal.

To properly frame these issues in the context of research into mental disorders of children and adolescents, the context of daily life for a child or adolescent with psychiatric, psychological, or behavioral problems should be considered. If we apply a liberal interpretation to the regulatory definition of minimal risk, which might be appropriate in some circumstances, such as in research into a childhood cancer that is uniformly lethal and for which we have no effective treatment, it may be problematic for certain studies of pediatric mental illness.

Because it may be impossible to know how a child with mental illness will interpret the experience, we may not be able to define satisfactorily minimal risk or a minor increment beyond. Thompson's (1990) view seems not too conservative when considering children and adolescents with mental disorders.

> More generally, it is clearer that in studies with special populations of children and youth—such as those who are incarcerated, have been maltreated, or are substance abusers—should not necessarily define standards of minimal risk in terms of the ordinary life experiences of children in these populations. (p. 7)

Of equal or greater complexity is defining and assessing risk in studies investigating factors that place seemingly healthy, normal minors at risk for mental disorders. Again, we may need to increase our level of suspicion that our standard assumptions of what is minimal risk or what is only a minor increment above such risk may be inadequate.

Regarding at-risk studies, Brock (1994) suggested that "direct benefit to the participants in the experimental group is virtually always intended. Therefore, prevention/educational intervention research has generally been regarded as humanitarian, socially relevant, and an unlikely candidate for ethical pitfalls or criticism" (p. 73). But after advocating for more such research of this kind, Brock (1994) listed a series of potential ethical land mines. For example, such studies, which involve minors without any diagnosis, often draw disproportionately from minority groups or underprivileged families. These investigations can include parents with conditions that not only put the children or adolescents at risk but diminish the parents' ability to serve as ethically valid surrogates. Even participation as a healthy normal subject may place a minor at risk for stigmatization and the effects of inappropriately set expectations as a result of being labeled by study participation. All of these possibilities, taken in the context of Evans' (1994) concerns about threats to trust, may pose potential harms to minor subjects that are difficult to quantify.

Empirical Studies of Children's and Adolescents' Understanding of the Research Process

Assessment of potential psychological harms to healthy or ill minors requires increased attention. Goldberg (1993) reviewed *Child Development Abstracts* from 1973 to 1993 and found only one article relevant to risk of psychological harm. Review of the bioethics literature adds only a few more citations (Haslam, 1993; Macklin, 1992; Melton, 1992; Thompson, 1992). There is a growing body of literature that should be read and contemplated by all investigators performing research with pediatric subjects and should serve as the beginning of more data collection about this issue. The casebook in this volume contains examples of ways in which harm has been minimized.

Nonetheless, no amount of reading or regulatory review will provide a formulaic means of risk calculation (Thomasma & Mauer, 1982). Instead, we need to proceed slowly, ask difficult and probing questions about how to minimize anticipated risks, and stretch our imaginations to contemplate previously unanticipated risks.

Moreover, we need to perform studies that will teach us about how healthy and ill children and adolescents perceive their experiences as research participants. Only as we learn more about how children and adolescents function within the research setting can we devise new strategies for minimizing existing risks and more accurately assess future studies.

At present, only a handful of such studies have been performed (Abramovitch, Freedman, Derbyshire, & Brunschot, 1995; Abramovitch, Freedman, Henry, & Brunschot, 1993; Susman, Dorn, & Fletcher, 1992). In what appears to be the first empirical investigation into the consent process for children in biomedical research, Susman and her colleagues (1992) at the National Institutes of Health (NIH), examined the assent capacity of children, adolescents, and young adults in cancer trials and studies of obesity. Although the minor subjects were reasonably clear on concrete information, such as time elements and freedom to ask questions, there was less understanding of the more abstract elements. These abstract elements included distinctions between scientific and therapeutic purpose and alternatives to study participation. Subsequent investigations (Abramovitch et al., 1993; Abramovitch et. al., 1995) have replicated these findings and support the conclusion that minor subjects do not fully grasp abstract aspects of the research process.

Especially in mental health research, where concerns about decisional capacity in adults are already heightened (Benson, Roth, Appelbaum, Lidz, & Winslade, 1988; DeRenzo, 1994a, 1994b), research into the assent process in mental disorders research with children and adolescents is needed. Unpublished data collected by the author and several NIH colleagues indicate that healthy normal children do not understand the research process and that we need to intensify our efforts to obtain fully informed assent from child subjects. We need to learn more about which elements of assent are understood and what conditions maximize understanding. The few data accumulated to date argue against assuming too great an appreciation in minor subjects, particularly those with, or those at risk for, psychosocial disturbances. Additionally, research is needed to follow up on the long-term, psychological well-being of minor subjects.

Surrogate Decision Making

Another area in which more attention is needed is surrogate decision making. When designing pediatric protocols, especially in mental health, investigators should give special attention to assessment and attempts to enhance sound surrogate decision making. Given the kinds of potential problems highlighted by Brock (1994), we might consider more seriously integrating support into protocols to assist parents and guardians to be more capable surrogates. Such support might include having mental health counselors and social workers provide an array of formalized services (Levine, Dubler, & Levine, 1991). IRBs should be asking about the support services investigators are building into their protocols for both minor subjects and their surrogates. Where such supports are not included but would be important for subject protection, IRBs should insist on the addition of ancillary services. Also, the socioeconomic characteristics of some surrogates in this study population may have worrisome implications for compensation of study participants that should be explored by IRBs.

Ethical Considerations of Ancillary Study Procedures

Another point to consider relates to study procedures conducted for safety and screening purposes that gather sensitive information. Here I refer to those protocols in which, for example, pregnancy and/or HIV testing, or screening for alcohol or illegal drug use are study exclusions. Whether testing for such conditions or substances is done at screening or somehow ascertained once a minor is in a study, investigators and IRBs need to clarify prospectively procedures for withholding or providing such information to minors and/or parents or guardians. Further, procedures must be in place to assure that appropriate counseling or medical services are either provided or handled on well-coordinated referral.

Genetic Testing in Minors in Research

Another issue that will demand increasing attention in the near future are the potential harms posed by the advent of genetics research (Wertz, Fanos, & Reilly, 1994). Consider the prospect for gene identification in mental disorders. Genetic analyses are already underway for conditions such as alcoholism, schizophrenia, and bipolar disorder, among others. It is likely that our ability to test for genetic susceptibility for mental disorders will outstrip our ability to prevent, treat, or cure these diseases. The proper use of genetic tests will be difficult to determine, given our limited management options for most mental disorders and their associated stigma. The layers of complexity in decision making about protocol design, child assent, and dissemination of clinically relevant information that may be obtained in the research setting in the population under discussion pose presently unanswerable questions. That such studies pose more than the minimal risk of taking a blood sample, however, is clear. Investigators must work with their IRBs, in consultation with experienced pediatric medical geneticists, clinical bioethicists, and others, to identify, at the protocol development stage, as many risks as possible so that reasonable safeguards can be instituted before subjects are enrolled.

Data and Safety Monitoring Committees

These are but a few examples of the many considerations that must take place each time a protocol is developed or reviewed. How these, and the many other necessary questions, are answered will have an impact beyond the specific study under consideration. This impact will extend to the need for future studies and the involvement of future minor subjects which is why expanded utilization of data and safety monitoring committees is gaining attention (Ashby & Machin, 1993; Pignon & Arriagada, 1994; Task Force of the Working Group on Arrhythmias of the European Society of Cardiology, 1994).

Although not new, data and safety monitoring committees have not been widely utilized in clinical research. These committees, where they do exist, are most often seen in large cancer and/or pharmaceutical trials. It may be useful, however, to begin thinking about having such bodies—or some variant—attached to smaller studies at more preliminary phases of the research (DeRenzo, 1995). At present, the standard procedure is for a protocol to run until the investigators have met the original endpoint(s). Setting more stringent stopping criteria to be assessed at prospectively set times by disinterested third parties, however, may hold out the prospect for involving fewer subjects and answering study questions more quickly. Given the controversy now taking place about the ethical acceptability of randomized clinical trials (Rothman & Michels, 1994; Royall, 1991), increasing the prospects for reducing study size and duration, especially in such scientifically and morally complex research as that of mental disorders of children and adolescents, could serve as an important addition to study design, safely speeding up the accumulation of data while increasing subject protections.

FUTURE DIRECTIONS

Clarifying Dual Roles

One reason for such protections is that the performance of biomedical human subjects research is a process of fitting round pegs into square holes. Clinical researchers and the other members of the research team are trained as clinicians first, researchers second. The primary clinical training that investigators bring to the research setting is duty-based. Clinical investigators are trained, and many will be so inclined by temperament, to focus on the care needs of individual, identified patients, not possible future patients. That may be why, at least in part, we have such a difficult time keeping clinical and scientific matters separate (Appelbaum, Roth, & Lidz, 1983; Bamberg & Budwig, 1992).

For example, it is difficult to keep our most basic terminology straight. We regularly call patient-subjects (or perhaps less starkly, patient-volunteers) *patients*. They are not, however, patients, in the ordinary sense most often understood by this term, and most commonly understood by the public and our research participants. Immediately on enrolling an individual into a study, even a study with expected direct benefit, we have added a new and distancing dimension to care. The individual we know as patient in the strictly clinical setting is more accurately referred to as patient-subject or patient-volunteer in the research setting.

Another similiar confusion is in our use of the words *therapy* or *treatment*. If we do not systematically add a word such as *investigational*, *study*, or *experimental* in front of the word treatment or therapy each time such words appear in our consent/assent documents and in our research explanations, we exacerbate the chronic blurring of research and clinical care—both for our patient-subjects and their families, as well as for ourselves. That the therapeutic misconception exists (Appelbaum et al., 1983) is a demonstrable fact; that we must work to minimize its existence is a moral requirement.

This refinement in our language is necessary to assist us in keeping in mind the inherent conflicts between the goals of clinical care and the goals of science. The research process, by its very nature, places the individual into a system of competing claims. At the broad, social level, there are conflicting claims between the good of the individual and the good of society. There may be times when individualized care of particular persons is sacrificed for the good of obtaining important knowledge to help future persons and advance the general well-being of society. At the level of the subject and the investigator, there are the conflicting claims created by the desires of individual subjects to derive direct benefit and the researcher's desire to provide such benefit, balanced against the drive to acquire knowledge of benefit to others, and the pursuit of his or her own intellectual interests.

As the research process becomes more open to public scrutiny, risk is high that the credibility of the research community will be reduced and public cynicism increased if this conflict is not acknowledged squarely. Further, when unaddressed, these conflicts threaten the well-being of research subjects. When research subjects are children, vulnerable not merely by age, but additionally by mental illness and its sequelae, it is imperative that we protect the subjects and the research enterprise by seeking creative solutions to the peculiarities these conflicts present. This is not to say that having conflicting goals diminishes the importance or necessity of human subjects research. It is, rather, that by becoming more punctilious in our acknowledgment of these competing claims, we become more alert to the potential harms. Only when we are alert to potential harms will we be vigilant in avoiding them and willing to exert the effort needed to arrive at creative ways of reducing them.

Encouraging Multidisciplinary Approaches

One general solution is to take a more sophisticated attitude toward implementing the spirit of multidisciplinary care. Especially in protocols involving psychiatrically and/or behaviorally disturbed or at-risk minors, making refined clinical determinations such as when to break a blind and remove a child from a study is optimized by wide clinical and moral input. That is, decisions such as when to shift a child from the status of patient-subject to patient is not simply a medical or scientific decision. It is a decision with a strong moral component. Particularly with subjects with mental disorders, it may be difficult to determine just what is, at any particular point in time, in a particular subject's best interest. Whatever the answer is will be value-laden. And when it comes to making value decisions, no member of the research or health care team's values should be considered more "right" than anyone else's. Rather, each will have an opinion based on his or her own ethical perspective and there may be several ethically permissible solutions to the same problem.

Some members of the team might be more consequentially driven than others. Some might shape recommendations within the context of perceived duties and obligations. Some may focus on relational and contextual aspects of the situation more than others. All can be expected to provide morally relevant considerations. Thus, optimal research decision making weighs and balances a wide spectrum of value assessments, jointly considering options. Through open discussion by all members of the research and care team, scientific progress can move forward in a way that maximally protects subject welfare and strengthens the integrity of the research process itself.

Although the shift to joint decision making is a well-accepted principle of modern systems administration, it is not yet well understood or appreciated within the biomedical research community. In the most recently issued guidelines of the Society for Research in Child Development (Committee for Ethical Conduct in Child Development Research, 1990), the report sets out as its first principle that investigators should avoid psychological as well as physical harm to children. While acknowledging that it is often difficult to characterize what might be psychological harm, the report emphasizes that it is the investigator's responsibility to do so.

This emphasis on avoiding psychological, as well as physical, harm is progressive, admirable, and necessary. That this appropriate focus on reducing and avoiding harm, however, is addressed only in terms of the investigator's responsibility is seriously flawed. Narrowly focusing on the investigator, and not mentioning the joint responsibilities of the rest of the research and care team members, perpetuates suboptimal decision making in the research setting and contributes to the ongoing confusion about clinical patients and clinical research subjects. Although the model of the doctor–patient relationship may still be an accurate picture of some clinical care settings, some might argue that this model no longer even represents the reality of modern clinical medicine. In the research setting, however, focusing on the primacy of the dyadic relationship can be counterproductive.

Commonly, associate investigators, research fellows, nurses, social workers, and bioethicists interact with subjects as or more frequently than do principal investigators. These associates and care providers, therefore, are the ones with actual knowledge of the setting in which the research is taking place and may have a greater appreciation for the specific circumstances and value preferences of the subject and her or his family. We need to accept honestly that the model of the doctor–patient relationship is not the model of clinical research, nor should it be. Rather, through the coordinated efforts of all members of a well-integrated multidisciplinary research team will we be able to make the kind of sound clinical and moral judgments posed by questions that arise in the management of subjects as vulnerable as children and adolescents with mental disorders. Further, it is not implausible to predict that if the particular ethical complexities posed by this kind of research are not addressed within the research setting, more research programs may be faced with court interventions like that now facing New York state (Hilts, 1995). In that case, roughly $52 million in New York state mental health research, monitored by the states' Office on Mental Health, is being threatened as a result of action on the part of a concerned public.

CONCLUSION

In summary, the larger question posed by the performance of research into mental disorders of children and adolescents involves distinguishing between considerations of individual welfare and the advancement of science. Although this is an important distinction in all human subjects research, it is more difficult when research involves children and adolescents with mental disorders. Where we draw the line between balancing the good of the subject and the good of others will be different for each protocol. There are no formulas for designing safe protocols that will produce useful and important data or for determining, for example, when a particular subject should be removed from a particular study.

Striking the optimal balance between good science and caring for humans with complex needs is a daunting task. The justification for involving vulnerable children in a research study must include scientific questions of the greatest importance. But we must not assume that important scientific questions will have simple or elegant answers. Perhaps, as Evans (1994) speculated, we need to rethink our assumptions about study design and endpoints:

> In essence, the fewer questions that a piece of research asks, the clearer the answers that may be obtained, assuming the research is well designed. A mark of scientifically poor research design is too many research aims. Therefore, a nontherapeutic research proposal that could, clinically speaking, be extended to address immediately therapeutic questions ought not to be so extended if we are to maximize scientific rigor. Here, the requirements of science tend to exclude broader clinical features that could be of therapeutic advantage to the children taking part in the research. (p. 554)

It is possible, however, that flexible research designs could be developed to allow direct benefit without jeopardizing the quality of the science.

Increasing the benefits might make us more comfortable about placing minors with mental disorders at risk for harms we cannot quantify. An example of where this trade-off may have occurred, and may demonstrate the value of making such a compromise, is in a study of children's willingness to report child abuse (Keary & Fitzpatrick, 1994). In this study, different methods for eliciting child abuse information were studied. Although the elicitation of the information may have been distressful for some of the child subjects, and by using different styles systematically it is possible that some children did not produce as much information as others, thus giving the investigators and others less information on which to intervene appropriately on these child-subjects' behalf, the study may have produced important direct benefits as well as generalizable results. If successfully replicated, these data may be useful in learning how best to elicit sexual abuse information safely from children in the future, while having provided direct benefit to the child subjects that they would not have received had the study not been performed.

We need to improve our methods and procedures for protecting research subjects as we collect and use research data rather than retard research through dogmatic adherence to particularized understandings of regulatory language (R. Levine, 1995). Also, the research development and review process, in and of itself, requires more thought and attention than it seems we have given it to date. At the institutional level, as at the protocol level, by perpetuating our limited vision of the scope and breadth of who should be involved in research discussions, particularly when the human subjects are vulnerable, we may fall short of moral excellence in our research performance. All relevant persons and institutional entities must take responsibility for discussing the moral aspects of the conduct of human subjects research. Our institutions must become not simply more tolerant of such discussions, but more welcoming.

The constraints and pressures on medical institutions suggest that the social effects of institutionalization and bureaucratization can be morally stultifying (Toulmin, 1990). This harkens back to the work of Max Weber, who envisioned the increased bureaucratization in institutions as an iron cage. Applying Weber's logic, Toulmin suggested the possibility that,

> In a fully differentiated and bureaucratized society, everybody's duties and responsibilities will be defined by job descriptions; ethical obligations will give way to functional imperatives; personal shame and

individual responsibility will be replaced by institutional excuses and evasions. When the claims of professional integrity and institutional survival come into conflict, victory will go to the stronger. In any head-on conflict, institutions are more powerful than individuals, and this will lead to the progressive devaluation of the moral claims of professionalism. (p. 23)

Although this bleak view may be representative of what can happen, it need not. The negative effects of bureaucratization can be mitigated by establishing a system for discussing these issues that empowers staff to voice moral concerns and generally elevates moral imagination within the institution.

One example of where such a system has been enacted is within the NIH's Human Genome Project. This model was designed to support parallel development of science and ethics. The initial plan for the Genome Project included significant funding for discussion and the study of ethical, legal, and social implications (ELSI) of genome research. The ELSI Program has funded, and continues to fund, important research in the extramural research community. Now that the Genome Project has evolved into the National Center for Human Genome Research (NCHGR), the NCHGR is creating an intramural NIH ethics infrastructure that is, moreover, being coordinated with other ethics components at the NIH, such as the NIH Clinical Center's Bioethics Program. This is an example well worth emulating.

Especially in research on mental disorders in children and adolescents, the need for increased and rigorous attention to the moral aspects of such studies is clear (Bulger et al., 1993). The vulnerability of these subjects require it; the public demands it. Increased attention, however, does not mean that the answers will come easily. There will never be any easy answers to the complex moral and scientific questions posed by research into the mental disorders of children and adolescents. The best that can be expected is that we bring to the process of such research the kind of wisdom about which Appelbaum (1994) spoke. He defined *wisdom* as including a special kind of understanding "that allows one to apply one's understanding to effecting solutions in the living world, and a capacity to place things into perspective, to bring a body of experience to bear on new events, to discern their meaning and their likely implications" (p. ix). As we continue to learn more about the prevention, treatment, and cure of these disabling conditions, we must place as much emphasis on examination and refinement of the moral questions such research poses as we do on the scientific questions yet to be answered.

REFERENCES

Abramovitch, R., Freedman, J. L., Derbyshire, A., & Brunschot, M. V. (1993). In G. Koren (Ed.). *Textbook of Ethics in Pediatric Research* (pp. 11–21). Malabar, FL: Krieger.

Abramovitch, R., Freedman, J. L., Henry, K., & Brunschot, M. V. (1995). Children's capacity to agree to psychological research: Knowledge of risks and benefits and voluntariness. *Ethics & Behavior, 5*(1), 25–48.

Ackerman, T. F. (1979). Fooling ourselves with child autonomy and assent in nontherapeutic clinical research. *Clinical Research, 27,* 345–348.

Annas, G. J., & Grodin, M. A. (1992). *The Nazi doctors and the Nuremberg Code: Human rights in human experimentation.* New York: Oxford University Press.

Appelbaum, P. S. (1994). *Almost a Revolution.* New York: Oxford University Press.

Appelbaum, P. S., Roth, L. H., & Lidz, C. (1983). The therapeutic misconception: Informed consent in psychiatric research. *International Journal of Law and Psychiatry, 5,* 319–329.

Ashby, D., & Machin, D. (1993). Stopping rules, interim analyses and data monitoring committees. *British Journal of Cancer, 68*(6), 1047–1050.

Bamberg, M., & Budwig, N. (1992). Therapeutic misconceptions: When the voices of caring and research are misconstrued as the voice of caring. *Ethics and Behavior, 2*(3), 165–184.

Bartholomew, W. G. (1976, December). Parents, children, and the moral benefits of research. *Hastings Center Report,* 44–45.

Benson, P. R., Roth, L. H., Appelbaum, P. S., Lidz, C. W., & Winslade, W. J. (1988). Information disclosure, subject understanding, and informed consent in psychiatric research. *Law and Human Behavior, 12*(4), 455–475.

Brock, D. W. (1994). Ethical issues in exposing children to risks in research. In M. A. Grodin & L. H. Glantz (Eds.), *Children as research subjects: Science, ethics & law.* New York: Oxford University Press.

Bulger, R. E., Heitman, E., & Reiser, S. J. (1993). *The ethical dimensions of the biological sciences.* New York: Cambridge University Press.

Committee for Ethical Conduct in Child Development Research. (1990, Winter). Report to the Society for Research in Child Development. *SRCD Newsletter,* pp. 5–7.

DeRenzo, E. G. (1994a, November–December). The ethics of involving psychiatrically impaired persons in research. *IRB: A Review of Human Subjects Research,* 7–9, 11.

DeRenzo, E. G. (1994b). The ethics of involving severely cognitively impaired persons in research: The continuing debate. *The Cambridge Quarterly of Health Care Ethics, 3*(4), 539–548.

DeRenzo, E. G. (1995). Commentary on responding to a request for genetic testing that is still in the lab. *Cambridge Quarterly of Health Care Ethics, 4*(3), 392–395.

Evans, M. (1994). Conflicts of interest in research on children. *Cambridge Quarterly of Healthcare Ethics, 3,* 549–559.

Fletcher, J. C., Quist, N., & Jonsen, A. R. (1989). *Ethics consultation in health care.* Ann Arbor, MI: Health Administration Press.

Freedman, B. (1975). A moral theory of informed consent. *Hastings Center Report, 5*(4), 32–39.

Gaylin, W. (1982). Who speaks for the child: No longer all or none. In W. Gaylin & R. Macklin (Eds.), *Who Speaks for the Child* (pp. 27–54). New York: Plenum.

Goldberg, S. (1993). Some costs and benefits of psychological research in pediatric settings. In G. Koren (Ed.), *Textbook of ethics in pediatric research* (pp. 63–73). Malabar, FL: Krieger.

Haslam, R. H. A. (1993). Research in children: Issues of risk and harm. In G. Koren (Ed.), *Textbook of ethics in pediatric research* (pp. 25–36). Malabar, FL: Krieger.

Hilts, P. J. (1995). Judge tells health department to stop experiments on patients. *The New York Times*, p. 52.

Hoffmaster, B., Freedman, B., & Fraser, G. (1989). *Clinical ethics: Theory and practice.* Clifton, NJ: Humana Press.

Institute of Medicine. (1989). *Research on children and adolescents with mental, behavioral and developmental disorders.* National Academy of Sciences. Report of a study of the Committee of the Division of Mental Health and Behavioral Medicine. Washington, DC: National Academy Press.

Katz, J. (1993). Human experimentation and human rights. *Saint Louis Law Review, 38*(1), 7–54.

Keary, K., & Fitzpatrick, C. (1994). Children's disclosure of sexual abuse during formal investigation. *Child Abuse & Neglect, 18*(7), 543–548.

La Puma, J., & Schiedermayer, D. (1994). *Ethics consultation: A practical guide.* Boston: Jones & Bartlett.

Levine, C., Dubler, N. N., & Levine, R. J. (1991). Building a new consensus: Ethical principles and policies for clinical research on HIV/AIDS. *IRB: A Review of Human Subjects Research, 13,* 1–17.

Levine, R. J. (1986). *Ethical and regulation of clinical research.* Baltimore, MD: Urban & Schwarzenberg.

Levine, R. J. (1989). Children as research subjects. In L. M. Kopelman & J. C. Moskop (Eds.), *Children and health care: Moral and social issues* (pp. 73–87). New York: Kluwer.

Levine, R. J. (1995). Research in emergency situations: The role of deferred consent. *Journal of the American Medical Association, 273*(16), 1300–1302.

MacKay, C. R. (1995). The evolution of the institutional review board: A brief overview of its history. *Clinical Research and Regulartory Affairs, 12*(2), 65–94.

Macklin, R. (1992). Autonomy, beneficence, and child development: An ethical analysis. In B. Stanley & J. E. Sieber (Eds.), *Social research on children and adolescents* (pp. 88–108). Newbury Park, CA: Sage.

McCormick, R. A. (1974). Proxy consent in the experimental situation. *Perspectives in Biology and Medicine, 18,* 2–20.

McCormick, R. A. (1976, December). Experimentation in children: Sharing in sociality. *Hastings Center Report,* 41–46.

Melton, G. B. (1992). Respecting boundaries: Minors, privacy and behavioral research. In B. Stanley & J. E. Sieber (Eds.), *Social Research on Children and Adolescents* (pp. 65–87). Newbury Park, CA: Sage.

Munir, K., & Earls, F. (1992). Ethical principles governing research in child and adolescent psychiatry. *Journal of the American Academy of Child and Adolescent Psychiatry, 31*(3), 408–414.

National Commission for the Protection of Human Subjects of Biomedical and Behavioral Research. (1977). *Appendix to report and recommendations: Research involving children.* Washington, DC: U.S. Government Printing Office.

Office for Protection from Research Risks. (1993). *Protection of human research subjects: Institutional review board guidebook.* Washington, DC: U.S. Government Printing Office.

Pence, G. E. (1980). Children's dissent to research—A minor matter? *IRB: A Review of Human Subjects Research, 2*(10), 1–4.

Pignon, J. P., & Arriagada, R. (1994). Early stopping rules and long-term follow-up in Phase III trials. *Lung Cancer, 10*(Suppl. 1), S151–S159.

Protection of Human Subjects. (1991). Title 45, Code of Federal Regulations, Part 46. *OPRR Reports.*

Ramsay, P. (1970). *The patient as person.* New Haven, CT: Yale University Press.

Ramsay, P. (1976). The enforcement of morals: Nontherapeutic research on children. *Hastings Center Report, 6*(4), 21–30.

Ramsay, P. (1977). Children as research subjects: A reply. *Hastings Center Report, 7*(2), 40–42.

Ramsay, P. (1980). "Unconsented touching" and the autonomy absolute. *IRB: A Review of Human Subjects Research, 2*(10), 9–10.

Range, L. M., & Cotton, C. R. (1995). Reports of assent and permission in research with children: Illustrations and suggestions. *Ethics & Behavior, 5*(1), 49–66.

Rothman, K. J., & Michels, K. B. (1994). The continuing unethical use of placebo controls. *The New England Journal of Medicine, 331*(6), 394–398.

Royall, R. M. (1991). Ethics and statistics in randomized clinical trials. *Statistical Science, 6*(1), 52–88.

Susman, E. J., Dorn, L., & Fletcher, J. C. (1992). Participation in biomedical research: The consent process as viewed by children, adolescents, young adults and physicians. *Journal of Pediatrics, 121,* 547–552.

Task Force of the Working Group on Arrhythmias of the European Society of Cardiology. (1994). The early termination of clinical trials: Causes, consequences, and control. *European Heart Journal, 15,* 721–738.

Thomasma, D. C. & Mauer, A. M. (1982). Ethical implications of clinical therapeutic research on children. *Social Science & Medicine, 16,* 913–919.

Thompson, R. A. (1990). Vulnerability in research: A developmental perspective on research risk. *Child Development, 61,* 1–6.

Thompson, R. A. (1992). Developmental changes in research risk and benefit: A changing calculus of concerns. In B. Stanley & J. E. Sieber (Eds.), *Social Research on Children and Adolescents* (pp. 31–64). Newbury Park, CA: Sage.

Toulmin, S. (1990). Medical institutions and their moral constraints. In R.E. Bulger & S.J. Reiser (Eds.), *Integrity in health care institutions: Human environments for teaching, inquiry, and healing.* Iowa City: University of Iowa Press.

Wertz, D. C., Fanos, J. H., & Reilly, P. R. (1994). Genetic testing for children and adolescents: Who decides? *Journal of the American Medical Association, 272*(11), 875–881.

11

Bridging Scientific and Ethical Perspectives: Toward Synthesis

Peter S. Jensen
Kimberly Hoagwood
National Institute of Mental Health
Celia B. Fisher
Fordham University

In producing this volume it has been our intention to assist researchers in meeting their responsibilities to conduct ethical, scientifically defensible, and humane research. Aware of the many obstacles that have impeded mental illness research in children and adolescents, we attempted to strike an appropriate balance between the objectives of enabling scientifically rigorous research, and the humanitarian standards of beneficence, respect for persons, and justice. Moreover, we have been guided by the perspective that, particularly in the case of children, we as investigators "do no harm."

In this context, the chapters and cases strive to lay out the ethical dilemmas that investigators confront in the course of balancing their dual roles as scientists and citizens. Throughout the casebook, the investigators considered the complex issues and special circumstances of the proposed research, the developmental and subject-specific factors unique for individual participants, and the local community context and setting in which the research was embedded. From this vantage point, the cases should be regarded as illustrative rather than demonstrative, and the volume should be considered a *casebook* rather than a *cookbook*. In some instances, the cases illustrate novel, creative solutions to difficult ethical problems, yet they cannot be readily extrapolated to another research question in another setting with another research participant population. In this regard, we suggest the need for caution. Indeed, an appropriate ethical analysis of any proposed research is only possible as each proposal is evaluated on its own merits, as DeRenzo notes in this volume. This, of course, is the responsibility of the institutional review board (IRB), where members of the local community can provide appropriate scrutiny concerning the protection of the individual research participants. Only this type of careful, case-by-case examination of any proposed research's unique circumstances can ensure that research programs are ethical in the most meaningful sense, rather than merely adhering to a bureaucratically mandated, routine format.

SPECIAL CHALLENGES
IN MENTAL HEALTH/ILLNESS RESEARCH
WITH CHILDREN AND ADOLESCENTS

Methodologic and Scientific Challenges. The field of mental health research with children and adolescents has been and continues to be hampered by the immaturity and relative lack of sophistication of the science. For example, few research-based treatments have been successfully demonstrated as safe and effective (as noted by Leonard et al., chapter 6 and Hibbs & Krener, chapter 5). This is due, in part, to the fact that the research tools needed to study young populations are complex to conceptualize, difficult to assemble, and often problematic to implement. Assessment tools must take into account the various vantage points of parents, children, and teachers, and accurate diagnosis is often difficult and cumbersome when diagnostic information does not converge on a single picture (as it rarely does). Further, although invasive procedures have been used often to examine biologic variables in adults, such procedures pose ethical and safety concerns with children and adolescents. Fortunately, new tools that limit children's exposure to risk are becoming available, but this process is slow at best.

Logistic, Financial, and Institutional Obstacles. In addition to the slow development of research tools and methods, additional obstacles to conducting research with children and adolescents include children's relative lack of autonomy, the dual requirement of assent and consent, institutions' concerns about greater liability with children, and the lack of financial incentives to conduct research with children. Seemingly, all of these obstacles co-conspire to ensure that children remain "therapeutic orphans," as noted by Leonard and colleagues (chapter 6). For example, despite thousands of medications being available over the counter or through prescription throughout the United States, only one in five of these medications has been rigorously examined to evaluate safety and efficacy in children. In the case of mental disorders in particular, thousands of adult subjects have been studied to determine safety and efficacy of antidepressant medications for depression, yet only several hundred children have been systematically enrolled in double-blind, placebo-controlled trials to establish the efficacy of these medications. Agents found to be safe and effective in adults may be neither in children and adolescents; nonetheless, despite the lack of safety and efficacy data for children, these agents are widely prescribed for developmental disorders. This poses a dilemma for clinicians, child patients and their parents, and is not easily resolved. Denying access to these medications may be inhumane; likewise, failing to advance this much needed research deprives the large class of persons under age 18 the benefits of scientific knowledge afforded to other groups more readily.

Despite the immaturity of the developmental sciences related to child and adolescent mental health and psychopathology, this area affords many research opportunities. Increasingly, investigators have become aware that the study of young populations promises to unlock the mysteries of the emergence of the severe adult psychopathologies. Thus, the developmental neurosciences are providing increased understanding of the effects of the environment on the developing brain. This developmental perspective on the emergence of psychopathology is the hallmark of state-of-the-art scientific approaches for studies of disorders such as schizophrenia, manic depressive disorder, autism, and other severe lifelong impairing conditions. From this viewpoint, research with children and adolescents is likely to be pivotal for understanding, treating, and preventing major mental disorders, not just in children and adolescents but in adults as well. We suggest that advancement of such research constitutes an ethical imperative, albeit not at the expense of any individual child's well-being or an unduly adverse risk–benefit ratio for a group of children.

Attitudinal Obstacles: Stigma. In addition to the immaturity of the science of mental health research with children and adolescents, other special issues characterize mental health-related studies in this population. Investigators and IRBs frequently hold subtle yet stigmatizing attitudes and opinions concerning research participants who may be at risk for or are afflicted by a mental disorder. Too often, the "presumption of incompetence" seems to shape the opinions and prejudices of investigators and IRB members. This "presumption of incompetence" stems from the undemonstrated belief that emotional, behavioral, and developmental disorders primarily impair participants' ability to comprehend information and meaningfully evaluate the risk–benefit ratio. There is, however, no empirical support for the assumption that children suffering from behavioral and emotional disorders (apart from those that frequently affect cognition, e.g., pervasive developmental disorders, autism, etc.) are less able than their age-matched counterparts to evaluate and participate in the assent and consent processes in research.

The "presumption of incompetence" also extends to prejudices regarding the ability of parents of children with such disorders to evaluate research participation vis-à-vis the best interests of their children. Thus, IRBs or investigators may feel the need to establish greater than usual protections for the disordered or disabled child from his or her presumably incompetent parent, (e.g., a consent auditor or parent monitor) during the course of the research. The stigmatization of parents of children with mental disorders in based in part on the same unsupported biases concerning the ability of at-risk or distressed persons to give fully informed consent, as well as the historical assumption that parents "cause" their child's mental disorder. That parents of children with mental disorders are incompetent to provide rational and fully informed consent has not been demonstrated.

Stigma also affects assumptions by investigators and IRBs about the kinds of questions and procedures to which children may be safely exposed in the course of research. For example, no evidence has demonstrated that asking children about suicidal feelings increases the likelihood of such feelings or gives a child passive permission to act out such suicidal impulses. Indeed, clinical experience suggests just the opposite; yet many IRBs assume that such questions may be dangerous or may lead to untoward consequences. In fact, asking children and families such personal, highly confidential questions is regularly seen as acceptable for the vast number of participating subjects and families (Lahey et al., in press).

The "Therapeutic Misconception": A Potential Area for Investigator/Participant Misunderstandings. Another issue that particularly touches on mental health-related research concerns "therapeutic research." In the United States, few services are available to treat children and adolescents as well as adults with mental disorders. As a rule, resources are sparse, and insurance companies and third-party payors have restricted full access to the range and level of mental health services thought to be necessary for adequate treatment for many conditions. In this context, parents may feel an even greater sense of urgency in obtaining care for their children. A university-based research program may appear to be a godsend, alleviating families' sense of urgency and concerns about helping their child. In such settings, parents may be subject to the "therapeutic misconception" (i.e., that participation with their children in the research will make active and effective treatments available; Appelbaum, Roth, & Lidz, 1983). Yet, given the current state of the science of clinical treatments of child and adolescent mental disorders, placebo treatments or other alternatives are critical in many, if not all, circumstances. Thus, in the context of the child's clinical needs, families may be severely disappointed if active treatment is not included as a part of their participation in a research program.

Furthermore, the clinical investigator must be aware of the conflict of interest inherent in therapeutic research: that his or her actions are shaped by two competing value systems: scientific responsibility and the protection of human welfare. Accordingly, he or she must be careful to avoid fueling the "therapeutic misconception" (either implicitly or explicitly), such that his or her actions are construed as solely for the benefit of the participant.

THE "ETHICAL COMPACT" BETWEEN INVESTIGATORS AND RESEARCH PARTICIPANTS

As others have noted, informed consent is best understood as a *process* rather than a piece of paper signed by the parent and child participants. In the deepest sense, what is required is a full and consensual understanding of the nature of the research program and its potential risks and benefits. This understanding should form the basis of an *ethical compact* between the investigator and the participant, and the information-sharing process should be couched in candor, respect, and mutual trust. This also requires that the investigator be aware of and fully communicate to prospective participants and their guardians his or her dual roles and the possibility for conflicts of interest in the course of attempting to satisfy both responsibilities. This requires acknowledgment that as a *scientist*, he or she is motivated to advance the state of knowledge, and as a *citizen*, he or she is motivated to act appropriately as a member of a compassionate society.

Full awareness of this conflict of interest on the part of the investigator can form the foundation for trust in the investigator–research participant relationship. Honest communication at the initial stages of a research partnership can serve as a firm basis for a relationship built on respect. Such mutual respect can in turn enhance the ethical compact by overriding what in many instances may appear to be unequal power relationships. This mutuality, candor, and shared participation in the research process is critical for research to proceed, and to maintain the public's trust and good will toward the goal of advancing science for the benefit of all. Clearly, this ethical position requires more than a single consent form signed under limited or less than optimal conditions. Truly informed consent is a *process* that begins with the initial consent procedures, continues through the duration of the research program, and ends with a thoughtful debriefing and a shared, final examination of the entire process. This process should be mutually and gladly undertaken by the investigator and the research participants.

These issues of informed consent as a *process,* the effects of stigma, and the lack of services and available alternatives, highlight the essential nature of trust between investigators and participant children and parents. Interestingly, during recent conferences hosted by the Institute of Medicine and the National Institute of Mental Health concerning ethical issues in mental health research, investigators and parents noted that there has been a recent erosion of trust between clinical investigators and families participating in research. For this reason, efforts to enhance communication and trust between investigators and patients and their families are essential. Initiatives must be developed to increase the level of agreement concerning the various methods to ensure fully informed and ongoing consent during the research process. It is important that in the conduct of their research, investigators aim not just for IRB approval, but to reach a higher standard: a plan to address human subjects issues that considers all possible ramifications of the research enterprise, embedded in ethical principles, and built on systematic efforts to increase trust in the investigator–participant relationship. Although IRBs cannot fully anticipate every eventuality that may arise during the course of research, if the investigator fully grasps the central nature of the *ethical compact,* he or she can make appropriate adjustments at critical points of the study, to ensure that the *informed consent process* continues during the course of the research, and that families' confidence in the research and the researcher increase during the course of their mutual collaboration. Although systematic approaches to addressing these issues have been developed (e.g., data safety and monitoring boards and ongoing reviews of side effects and treatment outcomes during the course of clinical trials), such formal mechanisms cannot replace the investigator's own concern for his or her research participants' well-being, and the active communication of these perspectives in interactions with families.

RECOMMENDATIONS

To address the issues noted here and to build on the perspectives outlined in this volume, we recommend several courses of action. First, new efforts are needed to strengthen the links among investigators, institutional review boards, families, and their communities. In the final analysis, the highest ethical standard cannot be obtained by an elegant, well-written, explicit consent form. Although such consent procedures are to be emulated whenever possible, they fall well short of an ethical standard that seeks to involve members of the larger "community of citizens" as research participants and collaborators in the goals of science and research. Although science should ultimately benefit the larger "community of citizens," all too often investigators complain that their research findings are not incorporated into available knowledge, nor do their findings actually change the standards of practice. Upon further consideration, this should not be too surprising; the terminologies used to define the research questions are usually very different from the policy objectives of program planners, or the more personal concerns of parents and families who are dealing with the immediate effects of a member who is suffering with a disabling disorder.

Research Participants as Community Partners. To address these difficulties in research dissemination, members of the communities whom the research is intended to benefit must increasingly be part of the early definition of the research questions, research procedures, selection of specific terminologies, and dissemination of research findings. This action perspective more closely joins the interests of scientists, research participants, and the larger community, and seems to us ethical in the deepest sense. Such an approach offers a more comprehensive means of strengthening collaborations between scientists and research participants, engendering trust, developing relevant research that is well-received by communities, and enhancing effective research dissemination. Such partnerships between scientists and the citizenry could yield a number of important benefits, including the development of consensus on levels of acceptable risk, the cultivation of a common will to address critical research gaps (particularly in the area of children and adolescents), and the reaffirmation of the importance of science in improving the lives of all citizens. In this regard, we note that several new program announcements in the National Institutes of Health have now inserted new scientific review requirements, which require that peer review committees evaluate research applications on the degree to which they have involved members of the communities whom the research is intended to benefit in the research conceptualization, design, informed consent forms, research language, and research dissemination plans. Although this may be controversial for some, this is a welcome and long overdue addition to the review of public health service research.

As Osher and Telesford (chapter 3) note, scientists need to be more aware of the language they use in the course of their research. Too often, language that is commonly used in scientific discourse may depersonalize and/or devalue research participants. From an ethical perspective, referring to a research protocol participant as "a schizophrenic" or another term that refers to a clinical condition, can be dehumanizing. Other more subtle yet equally distressing language difficulties can emerge when a child suffering from a crippling emotional disorder and his or her family learn that the child has "failed the protocol." Further involvement of patients and families in the development of consent procedures can remediate some of the language barriers that currently exist. Although these terms are used through no ill intent per se, many unfortunate examples abound, and it is quite easy to construct a lengthy list of scientists' poor habits of communication. Involvement of families as participants and partners in this process should improve the science and the likelihood of its translation into practice.

New Methods to Increase Children's and Families' Understanding. Given concerns about difficulties in younger children's understanding of research procedures, investigators must pay greater attention to the use of multiple modalities to inform subjects, establish consent, and continue the informed consent process. For example, efforts that rely on multiple sensory modalities (e.g., videotape, cartoons, pictures and sound, or multiple repetitions) may be advantageous. In the area of mental health assessment research, for example, investigators have noted that information can be presented, such that even young children can reliably report and respond to assessment protocols, if the information is carefully explained, developmentally appropriate, and relies upon multiple sensory modalities (Edelsohn, Ialongo, Werthamer-Larsson, Crockett, & Kellam, 1992; Ialongo, Edelsohn, Werthamer-Larsson, Crockett, & Kellam, 1995; Russell, 1990).

In addition, investigators may need to pay greater attention to the use of systematic "staged consent," particularly if consent procedures are long, complex, or if the research procedures take place over a longer period of time. Given children's ongoing development, longitudinal studies should consider systematic procedures over time to reaffirm consent. Children will often have some difficulty in saying "no," and the use of consent auditors or the explicit listing of a child's various alternatives during the consent process may be a useful means to establish and affirm consent in a developmentally appropriate fashion.

Developmentally Sensitive, Scientifically Sensible Designs. In the area of therapeutic research, investigators need to pay greater attention to developmentally appropriate, yet scientifically sensible designs. Given the nature of children's development and their needs over multiple settings and contexts, a child with a major emotional or behavior disorder may warrant more comprehensive treatment research approaches than simple placebo-controlled double-masked designs. Children develop simultaneously across multiple settings, and they are sensitive to input from all of these contexts. Ethical, yet feasible clinical research designs, in the case of medications, may require comprehensive treatment approaches with and without medications. Both of these treatment alternatives can be ethically justified as developmentally appropriate and sensible, given what we know about children's development. Such treatment strategies are likely to be more acceptable to families, offer a better basis for trust and shared commitment to the research process, and offer sensible and generalizable findings to inform public policy and health practices.

Increased Education and Communication Efforts Concerning New Technologies.   Increased communication of information about new technologies is needed. For example, although IRBs are more appropriately concerned about exposing children to undue risks, technologies are rapidly advancing. These new technologies are often less invasive and pose minimal risks, yet the procedures and terminologies may not be fully known to IRBs, patients, and families. Better communication of these methodologic advances is needed to educate patients and families as research participants, as well as IRBs that may not always be fully aware of safety issues.

Bridging Ethics and Science: A Science of Scientific Ethics.   Historically, the relationship of the discipline of ethics to science has been characterized as much by distance as by connectedness. Russell (1927) pointed out that the study of ethics consists in part of the study of what is good or bad. This question of what is good or bad, *independent* of its effects, has traditionally been viewed as lying outside the domain of science. Science, according to Russell, cannot contain any genuinely ethical precepts, because it is not concerned with questions of right or wrong, but with questions of truth or falsehood, and the two categories of questions are qualitatively distinct.

The relationship between science and ethics continues to pose problems for the social sciences. In 1993, a series of articles appeared in the *American Psychologist* addressing the question of whether psychology as a science of the mind is logically precluded from validating moral principles (Kendler, 1993, 1994). Arguments in the Russell tradition held that neither mentalistic nor behavioral conceptions of psychological science can offer the premises by which to make ethical judgments, because there is no logical connection beween what is established empirically and what ought to be. However, arguments for a closer relationship between science and moral thought begin with the understanding that a complete separation between empirical study and social knowledge is false, because it is impossible to extricate oneself from the social reality one is examining (Prilleltensky, 1994).

Thus, we suggest that the premises underlying research ethics as they are currently conceptualized in our society need to be viewed as historically situated and of recent origin, having come to the fore only since World War II. In fact, this system arose from medical conceptions of a provident yet paternal doctor–patient relationship, corresponding to the professional responsibilities a doctor had for the patient. Such a perspective is consistent with Christakis' (1992) contextualist view of research ethics, which recognizes the influence of culture upon questions of ethical standards in research. This contextual perspective extends beyond mere recognition of cultural differences or relativism, pointing instead to the ways in which culture shapes the form and content of ethical precepts, as well as the way ethical conflicts are handled.

Applying such a contextualist view of ethical issues to the relationship between science and ethics requires a realignment of the primary relationship. Ethics becomes a method for organizing thought, not simply a manual for identifying those standards by which right or wrong are configured. Ethical standards are conceived as embedded in systems of meaning that are culture-bound. As a consequence, ethics do more than regulate behavior; they provide a system for interpreting behavior. When ethics is seen as a system of interpretive thought, ethical conflicts offer a mode for engagement and negotiation (Christakis, 1992), and become a way of creating deeper meaning of the relationship between science and its use. In this model, research and ethics together form a system of interpretation, and offer the possibility of an evolving process whereby science is informed by ethical development, and ethical thought is informed by scientific advances.

In attempting to bridge this apparent gap between ethics and science, we close this volume on a note commonly sounded by researchers; more research is needed. Yet in this area, a new kind of research is required. As we have noted elsewhere, the science of scientific ethics must be developed and expanded (Fisher, 1993; Hoagwood, Jensen, & Leshner, in press). Better understanding of the determinants and circumstances under which children can comprehend and evaluate risks and benefits is needed. Likewise, fuller knowledge of the contextual factors affecting children's and families' consent to participate in research is essential. In particular, development of scales to assess children's ability to comprehend risk-benefit issues, studies of families' reactions to research procedures (e.g., random assignment, placebo controls), and empirical data on the impact of various forms of participant reimbursement, will advance both our science and our ethics.

We hope that this volume will spur further research, serving as a guide for current investigators, participating families, IRBs, and policymakers who shape the research enterprise. Research is not the province of science and scientists alone. Science, in the public trust and on behalf of the public health, is the province of us all.

REFERENCES

Appelbaum, P. S., Roth, L. H., & Lidz, C. (1983). The therapeutic misconception: Informal consent in psychiatric research. *International Journal of Law and Psychiatry, 5,* 319–329.

Christakis, N. A. (1992). Ethics are local: Engaging cross-cultural variation in the ethics for clinical research. *Social Science Medicine, 35,* 1079–1091.

Edelsohn, G., Ialongo, N., Werthamer-Larsson, L., Crockett, L., & Kellam, S. (1992). Self-reported depressive symptoms in first grade children: Developmentally transient phenomena? *Journal of the American Academy of Child and Adolescent Psychiatry,* 282–290.

Fisher, C. B. (1993). Integrating science and ethics in research with high-risk children and youth. *Society for Research and Development Social Policy Report, 7,* 1–27.

Hoagwood, K., Jensen, P. S., & Leshner, A. (1996). Ethical issues in research on child and adolescent mental disorders: Implications for a science of scientific ethics. In S. Henggeler & A. Santos (Eds.), *Innovative models of mental health treatment for clinical populations* (pp. 541–561). Washington, DC: American Psychiatric Press.

Ialongo, N., Edelsohn, G., Werthamer-Larsson, L., Crockett, L., & Kellam, S. (1995). The significance of self-reported anxious symptoms in first grade children: Prediction of anxious symptoms and adaptive functioning in fifth grade. *Journal of Child Psychology and Psychiatry, 36,* 427–437.

Kendler, H. H. (1993). Psychology and the ethics of social policy. *American Psychologist, 48,* 1046–1053.

Kendler, H. H. (1994). Can psychology reveal the ultimate values of humankind? *American Psychologist, 49,* 970–971.

Lahey, B., Flagg, E., Bird, H., Schwab-Stone, M., Canino, G., Dulcan, M., Leaf, P., Davies, M., Brogan, D., Bourdon, K., Horwitz, S., Rubio-Stipec, M., Freeman, D., Lichtman, J., Shaffer, D., Goodman, S., Narrow, W., Weissman, M., Kandel, D., Jensen, P., Richters, J., & Regier, D. (in press). The NIMH Methods for the Epidemology of Child and Adolescent Mental Disorders (MECA) Study: Background and methodology. *Journal of the American Academy of Child and Adolescent Psychiatry.*

Prilleltensky, I. (1994). Psychology and social ethics. *American Psychologist, 49*(11), 966–967.

Russell, B. (1927). Physics and perception. In *The Outline of Philosophy.* London: George Allen & Unwin.

Russell, J. A. (1990). The preschooler's understanding of the causes and consequences of emotions. *Child Development, 61,* 1872–1881.

Author Index

A

Abramovitch, R., 49, *56*, *258*, 275, *284*
Ackerman, T. F., *258*, 271, *284*
Adams, S., 94, 95, 97, *109*
Adelman, H. S., 7, 9, *13*, *262*
Adorno, T. W., 3, *13*
Akkerboom, J. C., 195, 196, *262*
Alexander, J. R., *258*
Allen, A. J., 77, *87*
Allmon, D., *263*
Alpert, J. J., 82, *87*
Aman, M. G., *258*
Amaya-Jackson, L., 115, *130*
Ambrosini, P. J., 76, 77, *87*
American Academy of Pediatrics, 73, 79, 80, 81, 86, *87*
American Association of Child and Adolescent Psychiatry, *258*
American Psychological Association, 44, *56*, 121, *130*, *258*
Amiel, S. A., 99, 105, *108*
Anthony, E. J., 6, *13*
Antonson, D. L., *265*
Applebaum, P. D., 207, *258*
Applebaum, P. S., 9, *13*, 53, *56*, 207, *264*, 275, 278, 283, *284*, 290, 297
Armstron, H., *263*
Arriagada, R., 27, *285*

B

Ashby, D., 277, *284*
Asher, S. R., 234, *258*
Atkins, M. S., *258*
Attikisson, C. C., 44, *56*, 57
Ayers, T. S., *261*

Babhulkar, S. S., 97, *108*
Bach, M. L., *258*
Bachman, D., 96, *110*
Baer, M. D., *258*
Baga, D., 97, *109*
Baldessarini, R., 74, 76, *88*, *87*
Balk, D. E., *258*
Bamberg, M., 277, 278, *284*
Barber, B., 107, *108*
Barkley, R. A., *258*
Baron, M., *258*
Barrera, M., *259*
Bartholomew, W. G., 271, *284*
Baumrind, D., 197, *259*
Bayer, R., *259*
Beauchamp, T. L., 232, *259*
Bech, K., *259*
Belanger, S., 9, 10, *13*, 123, 129, *131*, 143, 199, 205, 233, 234, *261*
Bellack, A. S., 9, *13*
Bell-Dolan, D. J., *259*
Belsky, J., *264*

299

Rajab, M., *265*
Ramsay, P., 92, *110*, 271, 273, *285*
Range, L. M., *286*
Rapoport, J. L., 7, 9, *14*, 77, *87*, 94, 95, 96, 99, *109*, 145, 152, *259*, *263*
Ratiner, C., *266*
Rau, J. M., 9, 10, *14*, 123, 129, *131*, 143, 199, 205, 233, 234, *261*
Regier, D., 290, *297*
Reich, W., *259*
Reilly, P. R., 106, *111*, 277, *286*
Reiser, S. J., 270, 283, *284*
Resnick, H. S., 115, *132*
Resnick, J. H., 197, *265*
Richards, P. G., 96, *110*
Richardson, D., 197, *266*
Richters, J., 290, *297*
Riolo, J. A., *259*
Ritchie, G. F., 94, 95, 99, *109*, *259*
Robbins, P. C., 207, *264*
Rogers, J. L., *265*
Roosa, M. W., *264*
Rosenbaum, A., 53, *56*, 207, *258*
Rosenblatt, A., 44, *56*, *57*
Rosendahl, S. W., 8, *13*, 176, 178, 179, 197, 199, 234, *261*
Rosengarten, H., 75, *88*
Rosnow, R. L., 9, *14*
Ross, L., 199, *263*, *265*
Rossa, M. W., *261*
Roth, L. H., 275, 278, *284*, 290, *297*
Rotherman-Borus, M. J., 8, 9, *14*, *131*, 262, *265*
Rothman, K. J., 79, *88*, 278, *286*
Rovet, J., 75, *88*
Royall, R. M., 278, *286*
Rubino-Stipec, M., 290, *297*
Rudd, M., *265*
Runyan, D. K., 115, 129, 130, *132*
Russell, B., 295, *297*
Russell, D. E. H., 115, *132*
Russell, J. A., 294, *297*
Rutter, M., *110*
Ryan, N. D., 76, 77, *87*, *88*

S

Saks, M. J., 116, *131*, 192, *264*
Saladino, R., 96, *110*

Sales, B. D., *260*
Sametz, L., *266*
Sarason, S., *265*
Sarkar, P., 97, *110*
Saunders, B. E., 115, *132*
Sauzier, M., 18, *132*
Scarr, S., *265*
Sceery, W., 77, *87*
Scherer, D. G., 100, *111*, 117, *132*
Schetky, D. H., *265*
Schiedermayer, D., 270, *285*
Schneider, H. G., 158, 178, *259*
Schoeman, F., *266*
Schooler, N. R., 9, *14*
Schwab-Stone, M., 290, *297*
Schwartz, T., 197, *265*
Scolnik, D., 75, *88*
Scott, D. J., *266*
Scott-Jones, D., 10, *14*, 51, *57*
Scrimger, J. W., 103, *109*
Sellden, H., *110*
Shaffer, D., 77, *87*, 290, *297*
Shanmugasundaram, T. K., 97, *110*
Shay, J., 105, *110*, *266*
Shipp, A. C., 3, *14*
Shirkey, H. C., 92, *110*
Sieber, J. E., 198, *266*
Sikora, D. M., *259*
Silva, M. C., *266*
Singer, E., 123, *132*
Small, A. M., 105, *110*, *266*
Smith, C., 115, *131*
Smith, M., 94, *110*
Smith, S. S., 197, *266*
Smith-Wright, D. L., 96, *111*
Snider, B. W., *265*
Snow, B., 118, *132*
Society for Research in Child Development, 121, *132*, 167, *266*
Socolar, R. S., 115, *130*
Sorenson, T., 118, *132*
Sorrell, J. M., *266*
Sotsky, S. M., 220, 221, *262*
Spencer, T., 74, *88*
Spiker, D., *266*
Sroufe, L. A., 100, *111*
Steingar, R., 74, *88*
Stern, A. E., 122, *131*
Stiffman, A. R., *266*
Stoff, D. M., *258*

Subject Index